AF321974

The Surgical Management
of the Diabetic Foot and Ankle

Dolfi Herscovici, Jr.
Editor

The Surgical Management of the Diabetic Foot and Ankle

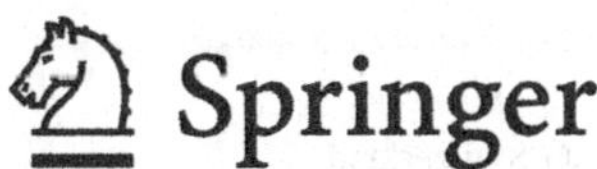

Editor
Dolfi Herscovici, Jr.
Foot and Ankle/Trauma Service
Tampa General Hospital
Florida Orthopedic Institute
Tampa, FL, USA

ISBN 978-3-319-27621-2   ISBN 978-3-319-27623-6   (eBook)
DOI 10.1007/978-3-319-27623-6

Library of Congress Control Number: 2016935692

Printed on acid-free paper

This Springer imprint is published by Springer Nature
The registered company is Springer International Publishing AG Switzerland

This book is dedicated to all of the healthcare providers currently taking care of, or will provide care to, the diabetic patient who presents with a problem to their foot or ankle. Hopefully, this information will give you more insight for managing these patients. It is also dedicated to those patients who have allowed us, as contributing authors, a chance to learn how to provide better options for the management of diabetic pathology and injuries, enabling diabetics to continue down the successful road to recovery. With the completion of this book, there are a few people I would like to specifically thank. First, I would like to thank the people who helped mentor me in the art and science of foot and ankle surgery: Randall E. Marcus, M.D.; V. James Sammarco, M.D.; and especially to G. James Sammarco, M.D. Thank you all for explaining things to me I did not understand and having the patience to answer all of my questions. Second, I would like to thank all of the authors for their hard work and patience with the edits. Thank you all for your contributions. Third, I would like to thank my four boys—Derek, Jake, Brad, and Troy—for putting up with me when I sequestered myself in my office editing the manuscripts and for understanding the demands that it took to complete this job. Lastly, I would like to thank my beautiful wife, Lisa, who through good times and bad has always been my biggest supporter, has played the task of my sounding board for ideas and suggestions, and has also played the role as my de facto editor.

Dolfi Herscovici, Jr., DO

Foreword

Diabetes, a disease of the world, is as old as the pyramids themselves. In fact, the earliest reference to the condition dates from the Ebers Papyrus, 1552 BCE, in which the patient was observed "… to eliminate urine which is too plentiful." This simple observation characterized the most obvious symptom of the disease. In India, a diabetic was noted to pass "honey urine" since the urine attracted ants and flies, and in the second century BCE the word diabetes, "to go through," was introduced. Two centuries later, symptoms leading to early death were recorded. By the fifth century CE in India, young thin diabetics were observed to die earlier than older heavier ones, and in China, patients were noted to be prone to infection. In Bagdad, diabetics were found to have sweet urine, increased appetite, gangrene, and sexual dysfunction.

During the Renaissance, recorded observations became more detailed. Paracelsus recognized that a white residue remained when diabetic urine was allowed to evaporate. In the Age of Enlightenment, Crowley observed that some patients with severe abdominal and pancreatic trauma developed diabetes. Dobson recorded sweetness in both urine and in blood serum, deducing that diabetes is a systemic disease.

In the nineteenth century science expanded the understanding of diabetes with many more investigators contributing findings. Chevreal associated the sugar in urine with glucose. Rollo added the descriptor "mellitus," meaning honey, to differentiate it from diabetes insipidus. Bernard created a model for diabetes in the laboratory, while Petters found acetone in the urine of patients in diabetic coma. Noyes described diabetic retinopathy. Allen deduced that diabetics used food inefficiently, noting that type 1 diabetics died early while those with type 2 survived longer. Following Langerhans' discovery of special pancreatic cells, Laguesse linked them to a substance he called hormone, Greek meaning "set in motion," which, in 1909, de Mayer named "insulin."

Prior to the twentieth century, natural medicines such as digitalis and opium, and techniques such as purging, special diets, starvation, physical therapies, and behavior modification, had failed to control the disease. But with advances in chemistry, extracts and other compounds began to appear. In Germany, Zuelzer used acomatol, a pancreatic extract, to treat diabetic coma. Other attempts followed including the early sulfonylureas.

In 1922, Frederick Banting, a Canadian orthopedist turned researcher, and his student, Charles Best, isolated the hormone insulin. The purified extract was administered to a severely diabetic 14-year-old boy resulting in a dramatic decrease in his blood sugar. When this was presented at a medical conference, there was a standing ovation. An avalanche of research soon followed with the rapid manufacturing of many different forms of insulin, thus saving the lives of millions. This discovery of insulin had propelled research into virtually all areas of medicine and surgery.

Better control of the disease, however, led to other problems, due to longer survival and a more active lifestyle of diabetics. Peripheral neuropathy, peripheral vascular and cardiac disease, and kidney and eye disease became more common. Neuroarthropathy of the weight-bearing extremities also increased in incidence. For example, a diabetic woman, while climbing stairs, would be surprised to see her foot begin to swell without pain, turn red, and then would be alarmed to watch her foot collapse within a few days. Her doctor would diagnose a "simple fracture" and treat it in "the standard manner." The deformity would then progress into "the worst arthritis you have ever seen." Closed or open treatment, using the current "acceptable standard of care," would result in nonunion or malunion with subsequent foot ulcers and osteomyelitis leading to possible amputation.

When Jean Martin Charcot described neuropathic deformity, he associated it with late-stage syphilis, but these patients were not syphilitic. Early case reports of diabetic Charcot foot and ankle neuroarthropathy now began to appear in medical literature more frequently. Treatment with nonsurgical modalities such as rest, limited weight-bearing, bracing, and modified footwear were standard. Surgical treatment generally consisted of soft tissue debridement and limb amputation.

In the 1950s Paul Brand, at the Carville National Leprosarium, began using total contact casting to off-weight neuropathic foot ulcers in patients with Hanson's disease. This soon became a modality also for treating diabetic foot ulcers. Total contact casting could help prevent or at least control collapse of an asensory foot or ankle. But it was not a panacea. In the 1980s, surgical treatment expanded beyond exostectomy, Achilles tenotomy, arthrodesis, and amputation to include reconstruction, as a means of limb salvage. Orthopedic researchers along with vascular surgeons became part of a broad group of diabetic specialists who contributed to reducing the need for major amputation. The introduction of external fixation as a part of the technique in controlling deep infection, reducing deformity, and maintaining limb viability has been remarkable. Likewise staged surgery, intramedullary rods, and locking screw-plate fixation are now in the orthopedic surgeon's armamentarium for salvaging severe foot and ankle collapse. Allografts, bone growth stimulators, bone growth hormone, bone substitutes, and wound suction devices are also used to fill bony gaps and promote wound healing.

The disease of diabetes has been a focus of physicians and surgeons for millennia. This book presents current information on diagnosis, treatment, and prevention of the foot and ankle orthopedic complications related to the disease. Advances in research will continue to improve our understanding of this common ailment. The experts offer the special knowledge and skills developed over recent decades here as a guide to orthopedic surgeons as they seek to improve care for their patients.

G. James Sammarco

References

Jacek Z, Shrestha A, et al. Chapter 1: The main events in the history of diabetes. In: Poretsky L, editors. Principles of diabetes mellitus. 2nd ed. New York: Springer; 2009.

Charcot J-M, Fere C. Affections osseuses et articulaires du pied chez les tabétiques (Pied tabétique). Archives de Neurologie. 1883;6:305–319 [in French].

Preface

According to the *National Center for Health Statistics*, in 1900 the life expectancy in the United States approached 47 years. Of the ten most common causes leading to death in 1900, six were due to infectious diseases with strokes, accidents, cancer, and senility contributing to the final four reasons that someone died. By 1949, the life expectancy had increased to 68 years, and diabetes mellitus was identified as the tenth most common cause leading to death. By 2013, the life expectancy increased to almost 79 years with diabetes then listed as the seventh most common cause leading to someone's death. This indicates that diabetes is certainly a disease of the late twentieth and early twenty-first centuries. In fact, a report from the *World Health Organization* recognizes diabetes as a growing epidemic affecting almost 350 million people worldwide. What does this mean to us, as physicians who treat and manage diseases of the musculoskeletal system? It means that because people are living longer, we can expect to see more patients present with chronic conditions or injuries that are specifically caused or affected by their diabetes.

Foot and ankle problems produce serious long-term complications, and any anatomical abnormality can progress to an ulceration, infection, or gangrene. These problems are often caused by a combination of such factors as peripheral neuropathy, vascular disease, immobile joints, an impaired ability to heal or fight infections, poor management of their diabetes, or outright denial of their medical problems. That these problems are costly to manage is implied because these patients often require lengthy and expensive hospitalizations, which may lead to an amputation.

When a diabetic patient presents with a significant foot or ankle problem, there are still many physicians who continue to offer only conservative care or amputation as option. In fact, this approach has not significantly changed over the last 30–40 years, even though it can ultimately lead to a poor outcome. There are a few reasons for this. First, the literature is replete with studies discussing higher rates and more significant complications in diabetics than in the control population. Second, most treating physicians rarely see these patients and thus have little experience in managing these problems. Third, there may be a significant hesitancy in offering a surgery, which can lead to a bad outcome and potential medicolegal issues. Fourth, physicians often fail to understand that the patients' associated comorbidities need to be preoperatively assessed and managed in order to avoid greater problems. Lastly, for a lot of surgeons their surgical approach that is used to manage a diabetic patient is similar to techniques used to care for a nondiabetic patient, often leading to failure of fixation and producing higher rates of morbidity and mortality. Given these reasons, it is understandable that physicians are tentative about managing these patients surgically.

This text has been put together to act as a reference guide, with up-to-date chapter references for the problems associated with the diabetic foot and ankle. It is also intended to function as a primer with the most current concepts of epidemiology, pathophysiology, workups needed, and treatments available for the diabetic who presents with abnormalities or injuries to their foot and ankle. In addition, a glossary has been provided so that the reader can understand some of the terms used throughout the text. A major strength of this book is that authors who were solicited are recognized as leading authorities when it comes to managing problems of the foot and ankle. This has been demonstrated in some of the treatment chapters with the authors providing their preferred step-by-step approach for the management of some of the more commonly encountered foot and ankle problems. By providing a better understanding of diabetes, and offering improved techniques for managing these patients, we should be able to demonstrate improved outcomes. This can produce happier patients and families, lower hospital usage, and decreased overall medical expenses, and it may also allow patients to maintain more active lifestyles and potentially return them into the workforce. As we advance through this century, it is hoped that the information provided in this text will help all healthcare professionals tasked with caring for the diabetic patient who presents with problems to their foot and ankle.

Temple Terrace, FL, USA   Dolfi Herscovici, Jr.

Acknowledgments

When I accepted the offer from Springer to put this book together, I knew that it would be a difficult project. Given the contributions from many authors, I knew that there were certain technical aspects that I needed to finish this project. With his input and skills, I would like to acknowledge my son Derek M. Herscovici for his assistance in helping me prepare and organize this text. Thanks for all your technical expertise downloading and formatting all of the incoming information sent to me and making sure that I had everything I needed to complete this book.

Contents

Contributors

Steven Anthony, DO Advanced Orthopedic Center, Port Charlotte, FL, USA

Erin A. Baker, MS Department of Orthopaedic Research, William Beaumont Hospital - Royal Oak, Royal Oak, MI, USA

John S. Early, MD Clinical Professor Orthopedic Surgery, University of Texas Southwestern Medical Center, Texas Orthopaedic Associates LLP, Dallas, TX, USA

Paul T. Fortin, MD Foot and Ankle Service, Department of Orthopaedic Surgery, William Beaumont Hospital - Royal Oak, Royal Oak, MI, USA

Erin Green, MD Division of Vascular Surgery, University of South Florida, Tampa, FL, USA

Dolfi Herscovici, Jr., DO Foot and Ankle/Trauma Service, Tampa General Hospital, Florida Orthopaedic Institute, Tampa, FL, USA

Joshua G. Hunter, MD Department of Orthopaedic Surgery and Rehabilitation, University of Rochester Medical Center and 2 Virginia Commonwealth University, Rochester, VA, USA

Brad Johnson, MD Division of Vascular Surgery, University of South Florida, Tampa, FL, USA

David E. Karges, DO Department of Orthopaedic Surgery, Saint Louis University, Saint Louis, MO, USA

Stephen L. Kates, MD Department of Orthopaedic Surgery and Rehabilitation, University of Rochester Medical Center and 2 Virginia Commonwealth University, Rochester, VA, USA

Bradley M. Lamm, DPM, FACFAS International Center for Limb Lengthening, Rubin Institute for Advanced Orthopedics, Baltimore, MD, USA

Dror Paley, MD, FRCSC Paley Advanced Limb Lengthening Institute, St. Mary's Hospital, West Palm Beach, FL, USA

Michael S. Pinzur, MD Department of Orthopaedic Surgery, Loyola University Health System, Maywood, IL, USA

Gregory Pomeroy, MD Orthopaedic Foot & Ankle, Mercy Hospital, Portland, ME, USA

Stefan Rammelt, MD, PhD University Center of Orthopaedics and Traumatology, Technische Universität Dresden, Dresden, Germany

V. James Sammarco, MD Reconstructive Orthopaedics and Sports Medicine, Cincinnati, OH, USA

Julia M. Scaduto, ARNP Foot and Ankle/Trauma Service, Tampa General Hospital, Florida Orthopaedic Institute, Tampa, FL, USA

Lew C. Schon, MD Department of Orthopaedic Surgery, MedStar Union Memorial Hospital, Baltimore, MD, USA

Sandeep P. Soin, MD Department of Orthopaedic Surgery and Rehabilitation, University of Rochester Medical Center and 2 Virginia Commonwealth University, Richmond, VA, USA

Eric W. Tan, MD Department of Orthopaedic Surgery, MedStar Union Memorial Hospital, Baltimore, MD, USA

Ross Taylor, MD, MBA Danville Regional Medical Center, LifePoint Health, Danville, VA, USA

Introduction, Demographics, and Epidemiology of Diabetes

Erin A. Baker and Paul T. Fortin

Introduction

Diabetes mellitus (DM, diabetes) is a condition caused by an inability of the insulin produced by the pancreas to adequately transfer glucose into cells via transporter recruitment. Depending on insulin secretion or lack thereof, the resultant transporter recruitment may be amplified or reversed, leading to uncontrolled hyperglycemia. The condition increases the risk of developing other comorbidities and complications, including hypertension, cardiovascular disease, cerebrovascular accident (CVA), skin infections and diseases, nephropathy, retinopathy and other ocular diseases, mental health status changes (e.g., depression, anxiety), neuropathy, and lower-limb compromise [1]. Diabetes is also implicated as the seventh leading cause and a contributing factor in mortality, with the condition recorded on 234,051 death certificates in the United States in 2010 [1].

The most common classifications of diabetes mellitus are polygenic forms Type I (T1DM) and Type II (T2DM). Type I is characterized by an absence of insulin production, due to autoimmune destruction of pancreatic beta cells, and may be immune-mediated or idiopathic. Type II is an acquired condition in which the pancreas either becomes insulin deficient or sufficient insulin is produced but cannot be effectively used, termed insulin resistance. More than 90 % of all diabetes diagnoses are of T2DM [2]. A subset of T2DM diabetes is gestational diabetes (GDM), which may present during the second or third trimesters of pregnancy and often persists after pregnancy.

In 2012, the American Diabetes Association (ADA) estimated economic costs of diabetes including hospital or emergency care, clinic visits, and medication, to approach $245 billion. This is an increase of $71 million (41 %) over a five-year period, in the United States and $548 billion globally [3–5]. Additionally, indirect costs, due to decreased productivity, disability, and premature mortality, were estimated at $69 billion in the United States. The National Diabetes Statistic Report (NDSR) concluded that medical expenses of diabetic patients are 2.3 times more than expenses of nondiabetic patients [4].

E.A. Baker, M.S.
Department of Orthopaedic Research, William Beaumont Hospital - Royal Oak, 3811 West Thirteen Mile Road, Ste 404, Royal Oak, MI, USA
e-mail: erin.baker@beaumont.org

P.T. Fortin, M.D. (✉)
Foot and Ankle Service, Department of Orthopaedic Surgery, William Beaumont Hospital - Royal Oak, 3535 West Thirteen Mile Road, Ste 744, Royal Oak, MI, USA
e-mail: pfortin@comcast.net

© Springer International Publishing Switzerland 2016
D. Herscovici, Jr. (ed.), *The Surgical Management of the Diabetic Foot and Ankle*,
DOI 10.1007/978-3-319-27623-6_1

Demographics

When categorizing countries into seven geographic regions (i.e., Africa, Middle East/North Africa, South East Asia, South/Central America, Western Pacific, Europe, North America/Caribbean), the International Diabetes Federation (IDF) estimated that the highest rates of prevalence of DM will be in Africa (93 %), the Middle East/North Africa (85 %) and South East Asia (64 %) by the year 2035 [5]. The IDF report has also defined the international cost of diabetes as 11 % of total healthcare expenses (i.e., expenses by health systems and patients), as approximating $612 billion. This expenditure is expected to increase to about $627 billion by 2035 [5].

An increased risk of DM has been linked to numerous demographic factors, including age, sex, race/ethnicity, socioeconomic/employment status, and environment/location. Although these factors have been reported to increase the risk of developing DM, it may be difficult to explain how their interactions lead to DM since at times no specific cause and effect may be found.

Age

The risk of developing DM appears to increase as patients get older. The Centers for Disease Control (CDC) has reported the incidence of DM (per 1000 people) between 1980 and 2011 in the United States (Table 1.1). For patients 18–44 years of age it reported a peak of 4.3 cases (per 1000 people) in 2008 and 2009 (tied). Within this age group there were 23,525 new cases of DM, 18,436 diagnosed as T1DM and 5089 as T2DM, in patients under 20 years of age. By 2014, the NDSR estimated 208,000 cases of DM had been diagnosed in Americans under 20 years of age, or about 0.25 % of that age cohort. The 45–64 age cohort showed a peak of 14.3 newly diagnosed cases (per 1000) in 2008, while patients 65–79 years of age had a peak incidence of 15.4 cases in 2011 with a 31-year average of 10.2 cases per 1000 people. In addition, it also reported that in patients greater than 65 years of age, the preva-

Table 1.1 Incidence (per 1000 people in age cohort) of newly diagnosed diabetes cases

Age cohort	1980 (first year)	2011 (most recent year)	31-year average	Range (year)
18–44	1.7	3.3	2.5	1.4 (1985)–4.3 (2008, 2009)
45–64	5.2	11.9	8.9	4.6 (1991)–14.3 (2008)
65–79	6.9	15.4	10.2	5.1 (1989)–15.4 (2011)

lence of diagnosed and undiagnosed diabetes approached 11.8 million, or 25.9 % for that age demographic [10].

Sex

The CDC also discussed the incidence of DM sorted by patient sex. In the female population, the incidence of newly diagnosed cases ranged between 2.8 (1988) and 5.9 (2011), with a 31-year average of 3.9 cases (per 1000 females per year). The male population showed similar data, with the incidence of new cases ranging between 2.6 (1981) and 7.0 (2010) (per 1000 males per year) with a 31-year average of 4.1 cases [6]. This indicates that since 1988 there appears to be an overall increase in the development of DM in both sexes.

Race/Ethnicity

In the United States, the rate of diabetes diagnoses were found to be the greatest in the adult American Indian and Native Alaskan populations, with an incidence of 15.9 % (per 1000) in 2014. For other races, the reported rates of diabetes diagnoses were 13.2 % for non-Hispanic blacks, 12.8 % for Hispanics, 9.0 % for Asian Americans, and 7.6 % in non-Hispanic whites. Within this subgroup of the Asian American population, the largest rates of diagnoses were identified in Asian Indians (13.0 %) and Filipinos

(11.3 %). A study of six Asian ethnic groups residing in California showed a higher prevalence of T2DM in second-generation Asian Chinese and Filipino men, and in first-generation Asian Filipino women and Korean women, compared to a Caucasian/White cohort [7]. In the Hispanic subgroup population, Puerto Ricans (14.8 %) and Mexican Americans (13.9 %) were identified as having the greatest rates of diabetes diagnoses [1].

The large differences, in prevalence of diabetes between various racial/ethnic groups, highlight environmental and genetic risk factors [8, 9]. Patterns of increased prevalence of diabetes have been established for ethnic groups migrating from rural/agricultural environments to urban or Westernized settings; however, any geographic location adjustment, not necessarily from rural to urban, has also shown an increase in prevalence [9]. For instance, second- and third-generation Japanese Americans, whose ancestors migrated to the Seattle, Washington area, demonstrated increased rates of diabetes (16–20 %) compared to the native Japanese population (4–5 %) for both sexes [10, 11]. Genetically, the Japanese population has shown a propensity for beta cell dysfunction, specifically Fujimoto et al. defined an association between the −30 beta cell GCK gene promoter, beta cell dysfunction, and abnormal glucose tolerance as well as other gene variants related to beta cell dysfunction. Combining environmental factors, such as increased caloric diet and decreased physical activity leading to obesity, in this genetically vulnerable population may ultimately lead to increased rates of diabetes, especially if these modifiable disease influencers are unchecked [11].

Other ethnic groups have also shown a similar genetic susceptibility to diabetes, including Mexican Americans, Latinos, African Americans, American Indians, and Pacific Islanders [8]. Epigenetic- and gene-based research has associated the rs10811661 T allele to T2DM in both Asian and European ethnicity groups [12]. Additionally, a study of eastern Asian Indian T2DM patients and controls found a significant relationship between the haplotype of two risk alleles of two genes, PON1 and PON2, in T2DM patients. PON1 and PON2 belong to a multigene family related to oxidative activities on chromosome 7 [13]. Therefore, for many ethnic groups with this genetic susceptibility, decreasing the prevalence of diabetes relies almost exclusively on lifestyle modification.

Socioeconomic/Employment Status

Socioeconomic status has also been shown to correlate with the risk of developing diabetes. In regions with depressed economic development, the prevalence of T2DM is elevated in the upper classes; however, in regions with increased wealth, the rates of T2DM are increased 2–4 times in groups with low socioeconomic status and may be exacerbated by healthcare access and quality, that are dependent on payment [2, 14, 15]. In the United States, Everson et al. discussed an inverse relationship for diagnoses of T2DM when comparing a patient's education level, occupation, and income [13–15]. There also appeared to be a higher prevalence of diabetes with the poverty income ratio (i.e., annual income divided by federal poverty line) and low socioeconomic status. Evaluating education in this same study, Everson at al. also reported that the prevalence of diabetes was almost three times greater in adults with less than 9 years of education than adults with at least a high school diploma [16–18]. These social determinants (e.g., education, employment security, housing, access to nutritious food) also relate to the development and progression of diabetes through the pathways of psychological, physiological, and behavioral responses (e.g., chronic stress, development of mental health conditions). After diabetes diagnosis, health disparity and disease progression may persist due to financial burden, insufficient access to quality healthcare and other resources to manage the disease, as well as employment- and education-limiting effects [15]. These disparities are illustrated by the high rates of uncontrolled diabetes (HbA$_{1C}$ ≥ 9 %), 48.7 % and 27.3 %, in patients insured with Medicaid and Medicare, respectively [19, 20]. Additionally, socioeconomic status may overlap with genetically vulnerable populations, and these groups may be confronted with the inability to overcome "obesogenic" environmental factors, resulting in increased rates of diabetes [2, 9].

Environment

Environmental causes have also played a role in developing and allowing DM to worsen. A spatial analysis study, integrating data from the CDC and United States Census Bureau, analyzed associations between diabetes prevalence and environmental factors including previously discussed primary factors such as race/ethnicity population percentages, education level, unemployment level, and poverty level. Also discussed were secondary factors including population density, percentages of obesity, physical inactivity, cycling/walking to work, and the consumption of food deserts. Excluding the aforementioned primary factors, the only significant finding in the secondary factors was a positive correlation between cycling/walking to work and diabetes prevalence [21]. In addition, a meta-analysis of long-term noise exposure demonstrated that populations exposed to day–evening–night noise levels, greater than 60 decibels (dB) in their primary residence, had a 16–22 % higher risk of developing Type 2 diabetes than populations exposed to less than 64 dB [17]. Increased risk was only found with exposure to increased noise in the residential environment, not occupational noise exposure. Additionally, animal-based studies of chronic noise exposure have described a decrease in plasma testosterone, which may be translatable to testosterone deficiency and increased risk of cardiovascular complications in men with diabetes [22–24].

Epidemiology

The National Diabetes Statistic Report (NDSR), an effort by the Centers for Disease Control and Prevention (CDC), National Institutes of Health (NIH), American Diabetes Association (ADA), and other organizations, was released in 2014 [1].

The report indicated that 29.1 million people in the United States, or 9.3 % of the entire population, were currently living with diabetes, with 21.0 million as diagnosed and 8.1 million as undiagnosed. In 2012, the new diagnoses in the one-year period were 1.7 million [1]. Internationally, the International Diabetes Federation (IDF) has reported that 387 million people (8.3 %) were living with diabetes as of 2014, with almost 179 million people (46.3 %) classified as undiagnosed cases [5].

Association Between Diabetes, Chronic Conditions, and Surgical Outcomes

The major complications associated with DM include cardiovascular disease (CVD), nephropathy, retinopathy, neuropathy, and foot care, according to the ADA. By far, CVD is the most expensive complication in terms of direct and indirect costs. The ADA has estimated that the annual cost of CVD in the diabetic population is approximately $17.6 million, which includes office, emergency, and outpatient visits as well as inpatient, nursing home, home health, and hospice care [25]. In addition, T2DM often presents with hypertension and dyslipidemia, which leads to microvascular complications. Nearly 80 % of patients in the T2DM population will eventually be diagnosed with microvascular disease, and the diabetic population has a two times greater risk of myocardial infarction and stroke compared to the general population [26, 27]. Nephropathy is also identified and is the leading cause of end stage renal disease occurring in 20–40 % of the DM population. Chronic albuminuria is an early diagnostic marker of nephropathy in T1DM, of disease development in T2DM, and increased risk of CVD [28–31]. Additionally, the osteoinductive factor may also be a biomarker for early diagnosis of diabetic nephropathy in T2DM patients [32]. Another vascular-related complication of DM is retinopathy, which affects almost all T1DM patients and more than 60 % of T2DM patients within 20 years of disease onset [33].

Various neuropathic conditions are also prevalent, including distal symmetric polyneuropathy (DPN), diabetic autonomic neuropathy, cardiovascular autonomic neuropathy (CAN), gastrointestinal neuropathies, and genitourinary tract issues. All of these conditions may present as focal or multifocal and range in severity [34]. The DPN and autonomic neuropathies are the most common in DM, with DPN being asymptomatic in 50 % of patients. This increases the risk of foot-related injuries and complications.

Additional comorbid conditions include obstructive sleep apnea, fatty liver disease, cancer, decreased testosterone levels in men, periodontal disease, and hearing impairment [31]. Musculoskeletal conditions affecting the DM population include carpal tunnel syndrome, adhesive capsulitis (e.g., frozen shoulder), tenosynovitis, decreased joint mobility, hip fractures, and osteoporosis [35].

In addition, mental health conditions, are observed in greater numbers of patients with DM and include schizophrenia, bipolar disorder, anxiety disorders, and major depressive disorders [36, 37]. Studies have estimated that 12–27 % of the diabetic population experiences depression at a rate two to three times that of the general population [36–42]. Also, patients with mental health disorders have been shown to have an increased risk of developing diabetes [36], with Mezuk et al. describing a 60 % increased risk following a diagnosis of depression [43]. All of these mental health issues may be caused by stress, adversity (especially early in development), inflammation, hypothalamic–pituitary–adrenal axis dysregulation, psychiatric medications, along with sex- and comorbidity-based differences based on the development of mental health conditions in the DM population [41, 42, 44]. It is estimated that approximately 50 % of patients demonstrate decreased psychological health at the time of diabetes diagnosis. An international survey indicated that diabetes-related distress affected 13.8–44.6 % of people with diabetes [45].

Lastly, diabetic patients have often demonstrated inferior surgical outcomes and increased complication rates. Although the exact pathophysiology is unknown, it is postulated that hyperglycemia results in nonenzymatic protein glycation and formation of advanced glycation end products that modify enzymatic activity, immunogenicity, produce a decrease in protein half-life, and cause a decrease in ligand binding [46]. Ultimately, these factors increase the risk of wound and bone healing complications in hyperglycemic patients with or without diabetes [47]. A number of studies have tried to delineate specific risk factor parameters in diabetic patients undergoing surgical intervention, but no consensus has been achieved [47]. However, several factors have been suggested, including poor glycemic control, loss of protective sensation, chronic renal failure, and peripheral vascular disease. Even poor glycemic control, in the nondiabetic patient, has been shown to be associated with an increased risk of complications [47]. Acott et al. reported a perioperative complication rate of 26.4 % in the diabetic population, compared to 14.1 % in the nondiabetic population. Additionally, mortality has been shown to be increased in the diabetic population compared to the nondiabetic population (4.2 % vs. 1.0 %) [48].

Summary

In the United States, newly diagnosed cases of DM have increased overall since the CDC began publishing reports in 1980. However, since 2006 the number of new cases diagnosed per year has not significantly changed [49]. Internationally, trends in DM diagnoses vary. The IDF has published rates of diabetes prevalence by country and has defined rates of national prevalence ranging from 1.29 % (Mali; comparative rate = 1.6 %) to 37.37 % (Marshall Islands; comparative rate = 37.1 %) (comparative rate adjusted for age differences between countries/regions to allow comparison) [5]. Low- and middle-income countries are impacted with the highest rates of DM prevalence, as 77 % of all people with DM live in one of these countries.

Social science, basic science, and clinical studies have researched and continue to investigate rates of diabetes diagnoses, etiologies and pathogeneses of diabetes as well as risk factors for diabetes. Published studies have identified five modifiable risk factors (obesity, physical activity level, diet, hypertriglyceridemia, and HDL cholesterol levels) related to incidence and methods to increase control of DM in the United states and the international population [50]. With a better understanding of DM, along with improved medical and surgical treatment options, the future care of diabetic patients will continue to decrease the morbidity and mortality associated with this patient population.

References

1. Centers for Disease Control Prevention. National Diabetes Statistics Report: estimates of diabetes and its burden in the United States, 2014. Atlanta, GA: US Department of Health and Human Services; 2014.
2. Blas E, Kurup AS. Equity, social determinants and public health programmes. Geneva: World Health Organization; 2010.
3. Nichols GA, Schroeder EB, Karter AJ, Gregg EW, Desai J, Lawrence JM, et al. Trends in diabetes incidence among 7 million insured adults, 2006–2011: the SUPREME-DM project. Am J Epidemiol. 2015;181(1):32–9.
4. American Diabetes Association. Economic costs of diabetes in the U.S. in 2012. Diabetes Care. 2013;36(4):1033–46.
5. International Diabetes Federation. IDF diabetes atlas. 6th ed. Brussels, Belgium: International Diabetes Federation; 2013.
6. Center for Disease Control and Prevention. Age-adjusted rate per 100 of civilian, noninstitutionalized population with diagnosed diabetes, by sex, United States, 1980–2011. 2015. http://www.cdc.gov/diabetes/statistics/incidence/fig3.htm. Accessed 8 June 2015.
7. Huang ZJ, Zheng C. Type 2 diabetes among 6 Asian ethnic groups in California: the nexus of ethnicity, gender, and generational status. J Health Care Poor Underserved. 2015;26(2 Suppl):16–35.
8. Triplitt C, Solis-Herrera C, Reasner C, DeFronzo RA, Cersosimo E. Classification of diabetes mellitus. In: De Groot LJ, Beck-Peccoz P, Chrousos G, Dungan K, Grossman A, Hershman JM, editors. Endotext. South Dartmouth, MA: MDText.com, Inc.; 2000.
9. van Tilburg J, van Haeften TW, Pearson P, Wijmenga C. Defining the genetic contribution of type 2 diabetes mellitus. J Med Genet. 2001;38(9):569–78.
10. Fujimoto WY, Boyko EJ, Hayashi T, Kahn SE, Leonetti DL, McNeely MJ, et al. Risk factors for type 2 diabetes: lessons learned from Japanese Americans in Seattle. J Diabetes Investig. 2012;3(3):212–24.
11. Fujimoto WY, Leonetti DL, Bergstrom RW, Kinyoun JL, Stolov WC, Wahl PW. Glucose intolerance and diabetic complications among Japanese-American women. Diabetes Res Clin Pract. 1991;13(1–2):119–29.
12. Bao XY, Xie C, Yang MS. Association between type 2 diabetes and CDKN2A/B: a meta-analysis study. Mol Biol Rep. 2012;39(2):1609–16.
13. Haldar SR, Chakrabarty A, Chowdhury S, Haldar A, Sengupta S, Bhattacharyya M. Oxidative stress-related genes in type 2 diabetes: association analysis and their clinical impact. Biochem Genet. 2015;53(4–6):93–119.
14. Baumann A, Schroder SL, Fink A. How social inequalities impact the course of treatment and care for patients with type 2 diabetes mellitus: study protocol for a qualitative cross-sectional study from the patient's perspective. BMJ Open. 2015;5(7), e008670.
15. Hill J, Nielsen M, Fox MH. Understanding the social factors that contribute to diabetes: a means to informing health care and social policies for the chronically ill. Perm J. 2013;17(2):67–72.
16. Everson SA, Maty SC, Lynch JW, Kaplan GA. Epidemiologic evidence for the relation between socioeconomic status and depression, obesity, and diabetes. J Psychosom Res. 2002;53(4):891–5.
17. Robbins JM, Vaccarino V, Zhang H, Kasl SV. Socioeconomic status and type 2 diabetes in African American and non-Hispanic white women and men: evidence from the Third National Health and Nutrition Examination Survey. Am J Public Health. 2001;91(1):76–83.
18. Maty SC, Everson-Rose SA, Haan MN, Raghunathan TE, Kaplan GA. Education, income, occupation, and the 34-year incidence (1965–1999) of type 2 diabetes in the Alameda County Study. Int J Epidemiol. 2005;34(6):1274–81.
19. Levy N, Moynihan V, Nilo A, Singer K, Bernik LS, Etiebet MA, et al. The mobile insulin titration intervention (MITI) for insulin adjustment in an urban, low-income population: randomized controlled trial. J Med Internet Res. 2015;17(7), e180.
20. Diabetes HbA1c {Poor control}. The U. S. Department of Health and Human Services. http://www.hrsa.gov/quality/toolbox/508pdfs/diabetesmodule.pdf. Accessed July 20th 2015.
21. Hipp JA, Chalise N. Spatial analysis and correlates of county-level diabetes prevalence, 2009–2010. Prev Chronic Dis. 2015;12, E08.
22. Dzhambov AM. Long-term noise exposure and the risk for type 2 diabetes: a meta-analysis. Noise Health. 2015;17(74):23–33.
23. Dzhambov A, Dimitrova D. Chronic noise exposure and testosterone deficiency—meta-analysis and meta-regression of experimental studies in rodents. Endokrynol Pol. 2015;66(1):39–46.
24. Grossmann M. Low testosterone in men with type 2 diabetes: significance and treatment. J Clin Endocrinol Metab. 2011;96(8):2341–53.

25. Hogan P, Dall T, Nikolov P, American DA. Economic costs of diabetes in the US in 2002. Diabetes Care. 2003;26(3):917–32.
26. Buse JB, Ginsberg HN, Bakris GL, Clark NG, Costa F, Eckel R, et al. Primary prevention of cardiovascular diseases in people with diabetes mellitus: a scientific statement from the American Heart Association and the American Diabetes Association. Diabetes Care. 2007;30(1):162–72.
27. Nichols GA, Brown JB. The impact of cardiovascular disease on medical care costs in subjects with and without type 2 diabetes. Diabetes Care. 2002;25(3):482–6.
28. Krolewski AS, Niewczas MA, Skupien J, Gohda T, Smiles A, Eckfeldt JH, et al. Early progressive renal decline precedes the onset of microalbuminuria and its progression to macroalbuminuria. Diabetes Care. 2014;37(1):226–34.
29. Garg JP, Bakris GL. Microalbuminuria: marker of vascular dysfunction, risk factor for cardiovascular disease. Vasc Med. 2002;7(1):35–43.
30. Klausen K, Borch-Johnsen K, Feldt-Rasmussen B, Jensen G, Clausen P, Scharling H, et al. Very low levels of microalbuminuria are associated with increased risk of coronary heart disease and death independently of renal function, hypertension, and diabetes. Circulation. 2004;110(1):32–5.
31. American Diabetes Association. Standards of medical care in diabetes—2014. Diabetes Care. 2014;37 Suppl 1:S14–80.
32. Wang S, Wang Y, Zheng R, Zhao Z, Ma Y. Osteoinductive factor is a novel biomarker for the diagnosis of early diabetic nephropathy. Int J Clin Exp Pathol. 2015;8(3):3110–5.
33. Fong DS, Aiello L, Gardner TW, King GL, Blankenship G, Cavallerano JD, et al. Retinopathy in diabetes. Diabetes Care. 2003;27 Suppl 1:S84–7.
34. Boulton AJM, Vinik AI, Arezzo JC, Bril V, Feldman EL, Freeman R, et al. Diabetic neuropathies: a statement by the American Diabetes Association. Diabetes Care. 2005;28(4):956–62.
35. Merashli M, Chowdhury TA, Jawad AS. Musculoskeletal manifestations of diabetes mellitus. QJM. 2015;108(11):853–7.
36. The Lancet Diabetes & Endocrinology. Poor mental health in diabetes: still a neglected comorbidity. Lancet Diabetes Endocrinol. 2015;3(6):393.
37. Deschenes SS, Burns RJ, Schmitz N. Associations between diabetes, major depressive disorder and generalized anxiety disorder comorbidity, and disability: findings from the 2012 Canadian Community Health Survey—Mental Health (CCHS-MH). J Psychosom Res. 2015;78(2):137–42.
38. Ali N, Jyotsna VP, Kumar N, Mani K. Prevalence of depression among type 2 diabetes compared to healthy non diabetic controls. J Assoc Physicians India. 2013;61(9):619–21.
39. Barnard KD, Skinner TC, Peveler R. The prevalence of co-morbid depression in adults with type 1 diabetes: systematic literature review. Diabet Med. 2006;23(4):445–8.
40. Nouwen A, Winkley K, Twisk J, Lloyd CE, Peyrot M, Ismail K, et al. Type 2 diabetes mellitus as a risk factor for the onset of depression: a systematic review and meta-analysis. Diabetologia. 2010;53(12):2480–6.
41. Anderson RJ, Freedland KE, Clouse RE, Lustman PJ. The prevalence of comorbid depression in adults with diabetes: a meta-analysis. Diabetes Care. 2001;24(6):1069–78.
42. Roy T, Lloyd CE. Epidemiology of depression and diabetes: a systematic review. J Affect Disord. 2012;142(Suppl):S8–21.
43. Mezuk B, Eaton WW, Albrecht S, Golden SH. Depression and type 2 diabetes over the lifespan: a meta-analysis. Diabetes Care. 2008;31(12):2383–90.
44. Pouwer F, Beekman AT, Nijpels G, Dekker JM, Snoek FJ, Kostense PJ, et al. Rates and risks for co-morbid depression in patients with type 2 diabetes mellitus: results from a community-based study. Diabetologia. 2003;46(7):892–8.
45. Chew BH, Shariff-Ghazali S, Fernandez A. Psychological aspects of diabetes care: effecting behavioral change in patients. World J Diabetes. 2014;5(6):796–808.
46. Ahmed N. Advanced glycation endproducts—role in pathology of diabetic complications. Diabetes Res Clin Pract. 2005;67(1):3–21.
47. Kotagal M, Symons RG, Hirsch IB, Umpierrez GE, Dellinger EP, Farrokhi ET, et al. Perioperative hyperglycemia and risk of adverse events among patients with and without diabetes. Ann Surg. 2015;261(1):97–103.
48. Acott AA, Theus SA, Kim LT. Long-term glucose control and risk of perioperative complications. Am J Surg. 2009;198(5):596–9.
49. Center for Disease Control and Prevention. Annual Number (in Thousands) of new cases of diagnosed diabetes among adults aged 18–79 Years, United States, 1980–2013. 2015. http://www.cdc.gov/diabetes/statistics/incidence/fig3.htm. Accessed 8 June 2015.
50. Anjana RM, Sudha V, Nair DH, Lakshmipriya N, Deepa M, Pradeepa R, et al. Diabetes in Asian Indians-How much is preventable? Ten-year follow-up of the Chennai Urban Rural Epidemiology Study (CURES-142). Diabetes Res Clin Pract. 2015;109(2):253–61.

Sandeep P. Soin, Joshua G. Hunter,
and Stephen L. Kates

Introduction

This chapter serves as a primer on the pathophysiology of both diabetes mellitus and Charcot arthropathy for the orthopedic surgeon. In regards to diabetes we will focus on the pathophysiology as it pertains to musculoskeletal manifestations of the disease process. The pathophysiology that underlies the development of diabetes is beyond the scope of this chapter. We will discuss both the historic theories of pathogenesis and identify modern theories and advancements in the understanding of Charcot arthropathy, a progressive disease that leads to degeneration of joints, especially to those of the foot and ankle.

Diabetes Mellitus

Diabetes mellitus is a disease of glucose metabolism. It has many different underlying etiologies, which have become increasingly important to understand as its prevalence has increased tremendously in both the United States and globally. It has been reported that over 29 million people have diabetes in the United States alone [1]. The many complications associated with diabetes can affect multiple end organ systems. The disease is one of the leading causes of death, blindness, renal failure, and amputation [1] and the cost associated with treating the disease and its associated complications surpassed $245 billion in 2012 [2].

There are two predominate types of diabetes: Type I, historically known as insulin-dependent diabetes, and Type II, formerly known as non-insulin-dependent diabetes. The fundamental difference between the two types is the way in which glucose metabolism is altered. In type I diabetes, insulin production is limited within the pancreas by an autoimmune process. In type II diabetes, insulin receptors are downregulated throughout the body resulting in insulin resistance. In either case, the result is deranged blood glucose control and periods of hyperglycemia. One focus of this chapter is to explore the pathogenesis of musculoskeletal complications in diabetes as it applies to both types I and II.

S.P. Soin, M.D. • J.G. Hunter, M.D.
S.L. Kates, M.D. (✉)
Department of Orthopaedic Surgery and Rehabilitation, University of Rochester Medical Center and 2 Virginia Commonwealth University, 1200 E. Broad St., Richmond, VA 23059, USA
e-mail: sandeep_soin@urmc.rochester.edu; joshua_hunter@urmc.rochester.edu; stephen.kates@vcuhealth.org

Charcot Arthropathy

Charcot arthropathy is a progressive and destructive disease process that affects the joints of the extremities in patients with neuropathic

© Springer International Publishing Switzerland 2016
D. Herscovici, Jr. (ed.), *The Surgical Management of the Diabetic Foot and Ankle*,
DOI 10.1007/978-3-319-27623-6_2

conditions [3]. Today it is most commonly associated with diabetes and is often found in the foot and ankle [3, 4]. Charcot arthropathy has historically been known as a rare disease; however, with increasing rates of obesity and increasing prevalence of diabetes, the impact of this devastating disease process, on both patients and healthcare dollars, will continue to increase [1, 2]. It is estimated that up to one in three patients with diabetic neuropathy will develop an arthropathy [5].

Charcot arthropathy was first described in the late 1868 by the neurologist Jean-Martin Charcot in patients with tabes dorsalis [6–8]. He described an acute onset of pain followed by joint destruction ultimately leading to impaired function. At that time, "Charcot's joint" was most commonly associated with syphilis and it was not until 1936 that the association to diabetes was made [7–9].

The disease process is often initiated by subtle or insignificant trauma to the joint of a neuropathic patient. The clinical and radiographic progression has been classically described by Eichenholtz as occurring in three distinct stages (see Fig. 2.1) [10]. Stage I (acute or developmental phase) is identified with swelling, erythema, warmth of the extremity and bony fragmentation on radiographs. This phase is often confused with a soft tissue infection, abscess or cellulitis, especially in the diabetic patient, leading to a delay in treatment. An important finding on physical exam is the resolution or improvement in erythema with elevation of the extremity [11] (See Table in the Appendix). The presence of dependent erythema is usually associated with Charcot arthropathy. It should also be noted that infection without the presence of a wound or ulcer is rare and that a diagnosis of a Charcot arthropathy should be strongly considered [11, 12]. Eichenholtz Stage II (coalescent or quiescent phase) is marked by improvement in swelling and erythema and consolidation of fracture fragmentation on radiographs. Stage III (reconstruction phase) is highlighted by ankylosis of joints and hypertrophy of the bone. Through the progression of the arthropathy, the patient may develop a deformity, instability, and dysfunction of the involved joint. Infection not only plays a role in confounding the diagnosis of Charcot

arthropathy, it is also a late complication. That is because the development of hypertrophic exostoses may cause an, altered gait and instability, and may lead to the development of an ulcer. These ulcers are challenging to manage due to both micro- and macro- vascular disease, along with an impaired immune function. This constellation of complications: deformity, dysfunction, and infection, creates significant problems for the orthopedic surgeon and unfortunately may be limb threatening.

Pathophysiology of Diabetes

The pathophysiology surrounding the complications of diabetes, as it pertains to the musculoskeletal system, will be reviewed. Intuitively and academically proven, diabetic patients are at higher risk for surgical site infections, foot ulcers, and poor bone healing. The underlying reasons can be explained in part by an impairment of the vascular system, nervous system, and immune system. These are summarized in Table 2.1.

Vascular System

Diabetes can lead to both microvascular and macrovascular disease through a dysfunction of endothelial cells and vascular smooth muscle [13]. Periods of hyperglycemia are a trigger for cellular dysfunction and dysregulation, by altering the normal coagulation pathways. This leaves vessels predisposed to thrombosis. The end product is reduced blood flow at the tissue level. This limits healing by allowing waste product accumulation and a lack of nutrient delivery. In the setting of infection, this vascular dysfunction will cause the delivery of antibiotic therapies to be limited. Please see Chap. 3 for further discussion of the vascular problems associated with diabetes.

Endothelial Cell Dysfunction

The endothelial cells, which line the vessels throughout the vascular system, play a crucial role in balancing blood flow. This is done on a local

Fig. 2.1 AP and lateral foot radiographs depicting the three Eichenholtz stages of Charcot neuroarthropathy. (**a**) Stage I—*acute phase*, note the prominent soft tissue swelling and early bony fragmentation, (**b**) Stage II—*coalescence phase*, improved swelling, beginning of callus formation, (**c**) Stage III—*reconstructive phase*, ankylosis of the midfoot and first tarsometatarsal joints

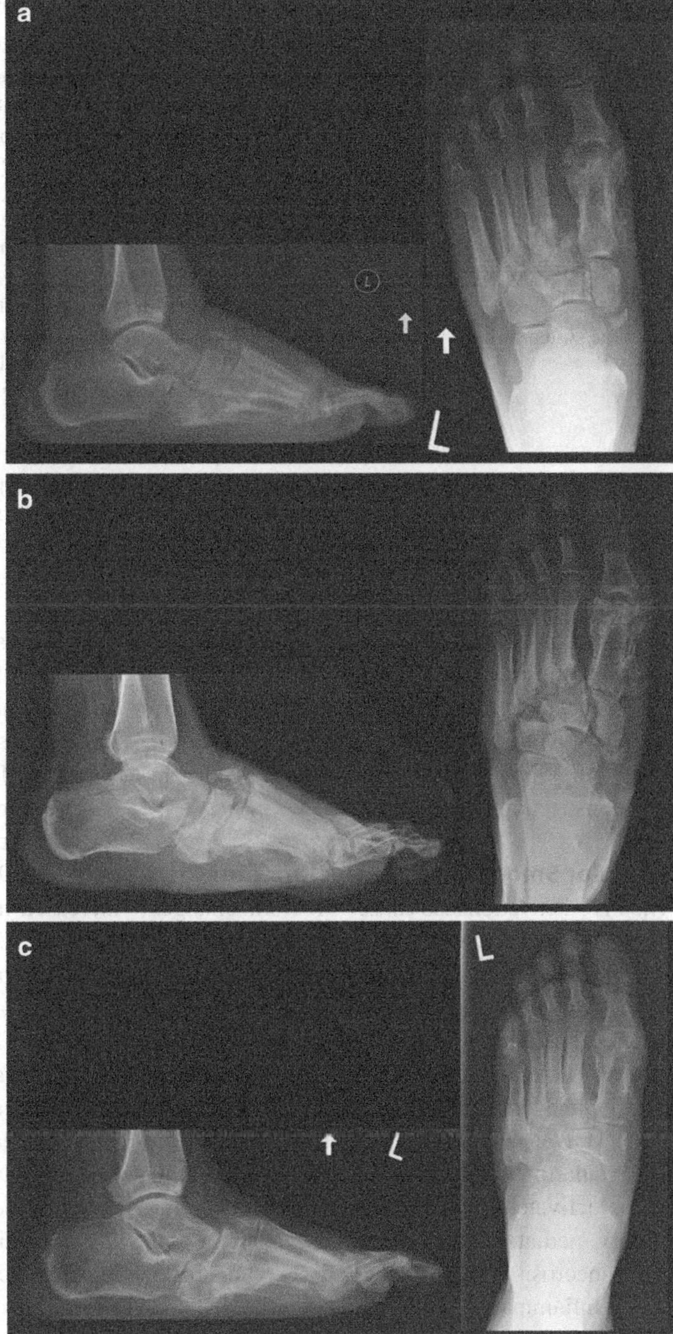

level through paracrine factors. High glucose levels decrease the levels of nitric oxide (NO), a locally active vasodilator [14]. The excess glucose is taken into the endothelial cell where protein kinase C (PKC) is activated in the mitochondria. The PKC activation is then accompanied by the production of radical oxygen species (ROS). It is through this mechanism that the majority of hyperglycemia-induced ROS are produced. Superoxide ions, a specific ROS, reduce the NO to peroxynitrite. Peroxynitrite easily passes through the membrane of endothelial cells

Table 2.1 Mechanisms of pathophysiology in diabetes mellitus by system

Vascular system	Endothelial cell dysfunction	NO imbalance, production of ROS
	Vascular smooth muscle dysfunction	PKC activation, ROS production, Monocyte activation, proinflammatory state, fibrosis
	Coagulation and platelet dysfunction	NF-kB activation → proinflammatory state, increased TF activation and increased PAI-1 Levels → thrombosis
Nervous system	Oxidative stress	Production of ROS, decreased synaptic NO, formation of AGEs, activation or RAGE, activation of NK-kB → proinflammatory state, mesenchymal stem cell apoptosis
	Microvascular disease	Neural hypoxemia, intraneural vascular hyalinization, thrombosis, loss of regulation of neural bloodflow
Immune system	Innate immune system dysfunction	Decreased complement, increased basal levels of TNF-a, IL-6, IL-8 via NF-kB activation, decreased inflammatory response from PBMCs in setting of stimulation, impaired PMN chemotaxis
	Adaptive immune system dysfunction	Monocyte/Macrophage dysfunction, IgG inactivation by glycosylation

NO nitric oxide, *ROS* reactive oxygen species, *NF-kB* Nuclear Factor Kappa-light-chain-enhancer of active B cells, *TF* tissue factor, *PAI-1* plasminogen activator inhibitor-1, *AGEs* advanced glycation end products, *RAGE* receptor for advanced glycation end products, *TNF-a* tumor necrosis factor alpha, *IL* interleukin, *PBMCs* peripheral blood mononuclear cells, *PMN* polymorphonuclear cells, *IgG* immunoglobulin G

and causes nitrosylation of the enzymes involved in the synthesis of NO. Through this mechanism, hyperglycemia leads to both reduction and impaired synthesis of NO, via the generation of ROS. The inability to regulate NO results in vasoconstriction [13, 14].

Vascular Smooth Muscle Dysfunction

The PKC activation also causes structural changes in the vascular architecture, induces the production of vascular inflammation, and causes the ROS to increase the transcription of proinflammatory genes. These genes include monocyte chemoattractant protein-1, vascular cell adhesion molecule-1, and intracellular adhesion molecule-1. When activated, these genes result in the adhesion of circulating monocytes to the endothelium. These activated monocytes then secrete inflammatory mediators, such as interleukin (IL)-1 and tumor necrosis factor alpha (TNF-a). The subsequent inflammatory state leads to fibrosis and dysfunction of the vascular smooth muscle, leading to narrowing of vessel caliber [15, 16].

Coagulation Dysfunction

In normal conditions, insulin inhibits platelet aggregation through tissue factor (TF) inhibition and decreased plasminogen activator inhibitor-1 (PAI-1) levels [17]. However, in type II diabetes,

insulin resistance is associated with increased cellular PAI-1 levels, thereby reducing tissue plasminogen activator levels, a known thrombolytic agent. This results in diabetic patients, especially those with type II diabetes, to become prothrombotic

There are multiple theories explaining the dysfunctional coagulation seen in the diabetic patient [13, 17–19]. Free fatty acid (FFA) levels are increased in most patients with type II diabetes. These FFAs bind to toll-like receptors, which are involved in activating the nuclear factor kappa-light-chain-enhancer of the active B cells (NF-kB) pathway. The NF-kB pathway is a proinflammatory pathway. This chronic low-grade inflammatory pathway induces the production of TF and causes an early trigger in the coagulation cascade. The proinflammatory state also causes endothelial cell dysfunction, as described above, which leads to endothelial cell damage. Once the damaged collagen is exposed to circulating platelets and coagulation factors, it leads to thrombosis. This is currently the best theory for this dysfunction.

Nervous System

Neuropathy is a common complication of diabetes. More than 60 % of diabetics have some signs and symptoms of neuropathy [5, 20]. These include loss of protective sensation, autonomic dysfunction, pain, and weakness. Diabetic neuropathy, coupled with the other complications of diabetes, sets patients up for ulceration, wound breakdown, and poor healing. The mechanisms by which diabetes and hyperglycemia lead to damage of the peripheral nervous system are explained in part by oxidative stress, inflammation, and microvascular disease. It is likely that a complex interaction between these mechanisms and multiple pathogenic processes ultimately leads to the clinical outcome of diabetic neuropathy.

Oxidative Stress

As noted with vascular dysfunction, hyperglycemia leads to an increased formation of ROS, which has a direct affect on NO production in endothelial cells. In the nervous system NO is a common neurotransmitter and ROS formation causes a reduction of the intracellular production of NO in neurons. This ultimately leads to dysfunction of the nerve.

Hyperglycemia also leads to the formation of advanced glycation end products (AGEs) by reducing reactions of protein amino groups [21, 22]. In addition to producing neurologic abnormalities, AGEs also have profound effects on the vasculature system and are deposited in collagen of soft tissues leading to muscle and tendon dysfunction. This contributes to altered gait patterns and predispose patients with peripheral neuropathies to microtrauma.

During its formation more ROS are liberated. This results in species that bind to the receptor for advanced glycation end products (RAGE), a transmembrane protein. This causes an activation of the NF-kB pathway. This leads to upregulation of the RAGE receptor, which increases the production of ROS, and leads to an increase in the numbers of proinflammatory mediators. This directs activated RAGE receptors towards apoptosis of mesenchymal stem cells [23]. Activation of this pathway sets the stage for chronic and unchecked inflammation.

Microvascular Neurologic Disease

It is believed that the vascular changes caused by hyperglycemia also lead to decreased endoneurial blood flow and nerve ischemia. Endoneurial blood flow is controlled through a process of arteriovenous shunting that is regulated by unmyelinated nerve fibers. When these regulatory nerve fibers are damaged there is a loss of regulation of blood flow to the nerve and hypoxemia is exacerbated. This is often associated with a decrease in motor neuron function. The structural changes that occur at the level of the intraneural vasculature include hyalinization and vessel wall thickening, similar to the changes that occur with microvascular disease. These changes include fibrin deposition, platelet activation, and thrombosis formation in the vessels supplying peripheral nerves.

Immune System

It has long been established that there is a degree of immune system dysfunction associated with diabetes. This dysfunction, coupled with that occurring to the vascular and nervous systems, predisposes diabetics to infections that can be difficult to treat and are potentially limb threatening. Diabetes has been associated with many derangements in the innate immune system but there has also been dysfunction noted in the adaptive immune system.

Innate Immune System

Diabetes has been found to affect the function of the innate immune system through multiple mechanisms [24, 25]. The innate immune system is a nonspecific host defense against pathogens. Its main components consist of physical epithelial barriers, phagocytic leukocytes, dendritic cells, a special type of leukocyte known as a natural killer (NK) cell, and circulating plasma proteins. In many cases it is the first line of defense against infection.

The complement system is a complex and integral part of the innate immune system that amplifies the response against a pathogen and ultimately results in cell death. Patients with diabetes have been shown to have a lower than normal serum concentration of complement factor 4 (C4), which is an important part of the complement pathway [26]. However, the clinical relevance of the reduced C4 levels in diabetics remains unclear.

As previously noted, hyperglycemia, and especially diabetes, increase production of ROS, which activates the NF-kB pathway and increases proinflammatory cytokines, predominately TNF-a, IL-6, and IL-8. These inflammatory cytokines play a critical role in regulation of the immune system in times of infection. However, due to persistent hyperglycemic conditions, the serum levels of these cytokines are chronically elevated [27, 28].

Due to chronically elevated cytokines, the response to an infection is decreased. Polymorphonuclear cells (PMNs) are the phagocytic cells of the innate immune system that predominate in the circulation. In order to gain access to a site of infection they undergo the process of chemotaxis. During this process, the cells migrate towards areas of infection or inflammation, following a chemical gradient of various cytokines. It has long been established that the PMNs of diabetic patients have defective chemotaxis [24]. Interestingly, the levels of inflammatory cytokines, produced from peripheral blood mononuclear cells of diabetic patients, do not increase as expected when stimulated with lipopolysaccharide (LPS), a component of gram-negative bacteria. One theory is that the constituently active monocytes of diabetic patient may grow tolerant to their stimulated environment and their response is often blunted in the setting of infection.

Adaptive Immune System

The adaptive immune system is responsible for historic immunity against pathogens. It is called into action against pathogens that are able to evade or overcome the innate immune defenses. When activated these components "adapt" to the presence of infection by activating, proliferating, and creating potent mechanisms for neutralizing or eliminating microbes. Diabetes has generally not been associated with derangements in the adaptive immune system; however, there are some observations that have been made that raise the concern of dysfunctional macrophage phagocytosis and antibody inactivation. One study has shown that patients with type I diabetes have a decreased antibody titer response to hepatitis B vaccination and have implicated impaired macrophage phagocytosis as the

mechanism [29]. This theory is supported by the macrophage/monocyte dysfunction that is due to chronically elevated inflammatory mediators.

There are two types of adaptive immune responses: humoral immunity, that is mediated by antibodies produced by B lymphocytes, and cell-mediated immunity, mediated by T lymphocytes. Immunoglobulin G (IgG) is a dominant antibody which confers adaptive immunity to individuals who have been exposed to antigens previously. In diabetic patients IgG can become nonenzymatically glycosylated. It is believed that these antibodies do not function as well as normal IgG. Using an animal model, one study examined asplenic rats inoculated with *Streptococcus pneumonia* that were treated with either normal or glycosylated IgG [30]. Those receiving normal IgG lived roughly twice as long than those receiving glycosylated IgG. It appears that glycosylation of IgG leads to inactivation and functional alteration of the adaptive immune system.

Pathophysiology of Charcot Arthropathy

Neurotraumatic and Neurotrophic Theories

Over time, many theories have been developed that have tried to explain the pathophysiology of Charcot arthropathy. Jean-Martin Charcot promoted the *French Theory*, in which it was believed that damage to the spinal cord or nerves resulted from an injury to vasomotor nerves, resulting in loss of the neural control over the vasculature [7, 31]. Volkmann and Virchow described the *neurotraumatic theory*, which described a process where the bones and joints changed due to repeated microtrauma in patients that cannot sense pain [7]. The *neurovascular or neurotrophic theory*, an advancement on Charcot's French Theory, described an autonomic neuropathy predominated by sympathetic denervation, leading to an increase in arteriovenous shunting and local blood flow by 30–60 %. This was thought to stimulate osteoclast activity and flush away the necessary minerals for bone formation, leading to the development of osteopenia.

Fig. 2.2 Summary figure depicting the major pathophysiologic steps and interactions between diabetes mellitus and Charcot neuroarthropathy. *ROS* reactive oxygen species, *AGEs* advanced glycation end products, *IL* interleukin, *TNF-a* tumor necrosis factor alpha, *RANK* receptor activator of NF-kB, *RANKL* receptor activator of NF-kB ligand, *OPG* Osteoprotegrin

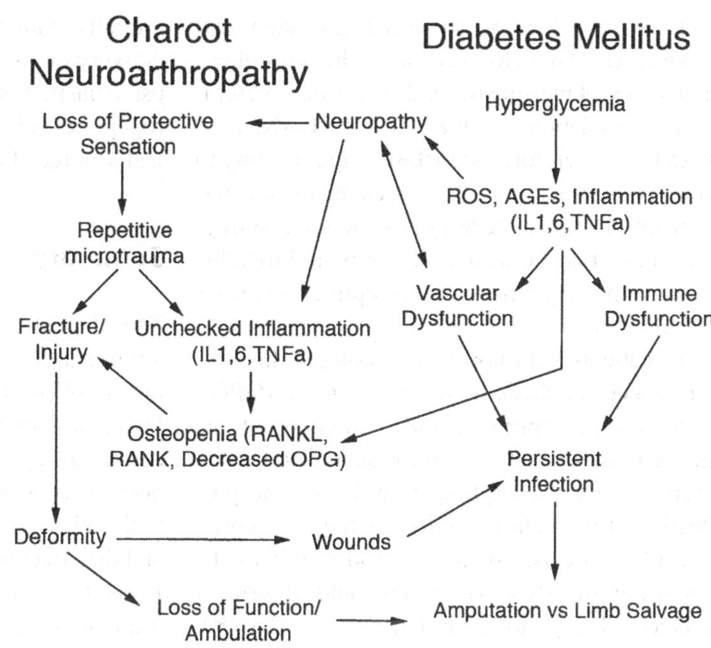

Modern Theory

The pathogenesis of Charcot arthropathy has proven to be complex and continues to be under investigation [31, 32]. However, it is clear that aspects of both the neurotraumatic and neurovascular theories contribute to the disease process. More recently, the role of inflammation, bone turnover, and neuropeptides have become the key topics discussed in the literature [32–35]. Charcot arthropathy has now become closely associated with diabetes, which is likely due to the rise in the prevalence of type II diabetes. Lately, more attention has been spent on the interaction between these two diseases. The degree of overlap between the two disease processes is depicted in Fig. 2.2.

Role of Inflammation and Bone Turnover

In normal physiologic conditions, inflammation is a natural response to injury. One hallmark of a proinflammatory state is pain, which limits the motion and stress an individual places on an injured extremity. However, in the setting of neuropathy, patients lack the ability to sense pain, leading to repetitive trauma to the injured extremity. In Charcot arthropathy, the resulting bone and

joint destruction described in the neurotraumatic model, was once thought to be a directly related to the trauma itself. However, the classic changes that are seen are actually related to an unchecked inflammatory cascade that results from the repetitive microtrauma. A finding that strengthens this theory is that Charcot patients have been shown to have significantly lower bone mineral density than non-Charcot diabetics with peripheral neuropathy [36]. This finding holds true for both the affected and unaffected limb, which supports a theory of inflammation-mediated bone resorption rather than solely trauma-related resorption.

A second item identified, that supports a theory of inflammation, is that the intraoperative tissue obtained from Charcot patients have been found to have positive immunohistological staining for IL-1, IL-6, and TNF-a, three hallmarks of inflammation [33]. Lastly, the theory is bolstered by the findings that proinflammatory cytokines lead to activation of the receptor activator of NF-kB ligand (RANKL). The increase in ROS production and nonenzymatic glycation results in the formation of more AGEs, which also activates RANKL. This triggers many downstream cellular pathways that are implicated in Charcot arthropathy. Activated RANKL interacts and binds with the receptor activator of NF-kB (RANK) and the receptor for advanced glycation end products (RAGE) This leads to further proinflammatory cytokine release and osteoclast maturation. Stimulation of the NF-kB, RANK, or RANKL is therefore osteoclastogenic, leading to bone resorption. It is this mechanism that has been implicated in the bony destruction and fragmentation that is seen in Charcot arthropathy, along with many other osteoresorptive conditions [35, 37–39].

In patients with normal physiology, this system is kept in check by osteoprotegerin (OPG). This is a glycoprotein, and a member of the tumor necrosis factor receptor superfamily, that regulates bone resorption by reducing the production of osteoclasts, inhibiting the differentiation of osteoclast precursors, and regulates the resorption of osteoclasts *in vivo* and *in vitro*. It acts as a decoy molecule that binds to RANKL preventing its activation of RANK. Normally OPG is upregulated via the NF-kB pathway, providing a check on uncontrolled osteoclast maturation. However, the repetitive microtrauma seen in Charcot neuroarthropathy leads to persistent inflammation and ultimately to an increased RANKL/OPG ratio.

Role of Neuropeptides

Neuropeptides are important to the overall health of a nerve, which play a role in bone metabolism. In Charcot patients, the nerves have lost the ability to transport cellular nutrients and neurotransmitters. The mechanism that contributes to bone loss and fragmentation is the loss of modulation of bone turnover by secreted neuropeptides. One such peptide is Calcitonin Gene-Related Peptide (CGRP). This peptide exists in two forms, alpha and beta, and is secreted from small sensory nerve terminals. It is intimately involved in osteoblastic activity and maturation. It binds to the CGRP receptor causing an increase in intracellular calcium in osteoblastic cells and stimulates proliferation and collagen synthesis. It has also been shown to cause the release of IL-10, an anti-inflammatory cytokine [34, 40, 41]. A second neuropeptide affecting bone metabolism is nitrous oxide (NO). This neuropeptide has been shown to induce apoptosis of osteoclast progenitor cells in animal models. With denervation, the delivery of NO is limited and cannot act to check osteoclastic bone resorption Together, these neuropeptides reign unchecked, leading to neurologically induced bone loss.

Summary

The clinical challenges associated with Charcot arthropathy are only compounded in the setting of uncontrolled diabetes. Progress has been made in laying a foundation for understanding the biochemical steps involved in the pathogenesis of diabetes. This includes a focus on problems associated with inflammation, bone resorption mechanisms, and the effect on the loss of certain neuropeptides. In addition, diabetic patients also face vascular and immune complications of diabetes, putting them at a greater risk of dysfunction and limb loss. Diabetic neuropathy also adds to the development of Charcot arthropathy but it appears that the pathophysiology associated with diabetes contributes to the overall process as well.

In order to gain a better understanding of the musculoskeletal manifestations associated with diabetes, one should focus on the derangement of the nervous, vascular, and immune systems. There are commonalities among these diverse systems and recent literature explores the affects of inflammatory pathways and proinflammatory cytokines. Understanding the pathogenesis of these devastating and costly diseases may help identify treatment options to preserve function and prevent limb loss.

References

1. Centers for Disease Control and Prevention. National diabetes fact sheet: general information and national estimates on diabetes in the United States. Atlanta, GA: Centers for Disease Control and Prevention; 2014.
2. American Diabetes Association. Economic costs of diabetes in the U.S. in 2012. Diabetes Care. 2013;36(4):1033–46.
3. Varma AK. Charcot neuroarthropathy of the foot and ankle: a review. J Foot Ankle Surg. 2013;52(6): 740–9.

4. Cameron NE, Eaton SE, Cotter MA, Tesfaye S. Vascular factors and metabolic interactions in the pathogenesis of diabetic neuropathy. Diabetologia. 2001;44(11):1973–88.

5. Cofield RH, Morrison MJ, Beabout JW. Diabetic neuroarthropathy in the foot: patient characteristics and patterns of radiographic change. Foot Ankle. 1983; 4(1):15–22.

6. Al-Nammari SS, Timothy T, Afsie S. A Surgeon's guide to advances in the pharmacological management of acute Charcot neuroarthropathy. Foot Ankle Surg. 2013;19(4):212–7.

7. Sanders LJ. The Charcot foot: historical perspective 1827–2003. Diabetes Metab Res Rev. 2004;20 Suppl 1:S4–8.

8. Kumar DR, Aslinia F, Yale SH, Mazza JJ. Jean-Martin Charcot: the father of neurology. Clin Med Res. 2011;9(1):46–9.

9. Wr J. Neuritic manifestations in diabetes mellitus. Arch Intern Med. 1936;57:307–66.

10. Eichenholtz SN. Charcot joints. Charles C Thomas: Springfield, IL; 1966.

11. Bowker JH, editor. The diabetic foot. St. Louis: Mosby; 1993.

12. Fernando Grover Páez SETS. Sara Pascoe González, and EGCMoz, García CEM. Intech: The Diabetic Charcot Foot; 2013.

13. Paneni F, Beckman JA, Creager MA, Cosentino F. Diabetes and vascular disease: pathophysiology, clinical consequences, and medical therapy: part I. Eur Heart J. 2013;34(31):2436–43.

14. Hink U, Li H, Mollnau H, Oelze M, Matheis E, Hartmann M, et al. Mechanisms underlying endothelial dysfunction in diabetes mellitus. Circ Res. 2001;88(2):E14–22.

15. Inoguchi T, Li P, Umeda F, Yu HY, Kakimoto M, Imamura M, et al. High glucose level and free fatty acid stimulate reactive oxygen species production through protein kinase C—dependent activation of NAD(P)H oxidase in cultured vascular cells. Diabetes. 2000;49(11):1939–45.

16. Brouwers O, Niessen PM, Haenen G, Miyata T, Brownlee M, Stehouwer CD, et al. Hyperglycaemia-induced impairment of endothelium-dependent vasorelaxation in rat mesenteric arteries is mediated by intracellular methylglyoxal levels in a pathway dependent on oxidative stress. Diabetologia. 2010; 53(5):989–1000.

17. Lemkes BA, Hermanides J, Devries JH, Holleman F, Meijers JC, Hoekstra JB. Hyperglycemia: a prothrombotic factor? J Thromb Haemost. 2010;8(8):1663–9.

18. Grant PJ. Diabetes mellitus as a prothrombotic condition. J Intern Med. 2007;262(2):157–72.

19. Beckman JA, Creager MA, Libby P. Diabetes and atherosclerosis: epidemiology, pathophysiology, and management. JAMA. 2002;287(19):2570–81.

20. Dyck PJ, Clark VM, Overland CJ, Davies JL, Pach JM, Dyck PJ, et al. Impaired glycemia and diabetic polyneuropathy: the OC IG Survey. Diabetes Care. 2012;35(3):584–91.

21. Zhao J, Randive R, Stewart JA. Molecular mechanisms of AGE/RAGE-mediated fibrosis in the diabetic heart. World J Diabetes. 2014;5(6):860–7.

22. Kurabayashi M. Vascular Calcification—Pathological Mechanism and Clinical Application—Role of vascular smooth muscle cells in vascular calcification. Clin Calcium. 2015;25(5):661–9.

23. Notsu M, Yamaguchi T, Okazaki K, Tanaka K, Ogawa N, Kanazawa I, et al. Advanced glycation end product 3 (AGE3) suppresses the mineralization of mouse stromal ST2 cells and human mesenchymal stem cells by increasing TGF-beta expression and secretion. Endocrinology. 2014;155(7):2402–10.

24. Mowat A, Baum J. Chemotaxis of polymorphonuclear leukocytes from patients with diabetes mellitus. N Engl J Med. 1971;284(12):621–7.

25. Geerlings SE, Hoepelman AI. Immune dysfunction in patients with diabetes mellitus (DM). FEMS Immunol Med Microbiol. 1999;26(3–4):259–65.

26. Vergani D, Johnston C, B-Abdullah N, Barnett AH. Low serum C4 concentrations: an inherited predisposition to insulin dependent diabetes? Br Med J (Clin Res Ed). 1983;286(6369):926–8.

27. Zozulinska D, Majchrzak A, Sobieska M, Wiktorowicz K, Wierusz-Wysocka B. Serum interleukin-8 level is increased in diabetic patients. Diabetologia. 1999; 42(1):117–8.

28. Mooradian AD, Reed RL, Meredith KE, Scuderi P. Serum levels of tumor necrosis factor and IL-1 alpha and IL-1 beta in diabetic patients. Diabetes Care. 1991;14(1):63–5.

29. Li Volti S, Caruso-Nicoletti M, Biazzo F, Sciacca A, Mandara G, Mancuso M, et al. Hyporesponsiveness to intradermal administration of hepatitis B vaccine in insulin dependent diabetes mellitus. Arch Dis Child. 1998;78(1):54–7.

30. Black CT, Hennessey PJ, Andrassy RJ. Short-term hyperglycemia depresses immunity through nonenzymatic glycosylation of circulating immunoglobulin. J Trauma. 1990;30(7):830–2. discussion 2-3.

31. Jeffcoate WJ. Charcot neuro-osteoarthropathy. Diabetes Metab Res Rev. 2008;24 Suppl 1:S62–5.

32. Bruhn-Olszewska B, Korzon-Burakowska A, Gabig-Ciminska M, Olszewski P, Wegrzyn A, Jakobkiewicz-Banecka J. Molecular factors involved in the development of diabetic foot syndrome. Acta Biochim Pol. 2012;59(4):507–13.

33. Baumhauer JF, O'Keefe RJ, Schon LC, Pinzur MS. Cytokine-induced osteoclastic bone resorption in Charcot arthropathy: an immunohistochemical study. Foot Ankle Int. 2006;27(10):797–800.

34. Offley SC, Guo TZ, Wei T, Clark JD, Vogel H, Lindsey DP, et al. Capsaicin-sensitive sensory neurons contribute to the maintenance of trabecular bone integrity. J Bone Miner Res. 2005;20(2):257–67.

35. Ndip A, Williams A, Jude EB, Serracino-Inglott F, Richardson S, Smyth JV, et al. The RANKL/RANK/OPG signaling pathway mediates medial arterial calcification in diabetic Charcot neuroarthropathy. Diabetes. 2011;60(8):2187–96.

36. Gutekunst DJ, Smith KE, Commean PK, Bohnert KL, Prior FW, Sinacore DR. Impact of Charcot neuroarthropathy on metatarsal bone mineral density and geometric strength indices. Bone. 2013;52(1): 407–13.
37. Larson SA, Burns PR. The pathogenesis of Charcot neuroarthropathy: current concepts. Diabet Foot Ankle. 2012;3.
38. Kaynak G, Birsel O, Guven MF, Ogut T. An overview of the Charcot foot pathophysiology. Diabet Foot Ankle. 2013;4:12. doi:10.3402/dfa.v4i0.21117.
39. Uccioli L, Sinistro A, Almerighi C, Ciaprini C, Cavazza A, Giurato L, et al. Proinflammatory modulation of the surface and cytokine phenotype of monocytes in patients with acute Charcot foot. Diabetes Care. 2010;33(2):350–5.
40. Irie K, Hara-Irie F, Ozawa H, Yajima T. Calcitonin gene-related peptide (CGRP)-containing nerve fibers in bone tissue and their involvement in bone remodeling. Microsc Res Tech. 2002;58(2):85–90.
41. Wang L, Shi X, Zhao R, Halloran BP, Clark DJ, Jacobs CR, et al. Calcitonin-gene-related peptide stimulates stromal cell osteogenic differentiation and inhibits RANKL induced NF-kappaB activation, osteoclastogenesis and bone resorption. Bone. 2010; 46(5):1369–79.

Evaluation and Management of Vascular Disease in the Diabetic Patient

3

Erin Green and Brad Johnson

Introduction

Diabetes is mentioned in early Egyptian manuscripts in 1500 BC [1] with atherosclerosis identified in 38 % of mummies of ancient Egyptians, demonstrating that both continue as problems of modern society [2]. Atherosclerosis in the diabetic occurs mainly in the popliteal and tibial vessels and is complicated by peripheral neuropathy and motor paralysis of the intrinsic muscles of the foot. These factors contribute to the finding that gangrene occurs 53 times more frequently in diabetic men and 71 times more frequently in diabetic women, as compared to their nondiabetic counterparts [3]. This chapter provides a fundamental understanding of the disease process while describing how to evaluate and manage these patients.

Pathophysiology

This section will provide a brief overview of the basic mechanism for plaque formation in diabetic patients while emphasizing those risk factors found in diabetics that promote it.

E. Green, M.D. • B. Johnson, M.D. (✉)
Division of Vascular Surgery, University of South Florida, Suite # 7005, 2 Tampa General Circle, Tampa, FL 33606, USA
e-mail: Bjohnson@hsc.usf.edu

In early atherogenesis, recruitment of inflammatory cells and the accumulation of lipids along the intima lead to the formation of a lipid core. If the inflammatory conditions persist, in the presence of dyslipidemia, then plaque formation will occur. Abnormalities in the components of the Metabolic Syndrome (Table 3.1) will increase those factors that promote plaque development [4]. One of those elements is diabetes and its associated hyperglycemia. Increased levels of glucose in diabetics cause the accumulation of glycated macromolecules which leads to the formation of advanced glycation end products (AGEs). The AGEs have been found to promote inflammation and are a key component of atherogenesis.

Thus, hyperglycemia increases AGEs, which in turn promotes inflammation and accumulation of smooth muscle cells in the arterial wall. These smooth muscle cells produce the growth factors leading to extracellular matrix formation and the generation of atherosclerotic fibrous plaques. Therefore, uncontrolled diabetes and its associated hyperglycemia can lead to plaque formation and peripheral arterial disease (PAD) at a younger age.

Studies have also shown that the duration of diabetes and use of insulin are associated with an increase in atherosclerosis and the development of PAD [5]. Due to these abnormalities, atherosclerosis develops at a younger age in diabetic patients and progresses rapidly if hyperglycemia is not well controlled. As a result, diabetic patients with PAD have a tenfold increase in the

© Springer International Publishing Switzerland 2016
D. Herscovici, Jr. (ed.), *The Surgical Management of the Diabetic Foot and Ankle*,
DOI 10.1007/978-3-319-27623-6_3

Table 3.1 Criteria for the metabolic syndrome[a]

Risk factor	Defining level
Abdominal obesity[b] (waist circumference[c])	
Men	>102 cm (>40 in.)
Women	>88 cm (>35 in.)
Triglycerides	≥150 mg/dL
HDL-C	
Men	<40 mg/dL
Women	<50 mg/dL
Blood pressure	≥130/≥85 mmHg
Fasting glucose	≥110 mg/dL

[a]Diagnosis is established when ≥3 of these risk factors are present

[b]Abdominal obesity is more highly correlated with metabolic risk factors than is increased body mass index (BMI)

[c]Some men developed metabolic risk factors when circumference is only marginally increased

HDL-C high density lipoprotein-cholesterol

Adapted from the Expert Panel on Detection, Evaluation, and Treatment of High Blood Cholesterol in Adults. JAMA. 285:2486,2001

rate of amputations compared to nondiabetics, often occurring at a much earlier age. This was identified in the Diabetes Control and Complications Trial (DCCT) which demonstrated that intensive glycemic control lead to a 42 % reduction in peripheral vascular events (i.e., revascularization procedures and amputations) [6]. Furthermore, aggressive glycemic control was also found to decrease the development of elevated total and low density lipoprotein (LDL) cholesterol, which have also been shown to contribute to atherogenesis.

Clinical Manifestations

In the majority of patients with PAD, the clinical manifestation of their disease process is calf cramping with ambulation and improvement of the cramping with rest. The term used to describe these symptoms is intermittent claudication and is the classic presentation of PAD. In patients with diabetes, the diagnosis of PAD can be more challenging as their peripheral neuropathy can cause blunting of their pain perception and prevent them from experiencing these classic symptoms. Diabetic patients tend to present with vague complaints of leg fatigue and decreased pace while walking. The difference in presenting symptoms ultimately leads to delay in diagnosis. Due to this, the lesions are usually more severe, diffuse, and tend to involve the distal vessels at the time of diagnosis. These lesions usually affect the tibial vessels (Image 3.1) and also produce significant occlusive disease of the metatarsal arteries. However, the calcification process in the metatarsal arteries is usually limited to proximal digital vessels and rarely involves distal digital vessels. This is an important concept to remember

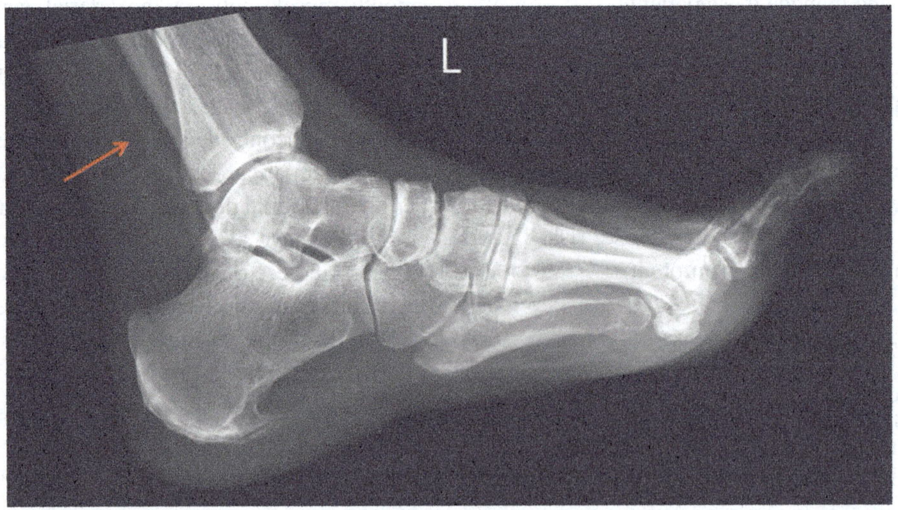

Image 3.1 Left foot plain X-ray. *Red arrow* indicates calcified posterior tibial artery in a diabetic patient with peripheral vascular disease. Also note calcified anterior vessel

during the evaluation of patients, since the calcification of tibial vessels limits the accuracy of the ankle-brachial index (ABI) while toe pressures (TP) will reflect the true blood perfusion of the foot.

The atypical presentation makes it difficult to determine the true prevalence of PAD in the diabetic population. In one study, ABIs were used to determine PAD in diabetic patients fifty years and older. The study identified the prevalence of PAD in this population to be approximately 29 %. It was also found that only a small percentage of these patients had classic symptoms of intermittent claudication [7]. Due to the atypical presentation combined with the fact that ABI is not as sensitive in diabetic patients, the actual incidence of PAD in this population is likely much higher.

Evaluation of Peripheral Arterial Disease

Prior to any surgical intervention, patients with diabetes and peripheral vascular disease must be assessed very carefully. This subgroup of patients can present with very complex pathology and this must be remembered during their evaluation. In addition, they often present with significant health problems, are at a high risk of poor wound healing, and can develop complications that may require numerous operations to salvage the extremity.

The first step in evaluation of any patient is a thorough history and physical exam. It is also important to determine how well the patient controls their diabetes and if they are followed closely by a primary care clinician. As previously discussed, diabetic patients tend to present with vague complaints of leg fatigue and slower walking pace. Patients should be asked how far they can walk before onset of symptoms and how their walking habits have been affected by their symptoms. This will give a clinician a good idea as to how active the patient has been and what impact their symptoms are having on how they live their life. It is also important to determine if the patient only has pain with ambulation or if the pain occurs at rest as well. Resting pain usually indicates a more severe problem and should be evaluated by a vascular surgeon immediately.

Once a complete history has been obtained, a thorough physical exam should be performed. Inspection of the patient's bilateral lower extremities is extremely important. All articles of clothing should be removed, especially socks, and the patient should be dressed in a gown to allow for complete examination. All pulses should be palpated, including bilateral radial, femoral, popliteal, dorsalis pedis, and posterior tibial pulses. If pulses are unable to be palpated, then a Doppler can be used to assess for arterial flow. Care should be taken to carefully inspect both feet to ensure there are no wounds or ulcerations. Motor and sensation should be tested grossly to determine the presence of diabetic neuropathy and the extent of involvement if present.

The next step of the evaluation is noninvasive testing such as ankle-brachial index, toe pressure, doppler analog waveform analysis, and duplex imaging. All diabetic patients should undergo evaluation with ankle-brachial index (ABI) and toe pressure (TP) measurements prior to any lower extremity orthopedic procedure. It is recommended that all noninvasive testing be performed by an accredited vascular lab to ensure validity. The ABI is performed by applying a blood pressure cuff superior to the ankle and then using a doppler to determine the systolic blood pressure of both the posterior tibial and the dorsalis pedis arteries. The highest value is then divided by the highest value of the brachial artery systolic blood pressure that has been measured from both upper extremities. A normal ABI is considered to be 0.9–1.1.

The ABI is highly valuable, since the ratio of the numbers has been shown to indicate the severity of arterial ischemia with progressively lower values corresponding to worsening PAD [8] (Table 3.2). However, it can be difficult to interpret in the diabetic patient due to the high prevalence of arterial wall calcification. An ABI ≥ 1.3 indicates poor compressibility of the vessel, usually secondary to highly calcified arterial walls. In this setting, the toe pressure can be used to further evaluate peripheral vascular disease (Image 3.2). To determine a toe pressure, a photoplethysmography (PPG) is placed onto the great toe in addition to a small sphygmomanometer. The great toe is usually the selected digit, but other toes can be used with accuracy if the patient has significant great toe wounds or has under-

Table 3.2 Ankle-brachial index

Ankle-brachial index (ABI)	Clinical status
1.0±0.10	Normal
0.59±0.15	Intermittent claudication
0.26±0.13	Ischemic rest pain
0.05±0.08	Impending tissue necrosis

ABI ≥ 1.3 is considered abnormal and indicated significant arterial wall calcification with incompressible tibial arteries. Adapted from Strandness and Zierler. See [8]

gone a previous amputation. The toe pressure is determined and then divided by the highest brachial systolic blood pressure, to give you the toe-brachial index (TBI). Again, the progressively lower values of TBI correspond to worsening PAD [8] (Table 3.3). The toe pressure can be used alone or in combination with the toe-brachial index to determine severity of arterial disease. In diabetics with noncompressible tibial vessels, toe pressures will reflect an accurate determination of foot perfusion. If the patient's ABI is 0.9–1.1 (indicating compressible tibial arteries) and the TP is greater than 80, then the patient can safely proceed for their scheduled orthopedic procedure. If ABI and/or TP are less

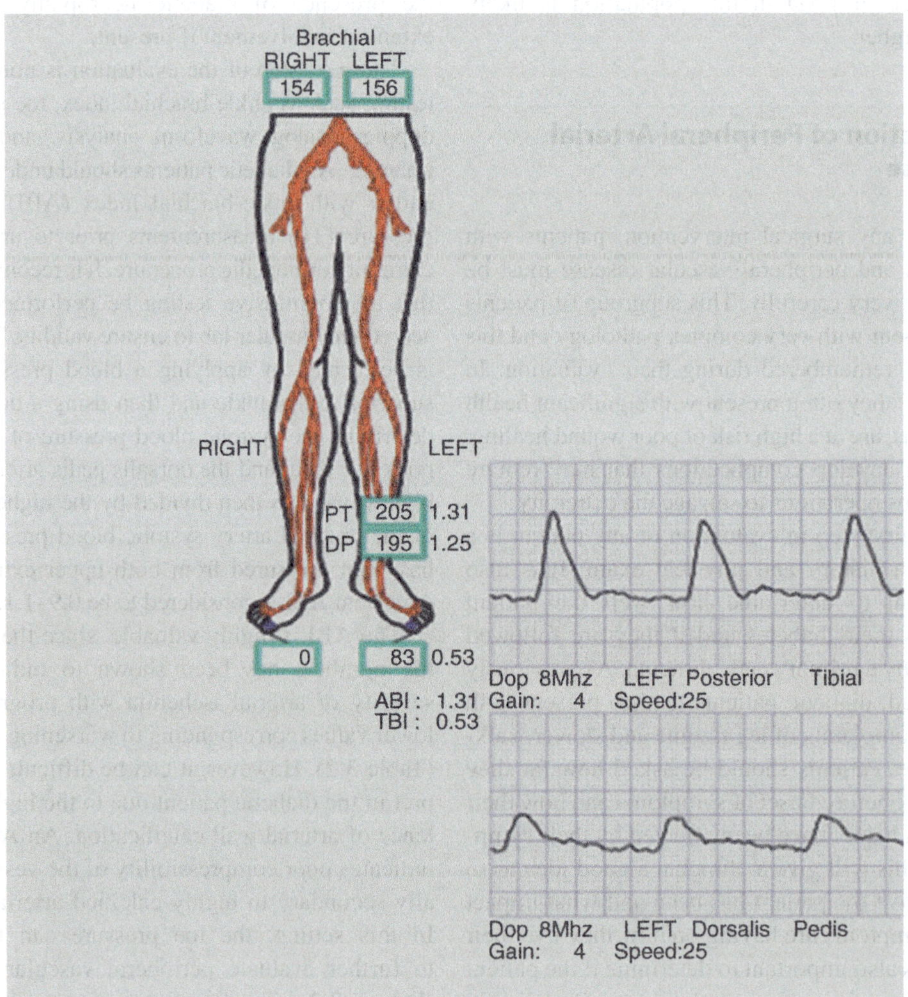

Image 3.2 Elevated ABI indicated the tibial artery is noncompressible, therefore, the ABI is not accurate. The TP can be used in this instance. A TP of 83 in this patient predicts good healing potential

than the previous mention numbers, then the patient should be referred to a vascular surgeon for further workup (Fig. 3.1).

Another noninvasive method for evaluating PAD in patients is the use of Doppler analog waveform analysis. This is usually obtained during the ABI and TP study as a combined exam. The Doppler probe is placed on the artery of interest and the waveform is determined. In this study, there are three types of waveforms that can be found: monophasic, biphasic and triphasic (Image 3.3). A triphasic waveform has a sharp upstroke, a short reversal inflow, and then a small forward flow. This waveform indicates a normal arterial flow with no lower extremity arterial disease. A biphasic waveform has a sharp upstroke followed by a loss in flow reversal. Once the upstroke becomes significantly blunted, the amplitude of the waveform is diminished and the waveform appears monophasic [8]. As proximal

PAD progresses, the waveform becomes biphasic and eventually monophasic.

A third noninvasive method of evaluating patients for PAD is the use of duplex imaging. In patients with a normal ABI, TP, and Doppler waveform (triphasic waveform), the duplex imaging does not need to be performed. Those patients have a normal vascular exam and can proceed for their orthopedic procedure. Patients with abnormal vascular studies should undergo duplex imaging. Arterial duplex scanning allows not only for anatomic imaging of the arteries, but also provides information about any areas of stenosis that may be causing vascular compromise. Duplex imaging can provide information from the abdominal aorta to the distal tibial vessels. The combination of visualization of lesions and waveform analysis allows for accurate detection of hemodynamically significant plaques (Image 3.4). In one study, arterial duplex mapping was able to detect hemodynamic significant lesions ($\geq$50 % stenosis) with a sensitivity of 89 % in the iliac vessels, 67 % in the popliteal artery, 90 % in the anterior and posterior tibial arteries, and 82 % for the peroneal artery [9].

In patients who present with findings suspicious for vascular compromise, further workup with computed tomography angiography (CTA) or angiogram is required. CTA is generally reserved for patients with a normal creatinine and

Table 3.3 Toe-brachial index and clinical status

Toe-brachial index (TBI)	Clinical status
0.64±0.20	Normal
0.52 =/−0.20	Intermittent claudication
0.23 =/−0.19	Ischemic rest pain or tissue loss

Adapted from Strandness and Zierler. See [8]

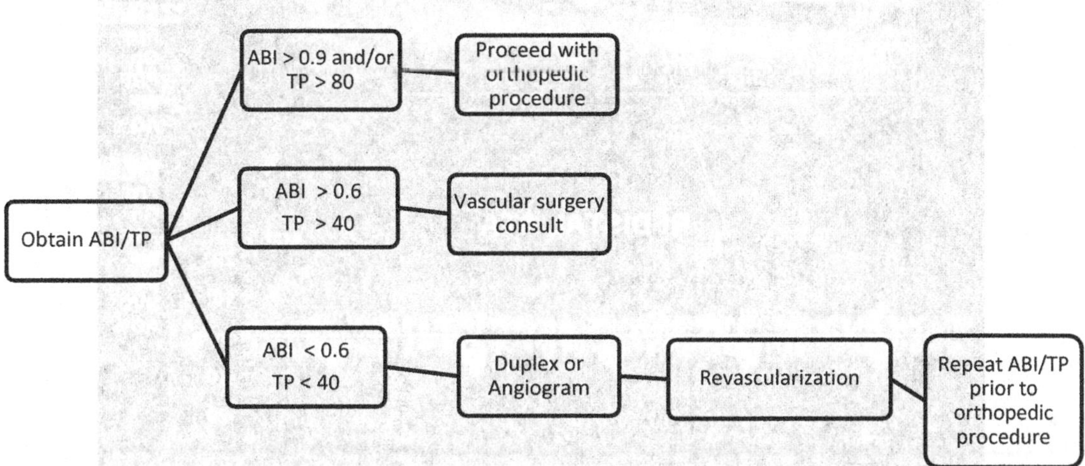

Fig. 3.1 Lower extremity orthopedic procedure algorithm

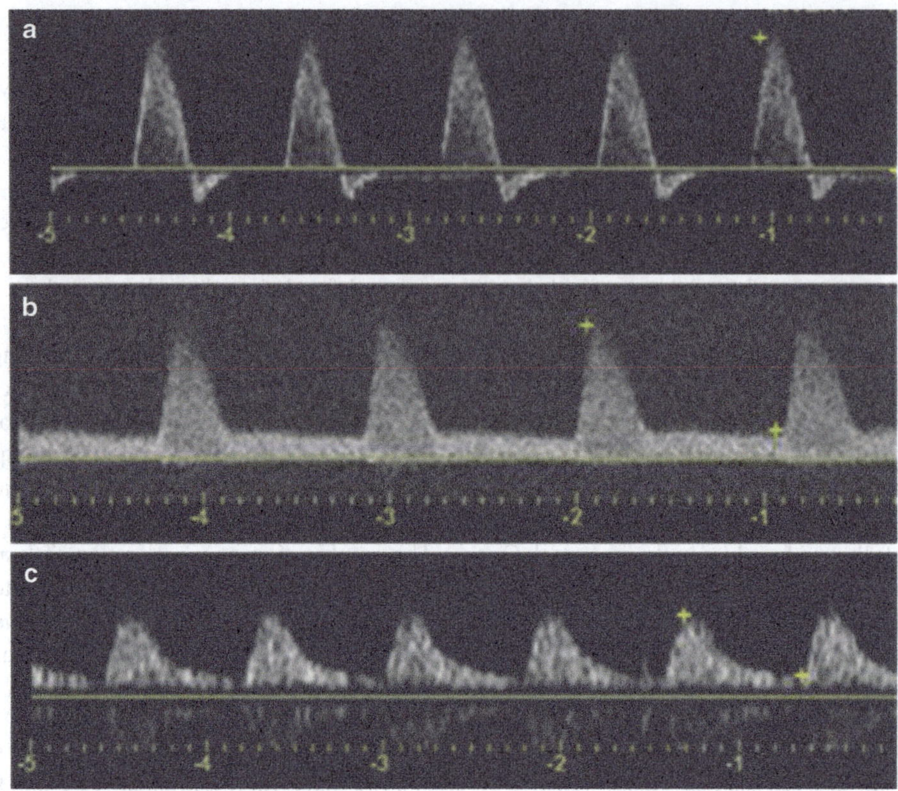

Image 3.3 Waveforms: (**a**) Triphasic. (**b**) Biphasic. (**c**) Monophasic

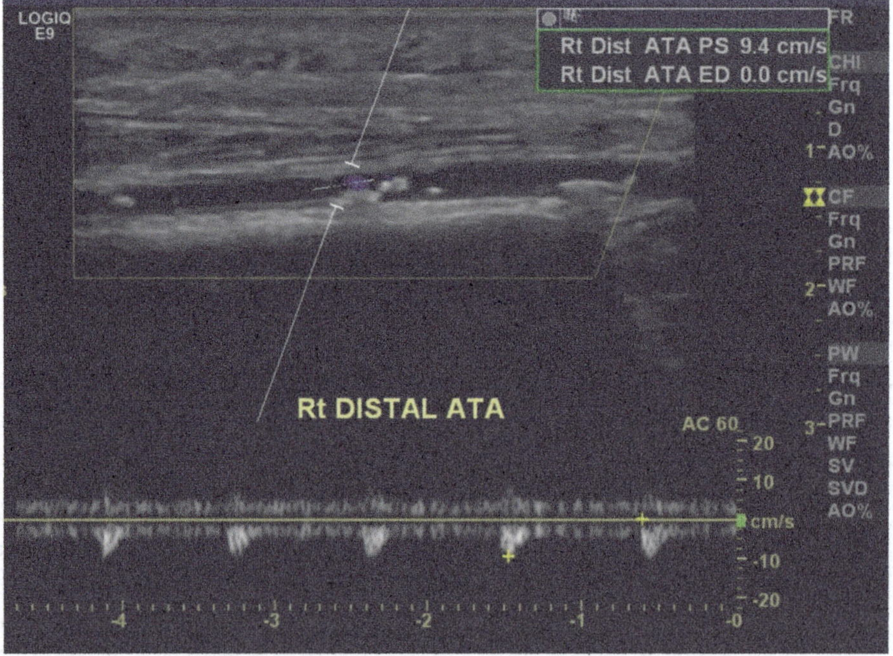

Image 3.4 Ultrasound demonstrating calcified anterior tibial artery with monophasic waveform

for whom there is a concern for multi-level vascular disease. The CTA provides an accurate picture of the inflow arteries (aorta, iliac, and femoral) yet, due to extensive calcification, may not accurately reflect which tibial and foot vessels are patent. Therefore, a digital subtraction angiogram should then be performed to determine tibial and foot vessel patency. If the creatinine is elevated, then an arterial duplex scan is done to determine the status of the inflow vessels, followed by a digital subtraction angiogram with limited contrast to determine patency of the tibial arteries. Another advantage to angiogram is the ability to treat lesions with endovascular interventions, such as balloon angioplasty or the placement of a stent. In either case, any hemodynamically significant lesions can be addressed by revascularization, either by using endovascular intervention or with the creation of a bypass.

Risk Factor Modification

Risk factor modification is an important aspect of long-term management of PAD, especially in the diabetic population. The progression of atherosclerosis affects the peripheral arterial system as well as the cardiovascular system and increases the risk of premature cardiovascular events. The major risk factors for atherosclerotic disease include diabetes mellitus, cigarette smoke, hyperlipidemia, and hypertension. The modification of these risk factors can function to improve the patient's symptoms and likelihood of limb salvage, along with reducing their cardiovascular risk.

Glycemic control in the diabetic population is a key aspect of their disease management, as evident in the previous section. Achievement of tight glycemic control is defined as a hemoglobin A1C value of less than 7 %. All diabetic patients should be managed closely by a primary care physician or endocrinologist, with close monitoring of their hemoglobin A1C. By achieving glycemic control, a decrease in microvascular disease progression may occur [10].

Tobacco smoking is one of the most important modifiable risk factors for reduction of atherosclerotic disease progression. The effects of cigarette smoke on the body are complex and multifactorial. One of the main components of cigarette smoke is nicotine, which has been shown to transiently increase blood pressure, stimulate coronary artery vasoconstriction, and impair endothelial function [11]. The combination of these effects leads to acceleration of plaque formation. The amount and duration of tobacco use has been directly associated with the development and progression of peripheral arterial disease [12].

In patients who require lower extremity bypass grafts, smokers have been found to have a threefold increase in graft failure if they continue to smoke [13]. By quitting smoking, patients can improve their symptoms along with decreasing their risk for critical limb ischemia and an amputation. The positive effects of smoking cessation, on arterial disease, can be seen in only a few short months as evident by improvement in ankle pressures and exercise tolerance [14]. Therefore, the subject of smoking cessation should be addressed in every clinical setting.

A third known risk factor is hyperlipidemia. Hyperlipidemia accelerates the atherosclerotic process and leads to diffuse vascular involvement. The addition of lipid-lowering medications has been shown to decrease a patient's risk of myocardial infarctions, stroke, and progression of peripheral vascular disease [15].

Lastly, treating hypertension is important in the management of patients with peripheral vascular disease. As noted with hyperlipidemia, hypertension is considered to be a risk factor for the development of a stroke and ischemic heart disease [16]. Therefore, aggressive blood pressure control is recommended in these patients. Although hypertension management is important for the cardiovascular risk reduction, data on the effects of antihypertensive agents on progression of peripheral vascular disease is unclear.

Management

All diabetic patients should undergo noninvasive testing with ankle-brachial index (ABI) and toe pressure (TP) measurements prior to any lower extremity orthopedic procedure. In diabetics with noncompressible tibial vessels, toe pressures will reflect an accurate determination of foot perfusion. If the patient's ABI is greater than 0.9 (indicating compressible tibial arteries) and the TP is greater than 80, then the patient can safely proceed for their scheduled orthopedic procedure. While the actual toe pressure required for healing mentioned in the literature can vary from 30 to 60 for diabetic patients, there is one study by Vitti et al. that clearly delineated appropriate values. In diabetic patients, they found that no primary amputation healed with a preoperative TP <40 mmHg and yet no failures occurred with a TP >68 mmHg [17]. Therefore, to err on the safe side, all patients with a TP <80 mmHg should be referred to a vascular surgeon.

In patients who present with physical findings suspicious for vascular compromise, a further workup using imaging with duplex or angiogram is required. Any hemodynamically significant lesions (>50 % stenosis) can be addressed by revascularization, either by using endovascular intervention, such as balloon angioplasty or the placement on a stent, or with the creation of a bypass. After the patient has been revascularized and recovered from their procedure, a repeat ABI and TP should be performed, prior to any lower extremity orthopedic operation, to ensure that adequate lower extremity perfusion has been achieved. Patients can undergo their orthopedic procedure 2–3 days after their revascularization.

All patients with peripheral vascular disease and diabetes, who require vascular surgery intervention, should be placed on an antiplatelet regimen after the procedure. The antiplatelet regimen may involve aspirin, blood thinners, or other types of antiplatelet agents depending on the severity of the lesion and the type of intervention required. If a stent has been placed, then the authors recommend that the patient remain on Plavix® for a minimum of 6 weeks without interruption. All diabetic patients with peripheral vascular disease should also be placed on aspirin for the duration of their lifetime, to reduce the patient's risk of stroke, myocardial infarction, and death [18]. If the patient is at high risk for bleeding during a specific orthopedic procedure,

the antiplatelet regimen can usually be held 7 days prior to surgery. The antiplatelet agent should then be restarted as soon as possible after the procedure.

Diabetics without PAD (ABI > 0.9 and or TP > 80) can undergo tourniquet use safely during an orthopedic procedure while those with PAD should not. If an orthopedic surgeon wishes to use a tourniquet, in these patients with PAD, they should undergo a preoperative evaluation by a vascular surgeon. It is the authors' recommendation that these patients should obtain an angiogram prior to the orthopedic procedure, which requires a tourniquet. If their blood flow is compromised after the orthopedic procedure, the authors will have to plan to revascularize the patient. If a patient has had a prior lower extremity bypass, and a tourniquet is required, the patient should be anti-coagulated with 5000 units of intravenous heparin prior to inflation. Once the tourniquet is deflated, heparin can be reversed with protamine sulfate.

Conclusion

While orthopedic surgeons often do not manage the diabetic patient's medical and vascular problems, understanding its implications will result in better patient care. The use of ABIs and toe pressures are easy and inexpensive tests that can help evaluate the patient and determine the correct path for management of their vascular insufficiency prior to any orthopedic procedure. If patients have significant vascular problems, they should be referred to a vascular surgeon. After appropriate vascular management, patients can usually proceed with their orthopedic procedures in a relatively safe manner.

References

1. Ripoll BC, Levtholtz I. Exercise and disease management. 2nd ed. Boca Raton: CRC Press; 2011. p. 25.
2. Thompson R, Allam A, Lombardi G. Atherosclerosis across 4000 years of human history. Lancet. 2013; 381:1211–22.

3. Bell ET. Atherosclerotic gangrene of the lower extremities in diabetes and non-diabetic patients. Am J Clin Pathol. 1957;28:27–36.

4. Creager MA, Dzau VJ, Loscalzo J. Vascular medicine. 1st ed. Philadelphia: Elsevier; 2006. p. 105.

5. Beks PJ, Mackaay AJ, de Neeling JN, de Vries H, Bouter LM, Heine RJ. Peripheral arterial disease in relation to glycemic level in an elderly Caucasian population: The Horn study. Diabetologia. 1995;38:86–96.

6. Effect of intensive diabetes management on macrovascular events and risk factors in the Diabetes Control and Complications Trial. Am J Cardio 1995; 75:894–903.

7. Hirsch AT, Criqui MH, Treat-Jacobson D, et al. Peripheral arterial disease detection, awareness and treatment in primary care. JAMA. 2001;286:1317–24.

8. Strandness E, Zierler RE. Duplex scanning in vascular disorders. 4th ed. Philadelphia: Lippincott Williams and Wilkins; 2010. p. 133–46.

9. Moneta GL, Yeager RA, Antonovic R, Hall LD, Caster JD, Cummings CA, Porter JM. Accuracy of lower extremity arterial duplex mapping. J Vasc Surg. 1992;15:275–84.

10. UK Prospective Diabetes Study (UKPDS) Group. Intensive blood-glucose control with sulphonylureas or insulin compared with conventional treatment and risk of complications in patients with type 2 diabetes (UKPDS 33). Lancet. 1998;352:837–53.

11. Benowitz NL. The role of nicotine in smoking-related cardiovascular disease. Prev Med. 1997;26(4):412–7.

12. Freund KM, Belanger AJ, D'Agostino RB, Kannel WB. The health risks of smoking. The Framingham Study: 34 years of follow up. Ann Epidemiol. 1993; 3:417–24.

13. Willigendael EM, Teijink JA, Bartelink ML, Peters RJ, Buller HR, Prins MH. Smoking and the patency of lower extremity bypass grafts: a meta-analysis. J Vasc Surg. 2005;42:67–74.

14. Quick CR, Cotton LT. The measured effect of stopping smoking on intermittent claudication. Br J Surg. 1982;69:S24–6.

15. Leng GC, Price JF, Jepson RG. Lipid-lowering for lower limb atherosclerosis. Cochrane Database Syst Rev. 2000;2, CD000123.

16. Chobanian AV, Bakris GL, Black HR, Cushman WC, Green LA, Izzo Jr JL, Jones DW, Materson BJ, Oparil S, Wright Jr JT, Roccella EJ, National Heart, Lung, and Blood Institute Joint National Committee on Prevention, Detection, Evaluation, and Treatment of High Blood Pressure, National High Blood Pressure Education Program Coordinating Committee. The seventh report of the Joint National Committee on prevention, detection, evaluation, and treatment of high blood pressure: the JNC 7 report. JAMA. 2003; 289:2560–72.

17. Vitti MJ, Robinson DV, Hauer-Jensen M, et al. Wound healing in forefoot amputations: the predictive value of toe pressures. Ann Vasc Surg. 1994;8:99–106.

18. Antiplatelet Trialists' Collaboration. Collaborative overview of randomized trials of antiplatelet therapy. I. Prevention of death, myocardial infarction, and stroke by prolonged antiplatelet therapy in various categories of patients. BMJ. 1994;308:81–106. Erratum in: BMJ 1994;308:1540.

Classification of Diabetic Foot Disease

Ross Taylor

Introduction

Disease classification provides a system that promotes the evidence-based treatment of complex and varied conditions through the dissemination of information, using common nomenclature. Useful classification systems have been developed to guide in the diagnosis and treatment of both Charcot arthropathy and ulcerative lesions of the foot. Classification of these two separate diabetic foot conditions is challenging as each are highly variable in location, etiology, and progression. Although there are many systems of classification for Charcot arthropathy and ulceration, only those that have contributed to the understanding of each condition are reviewed here. This chapter will discuss the classification of Charcot arthropathy and ulceration separately, as no classification system has been devised that incorporates both conditions.

Introduction to the Classification of Charcot Arthropathy

Neuropathic disintegration of the foot was first described in 1868 by the French neurologist Jean-Martin Charcot, who observed a rapidly

R. Taylor, M.D., M.B.A. (✉)
Danville Regional Medical Center, LifePoint Health,
142 South Main Street, Danville, VA 24541, USA
e-mail: Ross.Taylor@lpnt.net

destructive process involving the joints of patients presenting with neuropathy due to tertiary syphilis [1]. Jordan was the first to report Charcot's disease in the diabetic foot in 1936 [2]. Unlike tabes dorsalis, diabetic Charcot arthropathy almost exclusively affects the joints of the foot and ankle [3]. Today, diabetic neuropathy is recognized as the most common cause of Charcot arthropathy in the developed world.

Charcot arthropathy of the foot and ankle seemingly defies classification. It is by definition an inherently chaotic process. It may involve any joint in the foot and ankle, and it can present as multiple fractures, subluxations, and dislocations. Bizarre deformities may result, often leading to ulcerations and infections. Treatment of Charcot arthropathy is based on several factors, including the anatomic location, temporal progression, deformity, and the presence or absence of any coexisting ulceration and infection. In an attempt to facilitate our understanding of Charcot arthropathy and to standardize treatment options, numerous classification systems have been proposed.

Classification systems can be divided into two types: temporal and descriptive (anatomic). Temporal classification systems describe the stage of disease, and the only pure staging classification is the one published by Eichenholtz in 1966 [4]. Simultaneously published was an anatomic classification of Charcot arthropathy of the foot and ankle by Harris. Subsequent anatomic classification systems have been published by

© Springer International Publishing Switzerland 2016
D. Herscovici, Jr. (ed.), *The Surgical Management of the Diabetic Foot and Ankle*,
DOI 10.1007/978-3-319-27623-6_4

Cofield in 1983 [21]; Sammarco, and separately Schon in 1998 [29]; and Brodsky in 2006. The advantages of each will be reviewed in the subsequent sections.

Classification of the Charcot Foot and Ankle

Temporal Classification System of Eichenholtz

Perhaps the most widely referenced classification system of Charcot arthropathy was provided by Eichenholtz (Table 4.1). In 1966, he published his detailed monograph describing the clinical, radiographic, and pathologic findings in 68 consecutive patients with Charcot arthropathy of the foot and ankle [4]. Using this data, he established a classification system that described the temporal progression of the Charcot joint. Although the Eichenholtz temporal staging system is widely accepted, subsequent authors have pointed out that this system may not be inclusive of Charcot arthropathy at the earliest and latest stages of the disease. In fact, Classen et al. demonstrated that clinical symptoms, such as swelling, warmth, erythema, and even pain, frequently preceded the radiographic findings of Eichenholtz stage I by weeks or months, and that changes on bone scintigraphy could help detect early Charcot arthropathy [5]. Other authors have correctly identified that magnetic resonance imaging could detect the reactive osseous edema that precedes the changes in gross pathology [6–10]. Subsequently, in 1990 Shibata added a preceding fourth stage to Eichenholtz's classification, which was labeled as stage 0 [11]. Currently, the Eichenholtz classification is described as:

0: Foot at Risk
- Clinical—inflammation characterized by erythema, swelling, warmth, and instability
- Radiographic—absent bony changes, soft-tissue swelling may be observed
- Bone scintigraphy—increased radiotracer uptake in the involved joint
- MRI—bone and soft-tissue edema, joint effusion, noncortical stress fractures [10]

I: Stage of Development
- Known as the development-fragmentation, or acute stage, and was characterized by Eichenholtz as "debris, fragmentation, disruption, dislocation" of the joints
- Clinical—inflammation characterized by erythema, swelling, warmth, and instability
- Pathology—fragmentation of bone and cartilage. Pathognomonic of Charcot arthropathy, microscopy reveals bone debris embedded within the synovium
- Radiographic—osteopenia, fracture, subluxation and dislocation, periarticular fragmentation (Fig. 4.1a)

II: Stage of Coalescence
- This stage was initially described by Eichenholtz to demonstrate "sclerosis, absorption of fine debris, fusion of most large fragments"
- Clinical—decreased warmth, erythema, and swelling
- Radiographic—periosteal new bone formation, fracture healing, moderate joint destruction, osteopenia, and sclerosis (Fig. 4.1b)

III: Stage of Reconstruction and Reconstitution
- Eichenholtz described this stage as "lessened sclerosis, rounding of major fragment, with some attempts at reformation of joint architecture"
- Also referred to as the "chronic stage"
- Clinical—absence of inflammation, appears to be a stable deformity
- Radiographic—joint arthrosis, osteophytes, subchondral sclerosis, healing fractures, advanced deformity (Fig. 4.1c)

Although this classification system suggests that any deformity progression is minimal after stage II, more recent studies have refuted this finding. Hastings demonstrated that lateral arch collapse can progress for up to two years after the initiation of conservative treatment. This suggests that the period of instability may extend well beyond stage II, and that the stage III deformity, characterized by Eichenholtz as stable, may not be as static as once thought [12]. Additionally,

Table 4.1 Modified Eichenholtz classification of charcot arthropathy

	Clinical features	Radiographic features	MRI findings [12]	Treatment
Stage 0—Prodromal stage	• Swelling, warmth, and hyperemia • Instability	• Normal • Soft-tissue swelling may be seen	• Bone and soft-tissue edema • Joint effusion • Subcortical bone fractures may be seen	• Offloading and immobilization
Stage I—Stage of Fragmentation	• Swelling, warmth, and hyperemia • Increased instability • Deformity	• Fractures w bone fragmentation • Osteopenia • Subluxation, dislocation, and deformity	• Bone and soft-tissue edema • Joint effusion • Fractures • Subluxation, dislocation, and deformity	• Offloading and immobilization
Stage II—Stage of Consolidation	• Decreased swelling, warmth, and hyperemia • Decreased instability • Deformity	• Reabsorption of fracture fragments • Reduced osteopenia • Sclerotic bone • Subluxation, dislocation, and deformity • New bone formation	• Reduction in bone and soft-tissue edema • Reduced joint effusion • Callus formation • Subluxation, dislocation, and deformity	• Offloading and immobilization • Charcot restraint orthotic walker (CROW)
Stage III—Stage of Reconstruction	• Absence of swelling, warmth, and erythema • Stable deformity	• Rounding of remaining fracture fragments • Sclerosis • Subluxation, dislocation, and deformity with subsequent arthrosis	• Residual bone edema • Residual joint effusion • Subchondral erosions • Subluxation, dislocation, and deformity	• Custom inlay shoes with rocker-bottom sole for plantigrade foot • CROW for nonplantigrade foot versus surgical reconstruction

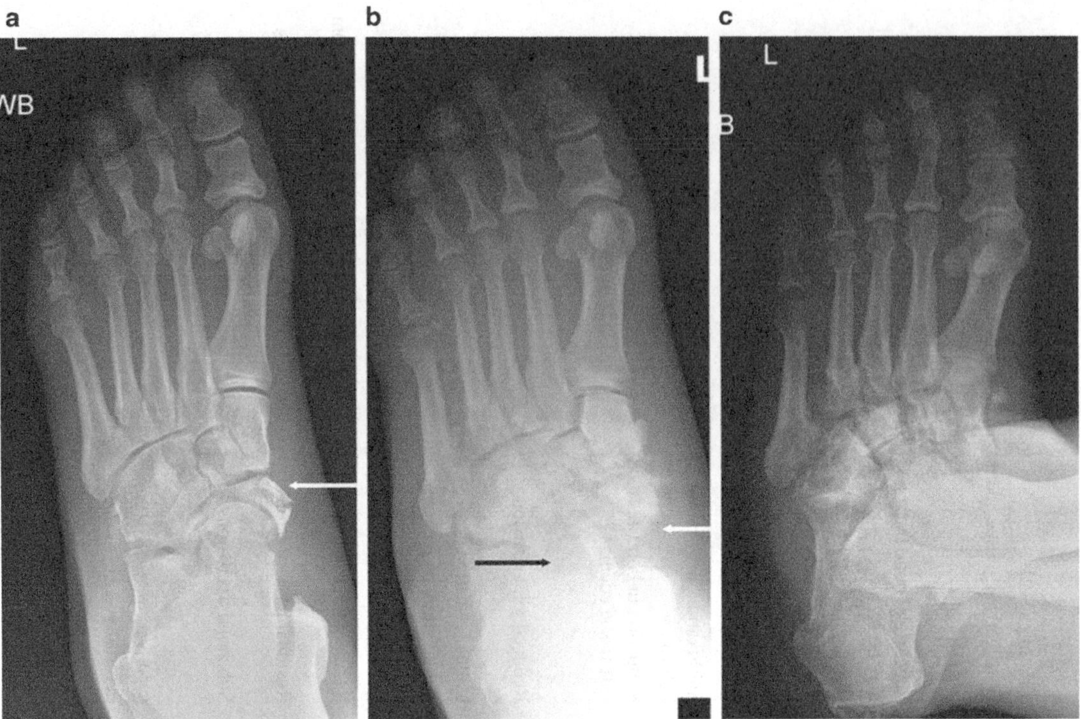

Fig. 4.1 Radiographic findings in Charcot arthropathy affecting the midfoot (**a**) stage of fragmentation—note fracture-subluxation of the talonavicular joint (*white arrow*) (**b**) stage of coalescence—note periosteal new bone formation and navicular fracture consolidation (*white arrow*). Talonavicular joint demonstrates destructive changes, osteopenia (*black arrow*), and adjacent sclerosis. (**c**) Stage of reconstruction—midfoot demonstrates advanced adduction deformity, and multiple healing fractures. Also notable is the involvement of the fifth metatarsophalangeal joint, which is in an earlier Eichenholtz stage. Multiple location involvement at varying stages is not uncommon

recurrence of Charcot at the same or adjacent joints, or regression to earlier temporal stages after the initiation of treatment is well described, with Osterhoff et al. reporting a recurrence in 23 % of the feet in his series [13–15, 16].

As imperfect as it may be, the Eichenholtz classification system is widely accepted. It has allowed for the meaningful discussion of treatment options based on the disease stage, it is used as to guide treatment, and it describes the progression of clinical and radiographic changes that occur in the Charcot foot and ankle. Arresting the Charcot process early, during stages 0 or 1, may prevent progression to instability and deformity leading to ulceration, infection, or other limb-threatening conditions as seen in later stages [16–18]. Although newer temporal classification systems based on MRI findings have been proposed, the utility of these has yet to be demonstrated [16–20].

Anatomic Classification System of Harris and Brand

Harris and Brand provided early insight into the process of neuropathic destruction of the foot. These authors may have been the first to associate elevated limb temperature with Charcot of the foot, by observing that warmth often accompanied the unstable neuropathic midfoot. Not only did Harris and Brand correctly suggest that an elevated limb temperature may indicate pending deformity and ulceration, but they also suggested that early intervention, in the form of total contact casting, may reduce the potential for fracture and deformity [20].

This classification system was devised based on the theory that a neuropathic fracture was initiated by trauma, and that collapse of the insensate foot occurred along one of several lines of weight-bearing force, or one of three "pillars."

These three are identified as posterior (calcaneus), central (talus), and anterior (navicular). This classification system proposes that these lines of force, or pillars, are altered by an initiating fracture, resulting in deformity and ulceration. Based on this theory, five anatomic patterns of neuropathic destruction were proposed. These three pillars consist of:

Posterior Pillar

- Fracture of the calcaneus, with flattening of the heel, hindfoot recurvatum, subtalar subluxation, and proximal migration of the posterior calcaneal tuberosity
- Leads to ulceration under the plantar aspect of the heel

Central Pillar

- Talus is the primary area of disintegration
- May be caused by a previous posterior pillar pattern with subtalar subluxation

Anterior Pillar, Medial Arch

- Deformity is initiated by a fracture of the navicular, which causes proximal migration of the cuneiforms (Fig. 4.1a)
- Flattening of the navicular leads to articulation between the talar head and the cuneiforms
- This leads to reversal of medial arch, with ulceration frequently occurring plantar to the head of the talus

Anterior Pillar, Lateral Arch

- Dislocation and fracture of the calcaneocuboid joint
- Results in a reversal of the lateral arch of the foot
- The medial arch is preserved
- Often dominated by sepsis due to ulceration under the base of the fifth metatarsal

Cuneiform: Metatarsal Base

- Initiated by fracture of the cuneiforms
- Leads to fracture propagation across the midfoot resulting in a "broad flail pseudoarthrosis"

Although this classification system is seldom cited today, it was the first accepted anatomic classification of Charcot arthropathy. Like later anatomic classification systems, Harris and Brand identified that breakdown of the lateral arch was the most malignant type of neuropathic deformity, with a propensity for ulceration and sepsis. This is also the only classification system that explains the pattern of breakdown of the neuropathic foot using the biomechanical concept of pillars, or weight-bearing lines of force. Nonetheless, the usefulness of this classification method has been limited due to a lack of clinical and radiographic correlations, and is mainly of historical interest.

Anatomic Classification System of Cofield

Cofield et al. classified radiographic changes based on three anatomic locations and correlated these changes with ulcer formation [21]. After evaluating 116 feet in 96 patients with diabetic neuropathy, they noted that all patients with radiographic changes of the phalanges, and most with metarsophalangeal radiographic changes had adjacent ulceration. Conversely, few of the patients with radiographic changes of the midfoot and hindfoot had any ulceration. They also noted that radiographic changes as well as ulcer formation were more common in patients with type II diabetes, as well as those with severe metabolic complications such as retinopathy and nephropathy. The described three patterns are:

- *Metatarsophalangeal or Phalangeal Involvement*: Observed in 78 of 116 feet, and almost always associated with ulceration (Fig. 4.2).
- *Tarsometatarsal (TMT) Joint Destruction*: Observed in 18 of 116 feet with a wide spectrum of radiographic changes seen at the tarsometatarsal joint. These range from mild degenerative changes to fragmentation and collapse. Ulceration was unusual in this group.
- *Destruction through the Head or Neck of the Talus, Navicular and Cuneiforms*: Identified in 20 of 116 feet, with similarity to the anterior pillar, medial arch pattern as described by Harris and Brandt. Charcot changes occurred

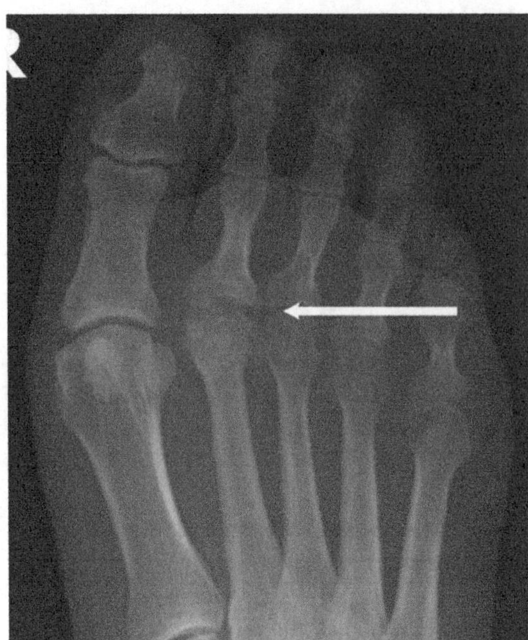

Fig. 4.2 Radiographs demonstrate chronic Charcot arthropathy affecting the 2nd metatarsophalangeal joint as described by Cofield

through the head or neck of the talus, navicular, and the cuneiforms. Ulceration rarely occurred in this group as well.

Anatomic Classification System of Sammarco and Conti

Sammarco and Conti classified the pattern of bony destruction in 22 patients with Charcot arthropathy of the midfoot [22]. Using anteroposterior (AP) and lateral radiographs, they defined 5-anatomic patterns of Charcot midfoot involvement. The authors noted that lateral midfoot involvement predisposed patients to ulceration, a finding that is confirmed in subsequent classification systems. This classification system consisted of:

Pattern 1
- Seen in 11 of 22 2 feet
- Identified as diastasis occurring between the first and second TMT joints
- On AP radiographs, fragmentation and collapse can extend laterally across the TMT joints. The forefoot is displaced lateral to the hindfoot, with the first metatarsal displaced only slightly lateral to a reference line along the talar neck
- Lateral radiographs demonstrate dorsal forefoot displacement

Pattern 2
- Observed in 4 of 22 feet
- Destructive changes are identified at the medial metatarsal-cuneiform joints without diastasis of the first and second metatarsals
- There is no involvement of the metatarsal-cuboid joints, and less lateral displacement of the metatarsals compared to pattern 1

Pattern 3
- Observed in 3 of 22 feet
- Arthropathy of the medial cuneiform-navicular joint with fragmentation of the middle cuneiform bone
- Destructive changes are identified in the lateral TMT joints

Pattern 4
- Observed in 2 of 22 feet
- Identified as bony destruction of the first metatarsal-medial cuneiform joint, with diastasis occurring between the first and second metatarsals
- Proximal and lateral extension occurs across the lateral intercuneiform joints and can involve the calcaneocuboid joint

Pattern 5
- Observed in 2 of 22 feet
- Consists of perinavicular bony destruction with distal intertarsal extension

Anatomic Classification of Brodsky

The Brodsky classification of Charcot arthropathy was developed from a series of 120 patients with Charcot arthropathy, who were treated at Ranchos Los Amigos Hospital in Los Angeles, CA., in the years prior to 1985 [23]. Based on a review of records and radiographs from this series of patients, Brodsky et al. classified Charcot arthropathy

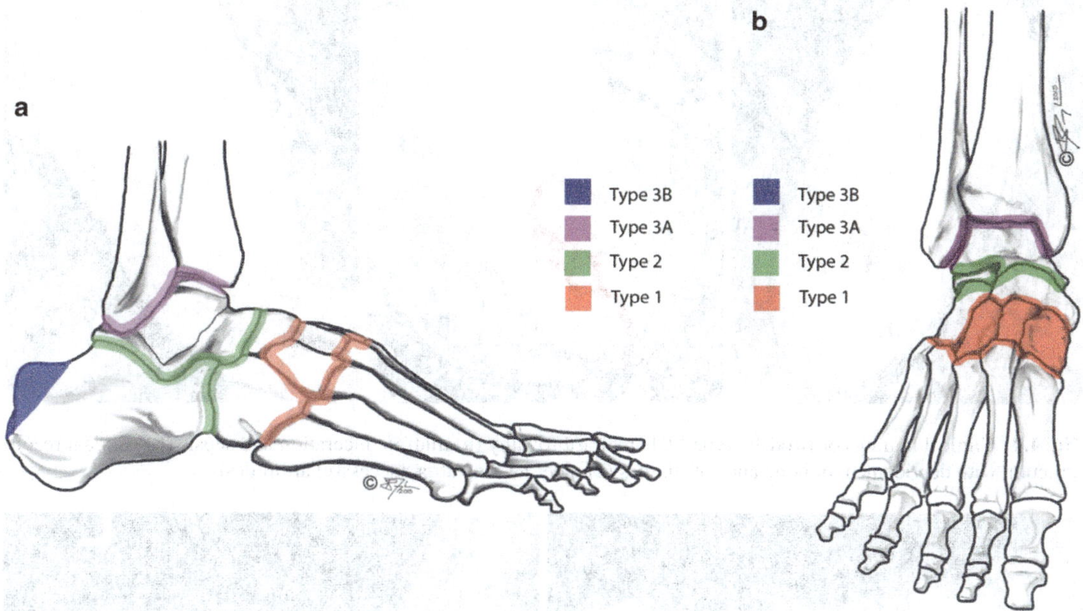

Fig. 4.3 Brodsky anatomic classification of Charcot arthropathy of the foot and ankle (**a**) lateral view (**b**) anterior view

according to the area of the foot in which maximum bony destruction occurred radiographically [24, 25] (Fig. 4.3). The utility of Brodsky's anatomic classification system lies in its simplicity. It remains the most widely quoted anatomic classification systems of Charcot arthropathy of the foot and ankle. This classification emphasizes that the more proximal the disease (the greater the Brodsky Type), the more unstable the involved joint, and the greater the potential for Charcot progression. This classification has been further modified by Trepman et al. to include types 4 and 5 [26]. The classification currently consists of:

Type I: Tarsometatarsal or Naviculocuneiform Joints

- This is identified in approximately 60 % of cases
- Typically presents later in the disease process than with Brodsky types II and III, and frequently presents during Eichenholtz stage II or III, when the foot is stable but deformed
- Frequently results in a fixed rocker-bottom foot with valgus angulation
- Often leads to the development of a plantar exostosis, which produces a risk of ulceration (Fig. 4.4)

Type II: Subtalar and or Chopart Joints (Fig. 4.5)

- Identified in 30–35 % of cases
- Typified by instability, this type is less likely to develop ulcerations than type I. Up to one-third can develop bony prominences
- Patients have persistent enlargement of the foot and often require periods of immobilization lasting up to 2-years
- The hindfoot tends to rest in a subluxed position, resulting in persistent valgus alignment

Type 3A: Ankle Joint

- Identified in 20 % of cases
- Charcot arthropathy involving the ankle is often initiated by a traumatic fracture in a neuropathic patient
- This type is characterized by a prolonged Eichenholtz stage I, and is the most unstable of all the Brodsky Types
- Produces chronic swelling and instability. May cause late varus or valgus deformities, leading to collapse and ulceration over the malleoli (Fig. 4.6)

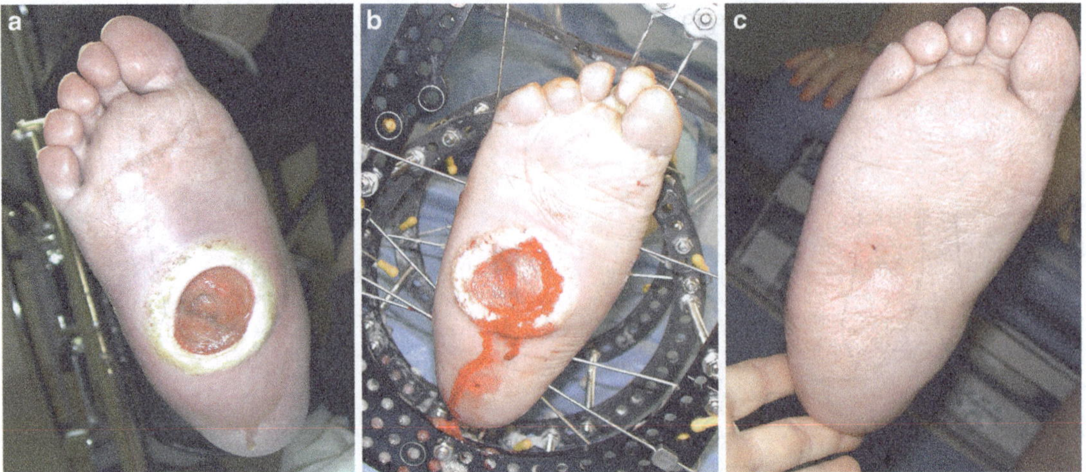

Fig. 4.4 Clinical findings of Brodsky type I Charcot arthropathy (**a**) midfoot ulceration and sepsis (**b**) surgical reconstruction with debridement of bone and soft tissues (**c**) ulcer healing after successful arthrodesis

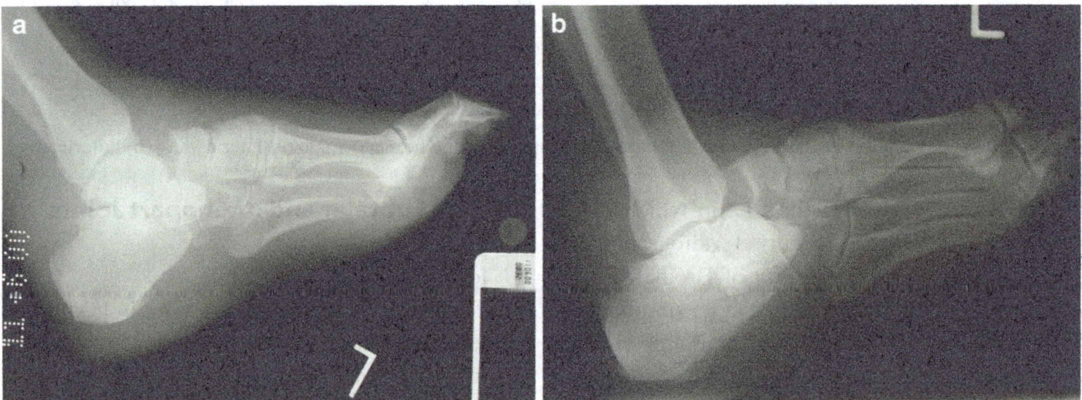

Fig. 4.5 Radiographic findings in Brodsky type II Charcot arthropathy (**a**) neuropathic fracture of the talus with subluxation of the subtalar joint and dislocation of the talonavicular joint (**b**) this highly unstable pattern progressed to flattening of the talus, extrusion of the talar head into the medial soft tissues, and a profound adduction–supination deformity with lateral rocker-bottom

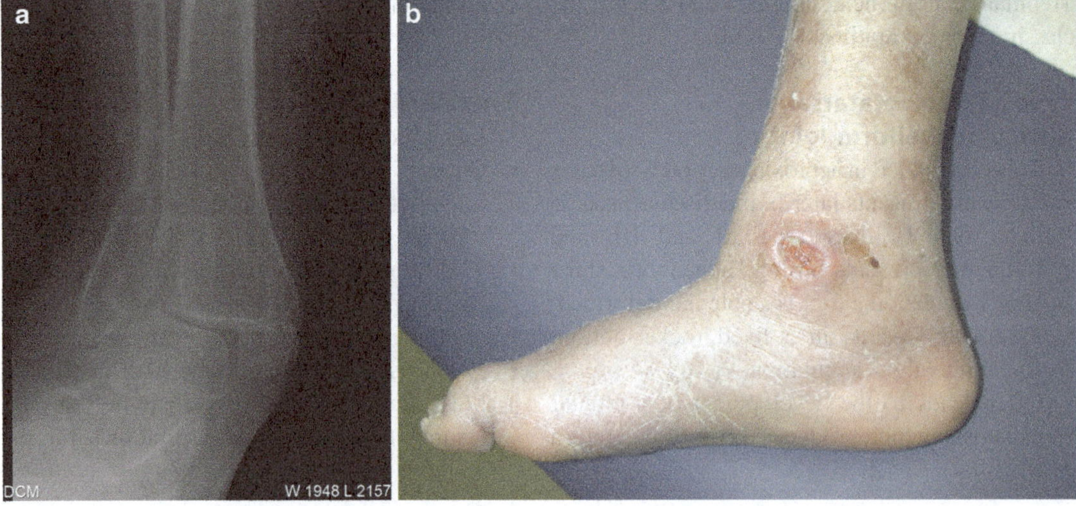

Fig. 4.6 Findings in Brodsky type 3A Charcot arthropathy (**a**) Anteroposterior (AP) radiograph obtained almost one year after presentation shows a severe valgus deformity (**b**) Associated ulceration over the medial malleolus

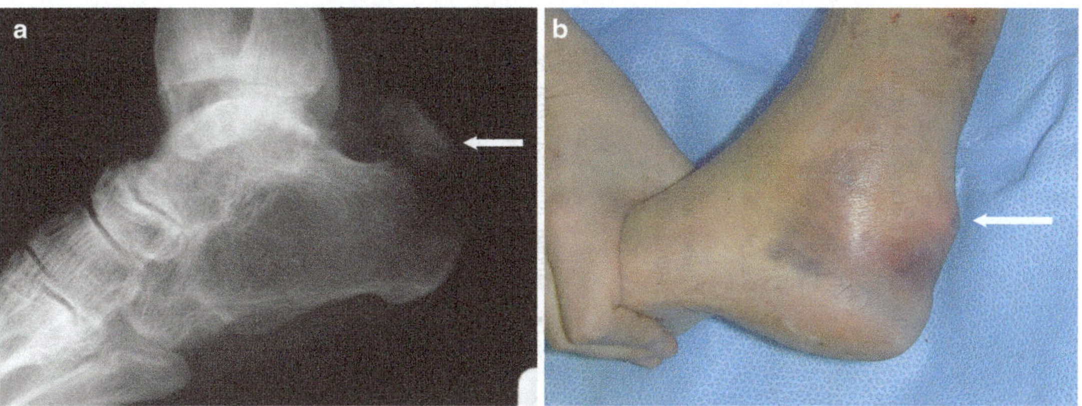

Fig. 4.7 (**a**) Lateral radiograph showing avulsion fracture of the calcaneal tuberosity (*white arrow*) as seen in Brodsky type 3B Charcot arthropathy (**b**) Clinical view showing associated soft-tissue compromise (*white arrow*)

Type 3B: Fracture of the Calcaneal Tuberosity

- Identified in fewer than 1 % of cases [23]
- This type results from bony avulsion of the Achilles tendon insertion (Fig. 4.7a)
- Causes distal foot changes and proximal migration of the tuberosity fragment
- Leads to distal collapse of the longitudinal arch of the foot
- May compromise skin in area overlying fracture, and may require immediate treatment in order to avoid skin necrosis [27, 28] (Fig. 4.7b)

Type 4: Combination of Areas

- Multiple simultaneous locations, often in different Eichenholtz stages (Fig. 4.1c)
- Concurrent involvement may be unilateral or bilateral

Type 5: Forefoot Involvement

- Only involves the forefoot
- Similar to Trepman et al. and Cofield et al., and it is often associated with ulceration and the development of osteomyelitis

Anatomic Classification System of Schon

Schon et al. established a detailed clinical and radiographic classification of acquired midtarsus deformities based on a series of 131 feet, including 86 with diabetic neuroarthropathy [29]. This system established four types of midfoot arthropathy based on the location of maximal deformity, as seen on AP and lateral weight-bearing radiographs (Table 4.2, Fig. 4.8). Concise radiographic parameters are used to define each deformity type, and the location of bony prominence for each deformity is provided. Like authors before them, Schon et al. recognized that collapse of the lateral column of the foot was associated with severe deformity and a poor outcome. Using this pretext, a novel measure of lateral arch collapse, using the lateral calcaneus-fifth metatarsal, was devised, which was shown to be decreased with lateral column involvement (Fig. 4.9a, angle C), and closely correlates with other measures of lateral column collapse including decreased calcaneal pitch (Fig. 4.9a, angle D), and reduced lateral radiographic arch height of the foot (Fig. 4.9a, measure E). From this same series of patients, Schon et al. devised a **clinical deformity severity stage** based on the degree of collapse of the longitudinal arch of the foot (Fig. 4.10).

These deformities consisted of three types:

- *Stage A*—minimal deformity, with arch still present
- *Stage B*—loss of medial or lateral arch with plantar or medial prominence
- *Stage C*—collapse of arch medially and laterally, with midfoot prominence that protrudes plantar beyond a line drawn between the heel and the ball of the foot

Table 4.2 Schon radiographic and clinical classification of acquired midtarsus deformities

Type	I—Metatarsocuneiform/metatarsocuboid or Lis-Franc pattern	II—Naviculocuneiform/metatarsocuboid pattern	III—Perinavicular pattern	IV—Transverse tarsal pattern
Frequency (%)	33	46	13	8
Location of maximum deformity	• First, second, and third metatarsocuneifom joints • Progresses to the fourth and fifth metatarsocuboid joints	• Medial naviculocuneiform joint • Progresses to the fourth and fifth metatarsocuboid joints	• Navicular and surrounding bones • Progresses laterally through the tarsometatarsal or calcaneocuboid joints	• Talonavicular joint • Progresses laterally through the calcaneocuboid joint • Earliest and most severe lateral column involvement
Type of deformity	• 81 % are abducted • Remainder are neutral or adducted	• 62 % are abducted • Minority were adducted or neutral	• Adduction • Lateral rocker-bottom deformity	• Abduction
Location of prominence	• Medial, plantar-medial • Centrally with progression	• Plantar-lateral and plantar-central, less commonly medial	• Plantar-central, or plantar-lateral	• Medial, plantar-medial, or plantar-central prominence
Distinctive radiographic features	• Relative preservation of lateral arch height • Greatest AP talo-1st metatarsal angle of all groups	• Greater loss of lateral arch height compared to type I; with calcaneal pitch an average of 0^c • Less abduction of the midfoot is seen compared to type I deformity, as indicated by a smaller AP talar-first metatarsal angle	• Largest lateral talo-first metatarsal angle of all the types • Lateral column involvement resulting in a lower calcaneal pitch than in type I • Lateral arch height significantly depressed	• Greatest talocalcaneal angle of all types • Loss of lateral arch height, as manifested by a negative calcaneal pitch, was the greatest of all four types

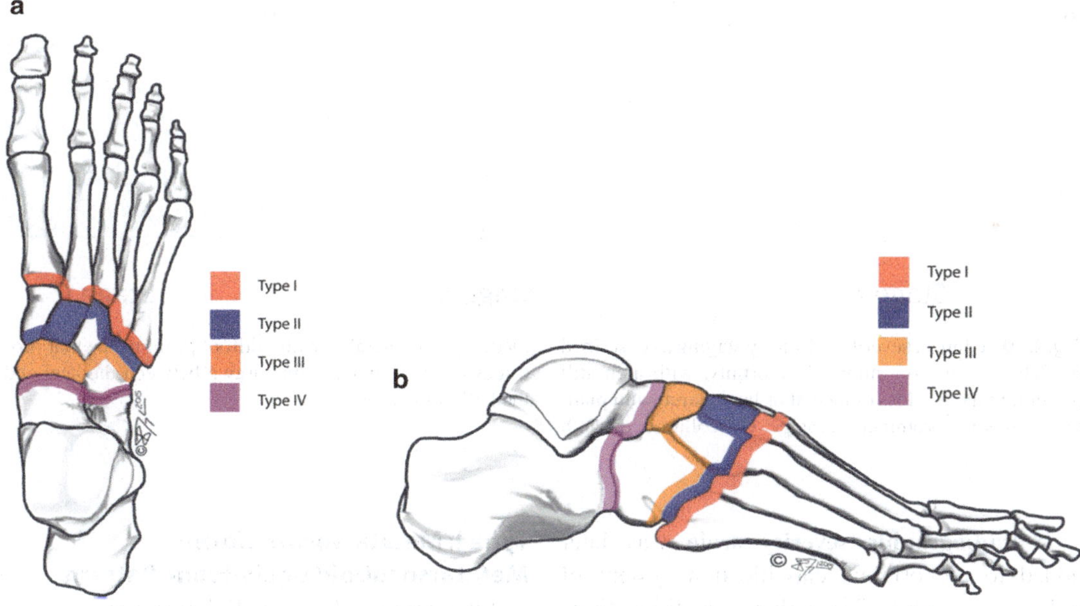

Fig. 4.8 Schon classification of acquired midtarsus deformity (**a**) dorsal view (**b**) lateral view

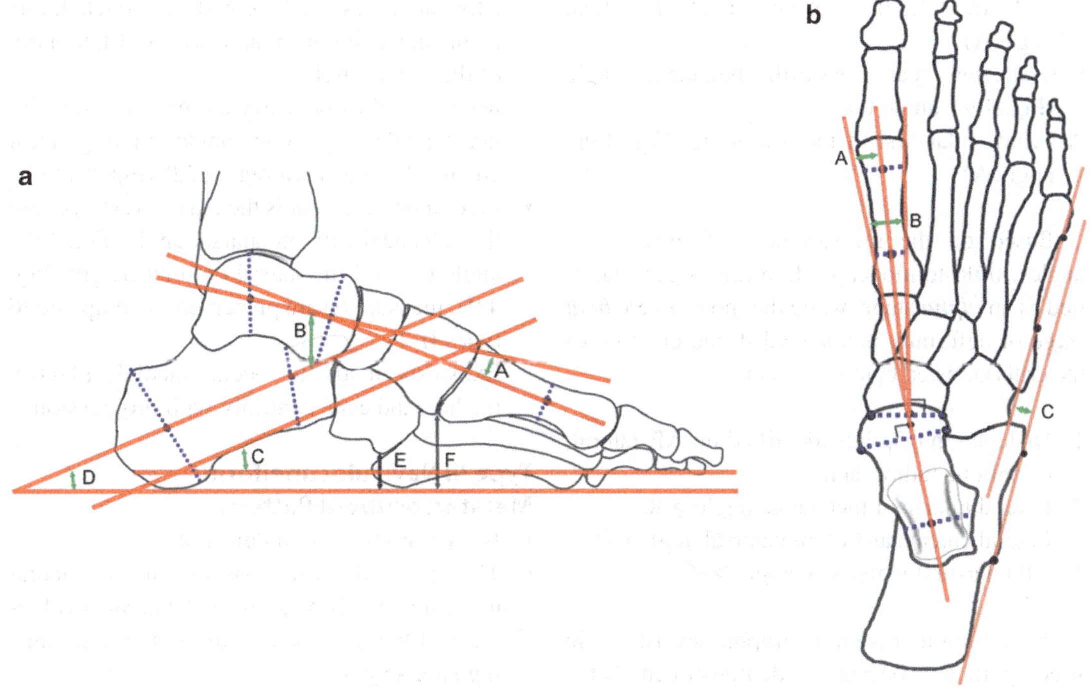

Fig. 4.9 Radiographic measurements and angles for quantifying midtarsal deformities (**a**) lateral radiographs: talar-first metatarsal angle (A); talocalcaneal angle (B); calcaneal-fifth metatarsal angle (C); calcaneal pitch (D); lateral column height (E); medial column height (F) (**b**) AP radiographs: talar-first metatarsal angle (A); talonavicular coverage angle (B); calcaneal-fifth metatarsal angle (C)

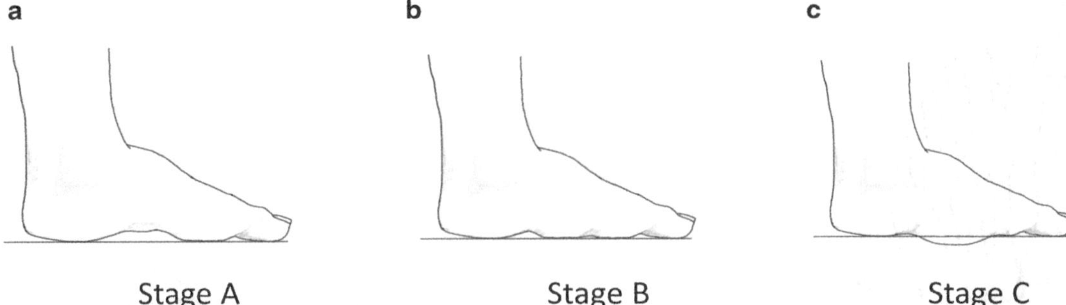

Fig. 4.10 Clinical severity deformity staging as described by Schon: Stage A—minimal deformity, with arch still present; Stage B—loss of medial or lateral arch with plantar or medial prominence; Stage C—collapse of arch medially and laterally, with midfoot prominence that protrudes plantar beyond a line drawn between the heel and the ball of the foot

A **radiographic severity scale** was later added to the original classification system of Schon et al. [30]. The authors identified three radiographic angles that were easy to measure, highly reproducible, and strongly correlated with clinical deformity:

Lateral view: talar-first metatarsal angle (Fig. 4.9a, angle A)
Lateral view: calcaneal-fifth metatarsal angle (Fig. 4.9a, angle C)
AP view: talar-first metatarsal angle (Fig. 4.9b, angle A)

Based on the measurement of these three angles, mild-to-moderate deformities are classified as an *alpha* stage, while the more severe *beta stage* of deformity is assigned if one or more of the criteria, listed below, are met:

1. Dislocation of joints identified on AP, lateral, or oblique radiographs
2. Lateral talar-first metatarsal angle $\geq 30°$
3. Lateral calcaneal-fifth metatarsal angle $\leq 0°$
4. AP talar-first metatarsal angle $\geq 35°$

The addition of the radiographic severity scale was significant, because it demonstrated that a beta stage deformity correlated with prognosis and treatment. Currently the classification of Schon et al. consists of:

Type I: Metatarsocuneiform/ Metatarsocuboid or Lis-Franc Pattern

- Encompasses 33 % of all deformities
- Bony destruction occurs at the first, second, and third metatarsocuneiform joints, and progresses laterally towards the fourth and fifth metatarsocuboid joints
- Clinically, these feet are widely abducted, due to medial column breakdown, and flattening of the medial arch
- Midfoot abduction, using the AP talo-1st metatarsal angle (Fig. 4.9b, angle A) is greatest among all groups, averaging 22° (Fig. 4.11)
- Lateral involvement is the least severe because the calcaneal-fifth metatarsal angle (Fig. 4.9a, angle C), and the lateral column height (Fig. 4.9a, measure E) are preserved as compared to types II–IV
- Exostosis tends to occur medial, plantar-medial, and even centrally with progression

Type II: Naviculocuneiform/ Metatarsocuboid Pattern

- Is seen in 46 % of all deformities
- The major deformity occurs at the medial naviculocuneiform joint, and lateral involvement of the tarsometatarsal joints occurs during later stages
- As measured by the AP talar-first metatarsal angle, (Fig. 4.9b, angle A) the majority of feet demonstrate forefoot abduction, although to a

lesser degree than with type I deformities. A minority of feet are adducted or in a neutral position

- The lower lateral column height (Fig. 4.9a, Measure E) demonstrates that the lateral arch height is decreased and that there is also a lower calcaneal pitch (Fig. 4.9a, Measure E Fig. 4.12) relative to feet with type I deformities

- Exostosis occurs most commonly on the plantar-lateral and plantar-central areas of the foot, less commonly medially

Type III: Perinavicular Pattern

- Identified in 13 % of all deformities
- The major deformity occurs medially at the navicular and surrounding bones, and progresses laterally through the tarsometatarsal or calcaneocuboid joints
- This pattern produces the most clinically significant deformity of all four types, with pronounced adduction and rocker-bottom deformity. The lateral talar-first metatarsal angle is the greatest of all types, and lateral column height is depressed (Fig. 4.13)
- Lateral column involvement results in a lateral rocker-bottom deformity and plantar-central or plantar-lateral bony prominence

Type IV: Transverse Tarsal Pattern

- Identified in 8 % of all deformities
- Bony destruction occurs through the Chopart (talonavicular-calcaneocuboid) joint, with maximum radiographic deformity occurring through the talonavicular joint

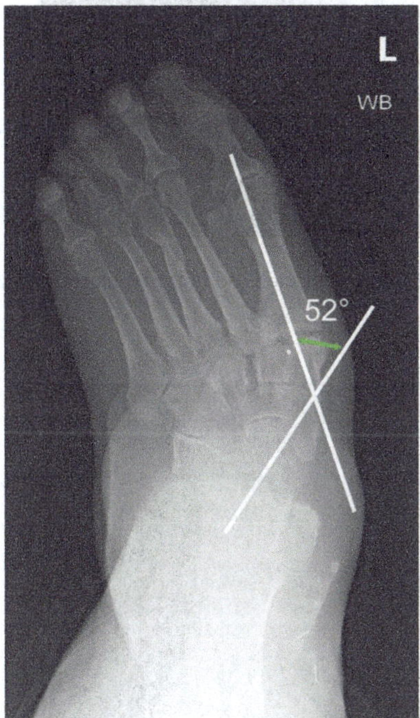

Fig. 4.11 AP radiographic findings in Schon type I midtarsus deformity. Note the severe midfoot abduction as manifested by exceptionally large AP talar-first metatarsal angle

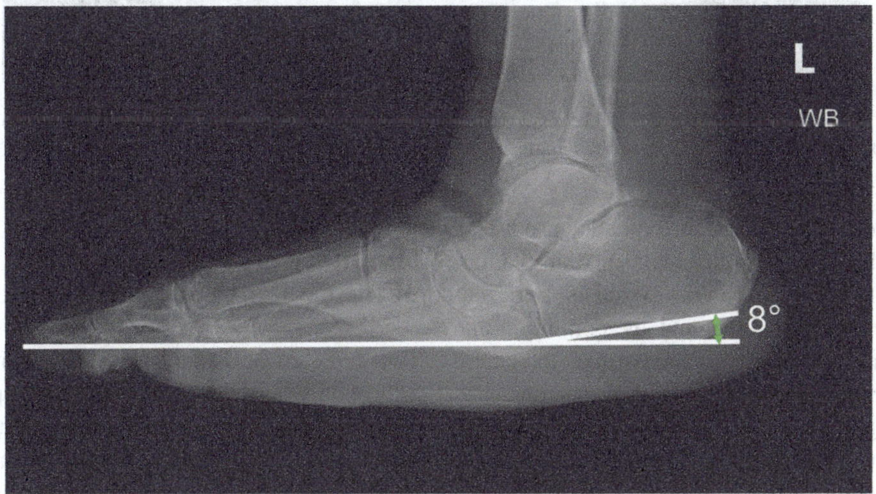

Fig. 4.12 Lateral radiographic findings in Schon type II midtarsus deformity. Note the rocker-bottom deformity as manifested by reversal of the normally positive calcaneal pitch angle

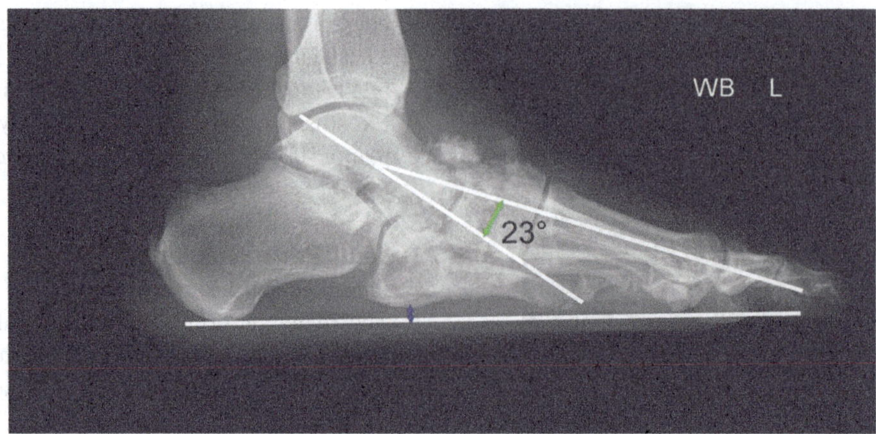

Fig. 4.13 Lateral radiographic findings in Schon type III midtarsus deformity. Increase in talar-first metatarsal angle (*green arrow*), depressed lateral column height (*blue arrow*)

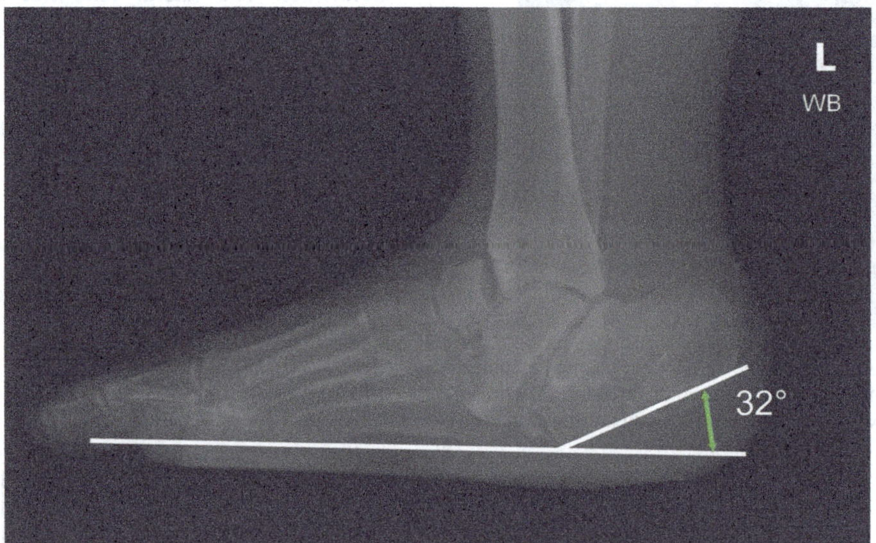

Fig. 4.14 Lateral radiographic findings in Schon type IV midtarsus deformity. Note the severe rocker-bottom deformity and extreme reversal of calcaneal pitch angle

- The deformity occurs proximally, producing an abduction deformity, with medial, plantar-medial, or plantar-central exostosis. Early lateral column involvement is common, and portends a poor prognosis due to lateral rocker-bottom deformity and ulceration
- Radiographically, talocalcaneal angle is greater than in types I–III, and loss of lateral arch height, as manifested by a negative calcaneal pitch, is the greatest of all four types (Fig. 4.14)

Summary of the Classification of the Charcot Foot and Ankle

Two types of classification systems for Charcot arthropathy have been reviewed- temporal and anatomic. Temporal classification systems provide reliable information about prognosis and expected progression of disease. The Eichenholtz system is the only temporal classification developed and describes the progression of Charcot arthropathy both clinically and radiographically. Most importantly, the Eichenholtz system provides general treatment guidelines, particularly when combined with anatomic systems of classification. Stage 0 added by Shibata, should be included when discussing the temporal classification of Charcot arthropathy, as this stage may represent an opportunity for early treatment, which may prevent progression to later stages [11].

As discussed, there are numerous anatomic classification systems. Although each system provides insights into Charcot arthropathy, the anatomic classification systems of Schon et al. and Brodsky et al. appear to be the most useful in guiding and discussing treatment. The classification by Schon et al. is important because it provides insight into specific patterns of Charcot arthropathy of the midfoot, and uses radiographic measurements to highlight the unique anatomic differences between distinct types of arthropathy. Additionally, the location of maximum bony prominence is correlated with each type of deformity, which may help guide treatment. However, the system of Schon et al. is useful only to classify disease of the midfoot.

The most comprehensive anatomic system developed however, is the one described by Brodsky et al. This system is simple to use and correlates well with the rate of progression through Eichenholtz's temporal stages. Additionally, it may help guide treatment, depending on the propensity for instability, deformity, and ulceration specific to each pattern. The weakness of this system lies in its simplicity, and unlike other anatomic classifications, Brodsky's classification does not distinguish between relatively benign forms of midfoot Charcot, such as isolated tarsometatarsal patterns, and those with a worse prognosis such as perinavicular patterns.

Classification of the Charcot foot should include both a temporal and anatomic system. The Eichenholtz temporal classification system should be used for staging, while either the Schon et al. or the Brodsky et al. anatomic classifications should be applied to describe the location of disease. Combining an anatomic and temporal classification allows the treating physician to make more accurate predictions regarding the

behavior of each case of Charcot arthropathy, while using such information to guide treatment. Furthermore, combined temporal staging and anatomic classification should facilitate future discussions in the scientific literature around this complex and difficult-to-generalize condition.

Classification of Ulcerative Lesions of the Diabetic Foot

Diabetic foot lesions have many classifiable parameters. These include size, location, depth, etiology, the presence of Charcot arthropathy, deformity, and the degree of neuropathy. Furthermore, multiple host factors, including glycemic control, nutritional status, and medical comorbidities, and local factors, such as ischemia and deep infections, may ultimately impact the timing and method of treatment of an ulcer. The precise classification of diabetic foot lesions would need to account for each of these variables and would create a classification system so complex as to defy common usage. Therefore, the most widely cited and used classification systems of diabetic foot ulcers strike a balance between precision and utility, and divide this diverse cohort into groups that allow for common treatment, such as mechanical offloading, surgical debridement, or vascular intervention. The four most commonly cited classification systems of diabetic foot ulcers consist of the: Wagner-Meggitt, Depth-ischemia, University of Texas, and the International Working Group on the Diabetic Foot (IWGDF) systems.

Wagner and Meggitt Classification of Diabetic Foot Lesions

The most widely referenced classification system of diabetic foot ulcers is the Wagner-Meggitt classification. F. William Wagner, Jr. M.D., and Bernard Meggitt, F.R.C.S. developed this system in the 1970s at Ranchos Los Amigos Hospital in Los Angeles [31]. This system classifies three independent conditions along the same continuum: ulceration, infection, and ischemia and

Table 4.3 Wagner–Meggitt classification of diabetic foot lesions (Fig. 4.16)

Grade 0	• No open lesions
	• History of previous ulceration, or predisposing bony prominence or deformity
Grade 1	• Superficial ulcer without penetration to deeper layers
Grade 2	• Exposed deep structures including tendon, joint capsule, or bone
Grade 3	• Deep tissue involvement with abscess or osteomyelitis
Grade 4	• Gangrene of some portion of toe, toes, or forefoot
	• Gangrene may be wet or dry, infected or noninfected
Grade 5	• Whole-foot gangrene

established six grades of diabetic foot lesions (Table 4.3) [32] (See Appendix, Table 2). The first three of these grades (0–2) are defined according to the depth of the lesion, which is determined by the type of exposed tissue, after excision of devitalized layers. Grade 3 ulceration is characterized by the presence of exposed bone and deep infection, while the final two grades (4 and 5) are defined by the presence and extent of ischemia. The Wagner-Meggitt classification is simple, widespread in its application, and it has formed a basis for the development of subsequent systems. Based on this system, Wagner established grade-specific treatment protocols [33]. Calhoun et al. demonstrated that when grade-specific treatment protocols were followed, outcomes were markedly improved [34]. Many of the treatment principles outlined by Wagner, using this classification, are still largely applicable today.

As insightful as it is, the Wagner-Meggitt classification is based on the misconception of progression. Wagner and Meggitt believed that a grade 0 lesion (at risk for ulceration) would eventually progress in severity to stage 4 (limited ischemia) without appropriate treatment [33]. Although progression and regression of lesions along the Wagner-Meggitt grades may occur for grades 0–2, there is little evidence to support the concept of regression once a grade 3 (ulceration with exposed bone and osteomyelitis) or even

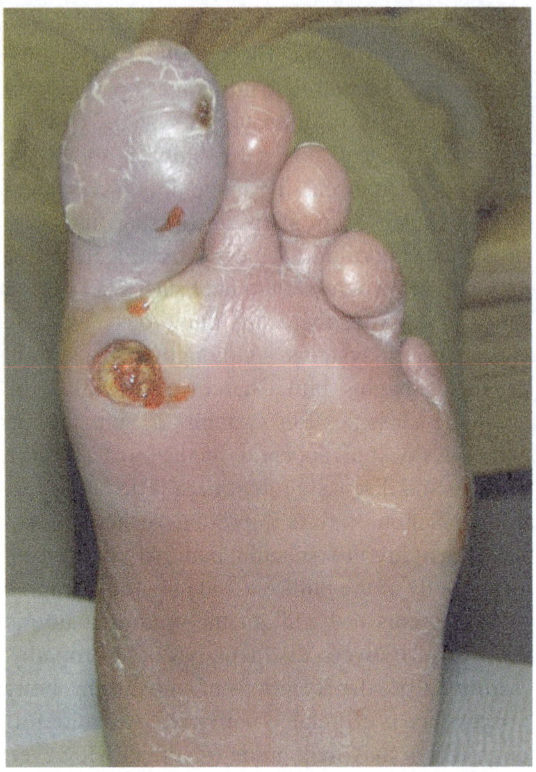

Fig. 4.15 Ischemia occurring in the presence of ulceration. This lesion would be graded according to the depth-ischemia classification system as Grade 2B (exposed deep structures including tendon or joint capsule, and ischemia without gangrene)

limited ischemia (grade 4) has occurred. However, Wagner and Meggitt did acknowledge that stage 5 lesions (whole-foot ischemia) were unique and not reversible. In reality, it is easy to appreciate that a deep infection (grade 3) can occur in the foot with a grade one lesion, or that ischemia (grade 4 and 5) may coexist with any of the lower grade lesions (Fig. 4.15). Therefore, resolution of this classification dilemma requires grading systems that independently account for infection and ischemia.

Depth-Ischemia Classification of Diabetic Foot Lesions

The depth-ischemia classification (DIC), by Brodsky et al., was developed to clarify initial decision-making when treating diabetic foot

Table 4.4 Depth-ischemia classification of diabetic foot lesions

Depth Classification	
Grade 0	• No open lesions, but foot is at risk
	• Predisposed to ulceration due to a combination of peripheral neuropathy and bony prominence
Grade 1	• Superficial wound without penetration to deeper layers by sight or probing
Grade 2	• Exposed deep structures including tendon or joint capsule
Grade 3	• Exposed bone and/or deep infection
	• Abscess and/or osteomyelitis
Ischemia Classification	
Grade A	• Not ischemic
	• Foot has excellent pulses, color, capillary refill, and hair growth
Grade B	• Ischemia without gangrene
	• Absence of one or more Grade A criteria
	• Absence of gangrene
Grade C	• Partial (forefoot) gangrene
Grade D	• Complete foot gangrene

Table 4.5 University of Texas classification of diabetic foot lesions

Depth Grade	
Grade 0	• Preulcerative or postulcerative lesion completely epithelialized
Grade 1	• Partial or full-thickness superficial ulceration
Grade 2	• Deep wound that involves tendon or joint capsule
Grade 3	• Wound that penetrates to bone
Infection and ischemia stage	
Stage A	• Clean wound
Stage B	• Nonischemic infected wound
Stage C	• Ischemic noninfected wound
Stage D	• Ischemic infected wound

lesions [35]. In contrast to the Wagner-Meggitt system, the depth-ischemia classification adds an alphabetic designation, which describes the degree of ischemia, based on clinical parameters. It also groups deep infections into a single grade (Grade 3). Emphasis is placed on the semiautonomous nature of ulceration and ischemia, creating a more precise classification of diabetic foot lesions (Fig. 4.15).

However, this system is similar to Wagner-Meggitt in many ways. First, it doesn't really distinguish lesion depth (Table 4.4). Secondly, it does not allow for the fact that a deep infection may occur in the setting of a more superficial-depth wound, or grade. Lastly, neither system accounts for deep abscess or osteomyelitis occurring in the setting of superficial ulceration.

University of Texas Classification of Diabetic Foot Lesions

The University of Texas Classification System (UTCS) expands on the depth-ischemia, as well as the Wagner-Meggitt classification systems

[35, 36]. The UTCS uses numeric staging of wound depth that is similar to the DIC, but provides greater specificity than previous systems. By using an alphabetic grading system, it accounts for the presence or absence of both ischemia and infection (Table 4.5). A recent study, using both the Wagner-Meggitt and the University of Texas systems to classify diabetic foot lesions in 194 patients, found that the UTCS, by accounting for ischemia and infection, more accurately predicted outcomes [37].

International Working Group on the Diabetic Foot Classification of Diabetic Foot Lesions

The most comprehensive classification of diabetic foot lesions was developed through the combined efforts of the International Working Group of the Diabetic Foot (IWGDF) and the Infectious Disease Society of America (IDSA) [38, 39]. This system was designed to facilitate research communication, and is therefore, somewhat cumbersome for routine clinical application. The classification is based on expert consensus and categorizes diabetic foot ulcers using the following parameters: *Perfusion*, *Extent* and size of the lesion, *Depth* and tissue loss, *Infection* severity, and *Sensation*. Within each category, lesions are graded according to objective measurements and

Table 4.6 International Working Group of the Diabetic Foot classification of diabetic foot ulcers

Perfusion	
Grade 1	No signs or symptoms of peripheral arterial disease (PAD) in the affected foot, in combination with: • Palpable dorsal pedal and posterior tibial artery or • Ankle-brachial index (ABI) 0.9–1.10 or • Toe-brachial index (TBI) >0.6 or • Transcutaneous oxygen pressure (tcpO2) >60 mmHg
Grade 2	Signs or symptoms of PAD, but not of critical limb ischemia (CLI): • Presence of intermittent claudication (in case of claudication, additional noninvasive assessment should be performed) or • ABI <0.9, but with ankle pressure >50 mmHg or • TBI <0.6, but systolic toe blood pressure >30 mmHg or • TcpO2 30–60 mmHg or • Other abnormalities on noninvasive testing, compatible with PAD (but not with CLI)
Grade 3	Critical limb ischemia, as defined by: • Systolic ankle blood pressure <50 mmHg or • Systolic toe blood pressure <30 mmHg or • TcpO2 <30 mmHg
Extent/size	
	• Determined after debridement
	• Measured in square centimeters by multiplying the largest diameter by the second largest diameter that is perpendicular to the first measure
Depth/tissue loss	
	• In setting where ulcer does not penetrate deep to skin, but deep infection is present by virtue of abscess or osteomyelitis, the infection is deemed to be deep, to the level of the involved structures
Grade 1	• Superficial full-thickness ulcer, not penetrating any structure deeper than the dermis
Grade 2	• Deep ulcer, penetrating below the dermis to subcutaneous structures, involving fascia, muscle, or tendon
Grade 3	• All subsequent layers of the foot involved, including bone and/or joint (exposed bone, probing to bone)
Infection	
	• Infection is a clinical diagnosis, based on the features described in this grading system, regardless of the results of wound culture
	• Three parameters are of importance when grading for infection, and directly impact treatment and outcome: involvement of skin, involvement of deeper structures, and systemic inflammatory response
Grade 1	Absence of signs or symptoms of infection
Grade 2	Infection involving the skin and the subcutaneous tissue only (without involvement of deeper tissues and without systemic signs, as described below). At least two of the following findings are present: • Local swelling or induration • Erythema >0.5–2 cm around the ulcer • Local tenderness or pain • Local warmth • Purulent discharge (thick, opaque to white, or sanguineous secretion) Other causes of an inflammatory response of the skin should be excluded (e.g., trauma, gout, acute Charcot arthropathy, fracture, thrombosis, venous stasis)
Grade 3	Deep infection as defined by: • Erythema >2 cm around ulcer plus at least one of non-erythema-bulleted items described in grade 2 or • Infection involving structures deeper than skin and subcutaneous tissues such as abscess, osteomyelitis, septic arthritis, fasciitis • Absence of systemic inflammatory response signs, as described in grade 4

(continued)

Table 4.6 (continued)

Perfusion	
Grade 4	Infection characterized by a systemic inflammatory response as defined by two or more of the following conditions:
	• Temperature >38° or <36 °C
	• Heart rate >90 beats/min
	• Respiratory rate >20 breaths/min
	• $PaCO_2 < 32$-mmHg
	• White blood cell count >12,000 or <4000/cu mm
	• 10 % immature (band) forms
Sensation	
	• The distinction between grades is the presence or absence of protective sensation, as determined by sensation to pressure and vibration
Grade 1	No detectable loss of protective sensation on the affected foot, as defined by the presence of sensory modalities described in grade 2
Grade 2	Loss of protective sensation on the affected foot is defined as the absence of perception of the one of the following tests in the affected foot:
	• Absent pressure sensation, determined with a 10-g monofilament, on two out of three sites on the plantar side of the foot
	• Absent vibration sensation, (determined with a 128-Hz tuning fork) or vibration threshold >25 V (using semiquantitative techniques), both tested on the hallux

criteria and is summarized by the acronym PEDIS (Table 4.6). Unlike previously discussed classifications, the infection category for this system accounts for systemic manifestations of diabetic foot infection, such as leukocytosis and acidosis, which are the end-result of untreated diabetic foot lesions and often portend a poor prognosis for limb salvage [39]. Although no study to date has verified the predictive power of this system, several studies have found that in the presence of ulceration, the IWGDF infection grade is predictive of amputation [40].

Summary of Ulcer Classifications

Numerous classification systems for diabetic foot lesions have been devised. The Wagner-Meggitt system is simple, easy to apply, and is the most commonly clinically referenced system for the classification of diabetic foot ulcers. The problems, however, are that this system assumes a progression of the ulcer, a reversal that may or may not occur, and also does not account for ischemia and infection occurring independent of wound depth. The depth-ischemia classification system accounts separately for ischemia, while the UTCS accounts separately for both ischemia and infection. Because each of these systems does address ischemia and infection, through alphabetic designations, these both may provide greater treatment-relevance and predictive power. Finally, the IWGDF classification system does focus on variables that are not addressed by other classifications, but its use as a research tool may make it too cumbersome for routine clinical use. From the author's perspective, each system has merit and additional research is needed in order to validate each of these systems. Therefore, when deciding on a system, pick one that is easy to use and remember and then use it consistently.

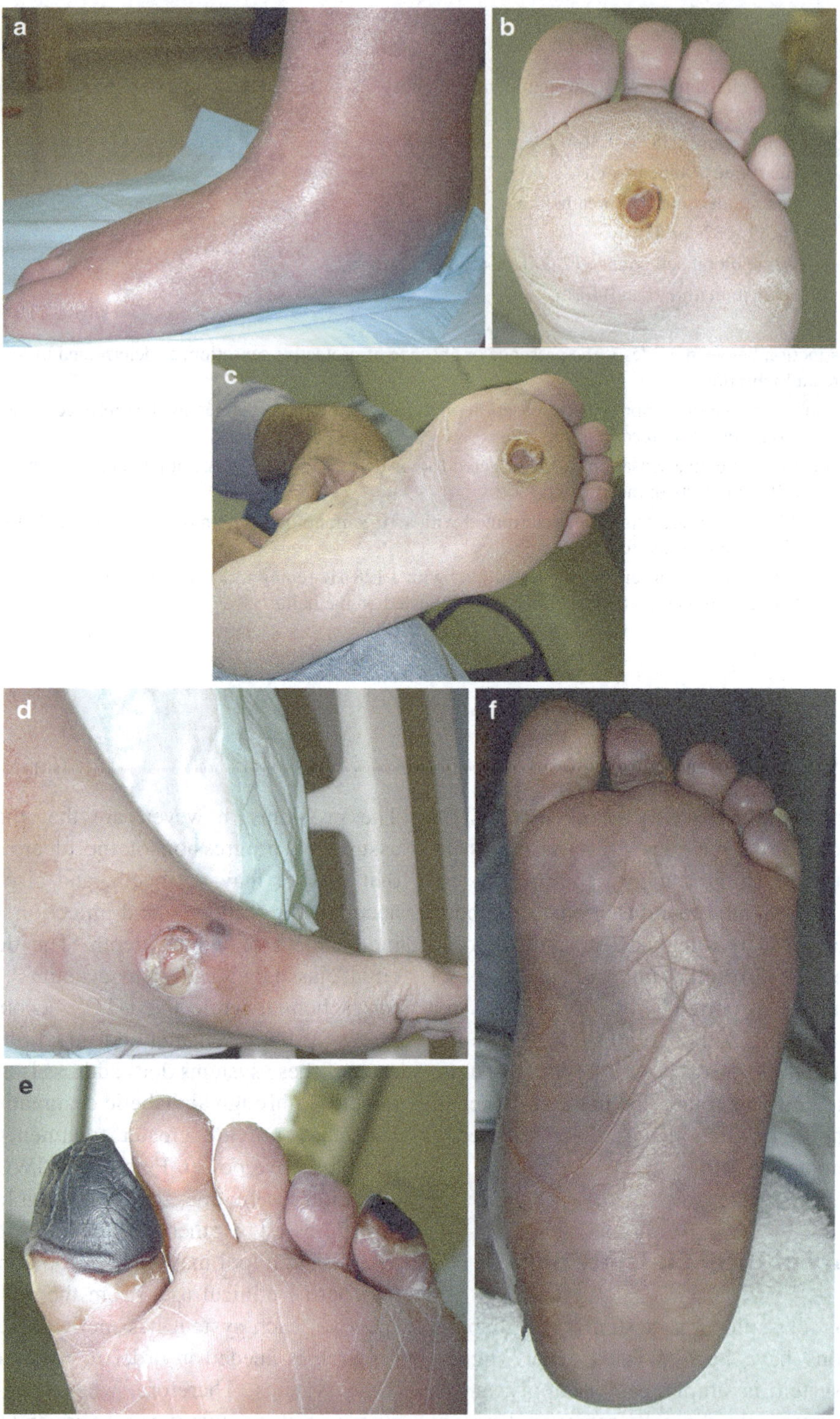

Fig. 4.16 Wagner-Meggitt classification of diabetic foot lesions (**a**) Grade 0: deformity created by an underlying Charcot arthropathy has created a preulcerative bony prominence beneath the subluxed talar head. (**b**) Grade 1: superficial ulceration (**c**) Grade 2: ulceration which probed to the MTP joint capsule, but absent signs of infection. (**d**) Grade 3: ulceration with exposed bone and deep infection. (**e**) Grade 4: gangrene limited to forefoot. (**f**) Grade 5: early whole-foot gangrene

References

1. Charcot J. Sur quelaques arthropathies qui paraissent depender d'une lesion du cerveau ou de la moele epiniere. Arch Des Physiol Norm Path. 1868;1:161–71.
2. Jordan W. Neuritic manifestations of diabetes mellitus. Arch Intern Med. 1936;57:145–87.
3. Johnson JT. Neuropathic fractures and joint injuries. Pathogenesis and rationale of prevention and treatment. J Bone Joint Surg Am. 1967;49:1–30.
4. Eichenholtz SN. Charcot joints. Springfield: C.C. Thomas; 1966.
5. Classen JN, Rolley RT, Carneiro R, Martire JR. Management of foot conditions of the diabetic patient. Am Surg. 1976;42:81–8.
6. Kiuru MJ, Pihlajamaki HK, Hietanen HJ, Ahovuo JA. MR imaging, bone scintigraphy, and radiography in bone stress injuries of the pelvis and the lower extremity. Acta Radiol. 2002;43:207–12.
7. Kiuru MJ, Pihlajamaki HK, Ahovuo JA. Bone stress injuries. Acta Radiol. 2004;45:317–26.
8. Dutta P, Bhansali A, Singh P, Mittal BR. Charcot's foot: advanced manifestation of diabetic neuropathy. Postgrad Med J. 2004;80:434.
9. Moore TE, Yuh WT, Kathol MH, el-Khoury GY, Corson JD. Abnormalities of the foot in patients with diabetes mellitus: findings on MR imaging. AJR Am J Roentgenol. 1991;157:813–6.
10. Chantelau E, Poll LW. Evaluation of the diabetic charcot foot by MR imaging or plain radiography—an observational study. Exp Clin Endocrinol Diabetes. 2006;114:428–31.
11. Shibata T, Tada K, Hashizume C. The results of arthrodesis of the ankle for leprotic neuroarthropathy. J Bone Joint Surg Am. 1990;72:749–56.
12. Hastings MK, Johnson JE, Strube MJ, et al. Progression of foot deformity in Charcot neuropathic osteoarthropathy. J Bone Joint Surg Am. 2013;95:1206–13.
13. Christensen TM, Gade-Rasmussen B, Pedersen LW, Hommel E, Holstein PE, Svendsen OL. Duration of off-loading and recurrence rate in Charcot osteoarthropathy treated with less restrictive regimen with removable walker. J Diabetes Complications. 2012;26:430–4.
14. Fabrin J, Larsen K, Holstein PE. Long-term follow-up in diabetic Charcot feet with spontaneous onset. Diabetes Care. 2000;23:796–800.
15. Rudrappa S, Game F, Jeffcoate W. Recurrence of the acute Charcot foot in diabetes. Diabet Med. 2012;29:819–21.
16. Osterhoff G, Boni T, Berli M. Recurrence of acute Charcot neuropathic osteoarthropathy after conservative treatment. Foot Ankle Int. 2013;34:359–64.
17. Edmonds M, Watkins PJ. The Charcot joint: understanding its natural history leads to new treatment and prevention. Diabet Med. 1984;1.
18. Pinzur MS, Lio T, Posner M. Treatment of Eichenholtz stage I Charcot foot arthropathy with a weightbearing total contact cast. Foot Ankle Int. 2006;27:324–9.
19. Chantelau EA, Grutzner G. Is the Eichenholtz classification still valid for the diabetic Charcot foot? Swiss Med Wkly. 2014;144:w13948.
20. Harris JR, Brand PW. Patterns of disintegration of the tarsus in the anaesthetic foot. J Bone Joint Surg. 1966;48:4–16.
21. Cofield RH, Morrison MJ, Beabout JW. Diabetic neuroarthropathy in the foot: patient characteristics and patterns of radiographic change. Foot Ankle. 1983;4:15–22.
22. Sammarco GJ, Conti SF. Surgical treatment of neuroarthropathic foot deformity. Foot Ankle Int. 1998;19:102–9.
23. Brodsky JW. Personal communication. Accessed 15 Mar 2015.
24. Johnson J, Klein SE, Brodsky JE. Diabetes. In: Coughlin M, Saltzman C, Anderson RB, editors. Mann's surgery of the foot and ankle. 9th ed. Philadelphia: Elsevier; 2014. p. 1396–8.
25. Brodsky J, Wagner F, Kwong P. Patterns of breakdown in the Charcot tarsus of diabetes and relation to treatment. Foot Ankle. 1986;5:353.
26. Trepman E, Nihal A, Pinzur MS. Current topics review: Charcot neuroarthropathy of the foot and ankle. Foot Ankle Int. 2005;26:46–63.
27. Biehl 3rd WC, Morgan JM, Wagner Jr FW, Gabriel R. Neuropathic calcaneal tuberosity avulsion fractures. Clin Orthop Relat Res. 1993;12:8–13.
28. Hess M, Booth B, Laughlin RT. Calcaneal avulsion fractures: complications from delayed treatment. Am J Emerg Med. 2008;26:254.
29. Schon LC, Weinfeld SB, Horton GA, Resch S. Radiographic and clinical classification of acquired midtarsus deformities. Foot Ankle Int. 1998;19:394–404.
30. Schon LC, Easley ME, Cohen I, Lam PW, Badekas A, Anderson CD. The acquired midtarsus deformity classification system—interobserver reliability and intraobserver reproducibility. Foot Ankle Int. 2002;23:30–6.
31. Brodsky JW. Classification of foot lesions in diabetic patients. In: Pfeifer JHB, editor. Levin and O'Neal's the diabetic foot. Philadelphia: Mosby Elsevier; 2008.
32. Wagner FW. A classification and treatment program for diabetic, neuropathic and dysvascular foot problems, vol. 28. Rosemont: AAOS; 1979. p. 143–65.
33. Wagner Jr FW. The dysvascular foot: a system for diagnosis and treatment. Foot Ankle. 1981;2:64–122.
34. Calhoun JH, Cantrell J, Cobos J, et al. Treatment of diabetic foot infections: Wagner classification, therapy, and outcome. Foot Ankle. 1988;9:101–6.
35. Brodsky JW. Outpatient diagnosis and management of the diabetic foot *AAOS*. Instr Course Lect. 1993;42:121–39.

36. Lavery LA, Armstrong DG, Harkless LB. Classification of diabetic foot wounds. J Foot Ankle Surg. 1996;35:528–31.
37. Oyibo SO, Jude EB, Tarawneh I, Nguyen HC, Harkless LB, Boulton AJ. A comparison of two diabetic foot ulcer classification systems: the Wagner and the University of Texas wound classification systems. Diabetes Care. 2001;24:84–8.
38. Schaper NC. Diabetic foot ulcer classification system for research purposes: a progress report on criteria for including patients in research studies. Diabetes Metab Res Rev. 2004;20 Suppl 1:S90–5.
39. Lipsky BA, Berendt AR, Deery HG, Embil JM, Joseph WS, Karmicher AW, LeFrock JL, Lew DP, Mader JT, Norden C, Tan JS. Diagnosis and treatment of diabetic foot infections. Clin Infect Dis. 2004;39:885–910.
40. Pickwell K, Siersma V, Kars M, et al. Predictors of lower-extremity amputation in patients with an infected diabetic foot ulcer. Diabetes Care. 2015;38(5):852–7.

Nonoperative Care and Footwear for the Diabetic Foot and Ankle Patient

David E. Karges

Introduction

The foot is a dynamic structure. Normal gait begins as the hindfoot strikes the ground causing the gastrocnemius-soleus complex and tibialis posterior muscles to contract. This produces inversion of the heel and locks the midtarsal joints, which creates a rigid lever that promotes body locomotion. As the body axis advances over the midfoot, momentum is generated with the power of toe-lift propelling the forefoot and body forward. When the foot is lifted from the ground it ends the gait-cycle. While swinging the ipsilateral foot forward, the midtarsal joints unlock and the contralateral foot begins its cycle. In the neuropathic patient, this pattern can be significantly altered, producing eccentric pressures to the foot and ankle.

In the United States, diabetes is the foremost cause of neuropathic joint disease and the foot is the most common location, seen in approximately 8.5/1000 people with diabetes per year [1]. As part of the disease process, these patients lose peripheral sensation, proprioception, and fine motor control [2]. Because the patient doesn't experience any pain, greater than 50 % of patients present with neuropathic collapse of the foot or ankle, most often due to a minor traumatic event. The resultant inflammatory process increases blood flow, produces more resorption of bone, and renders this region weak and susceptible to further injury. Continued weight-bearing leads this altered anatomy producing more bony destruction, which ultimately affects gait. In this population, approximately 60 % of foot problems affect the tarsometatarsal joints, 30 % affect metatarsophalangeal joints, and the remaining 10 % affect the ankle and hindfoot [3]. These patients also present with autonomic neuropathy which leads to chronically dry and harden skin [4]. Over time, the epidermal skin cracks allowing for the entry of bacteria to the dermal layer. This leads to further breakdown of skin, allowing for the development of wounds and infection. Additionally, diabetic motor neuropathy occurs and produces contractures of the foot leading to flexion of digits, hyperextension of metatarsophalangeal joints, equinus of the ankle and transverse tarsal joints, and varus and valgus deformities of the hindfoot. These deformities also contribute to tissue breakdown and formation of ulcers.

Avoiding complications and accommodating for the loss of protective sensation and autonomic dysfunction is indeed challenging. Since the neuropathy cannot be reversed, the nonsurgical treatment focuses on managing the areas of the foot

D.E. Karges, D.O. (✉)
Department of Orthopaedic Surgery, Saint Louis University, 3635 Vista Ave., Desloge Towers 7th Fl., Saint Louis, MO 63110, USA
e-mail: kargesd@slu.edu

© Springer International Publishing Switzerland 2016
D. Herscovici, Jr. (ed.), *The Surgical Management of the Diabetic Foot and Ankle*,
DOI 10.1007/978-3-319-27623-6_5

and ankle with soft tissue and bone prominences. By applying cushioning shoewear, custom contouring of insoles, and the addition of daily inspection of feet, this chapter will offer nonoperative approaches that can be used to treat and manage these patients.

Evaluation and Diagnosis

The typical patient presents with a painless deformity, erythema, warmth, and swelling. Patient history is an important initial step and should include asking about the mechanism of injury, timeline of any foot pain, and whether patients have had any soft tissue ulceration, foot deformities, or a history of infection. One should also inquire about any previous surgical management to the foot and ankle, possible treatment complications, history of immobilization, their ability to ambulate, need of special shoes, if braces are used, and whether or not they require any ambulatory aids. Other important information should include the patient's duration of diabetes, how their diabetes is currently managed (insulin dependant or non-insulin dependant), the duration of their diabetic treatment, whether they monitor and record daily blood glucose levels, and whether or not they have scheduled serum A1c (goal of <7.0 %) measurements. Lastly, knowledge of the patient's family and friend support structure is important to understand and help in their daily ability to follow a treatment plan.

The physical examination should begin with a complete evaluation of the foot and should assess the skin, nails, vascular status, musculoskeletal alignment, and whether or not protective sensation exists. Sensory neuropathy is assessed using Semmes-Weinstein monofilaments and protective sensation is confirmed when the patient can accurately detect pressure from a 5.07 monofilament to the forefoot. All corns, calluses, signs of pre-ulcerative skin conditions (such as blisters) and any pain, it is important to remember acute neuroarthropathy can be painful in up to 33 % of patients. If pain exists in either the acute or chronic diabetic patient, even in the absence of any foot ulceration, the presence of an infection should be suspected. However, unless a fracture

or dislocation is in the location of an active, or previous ulcer or open wound, the chance of osteomyelitis is uncommon. Lastly, distal vascular perfusion is assessed by the presence or absence of dorsalis pedis and posterior tibial artery pulses. Skin that is delicate, hairless, and shiny all indicate that there is a decreased perfusion to the extremity. If peripheral arterial disease is suspected, evaluation and measurement of foot and ankle perfusion may be required. The two easiest methods are arterial Doppler ultrasound and transcutaneous oxygen tension ($TcPO_2$) measurement. Literature suggests that both tests are equivalent as predictors of healing ulcerations and in their ability to determine levels of amputation preoperatively [4]. Patients with diabetic neuroarthropathy routinely present with Doppler indices greater than 0.6 [5]. Transcutaneous oxygen tension measurements ($TcPO_2$) assess the partial pressure of oxygen diffusing through skin with a special temperature-controlled oxygen electrode. A value of 30 mmHg is predictive of adequate circulation for soft tissue healing. Caution is recommended when interpreting $TcPO_2$ levels for the values are affected by edema and cellulitis [6, 7]. In addition, measuring toe pressures have been shown to be one of the most accurate predictors to healing if the pressures are at least 40 mmHg [8]. Further discussions can be found in the chapter on the Vascular Evaluation and Management of Vascular Disease in the Diabetic Patient.

After the history and physical examination, diagnostic studies are an essential part of patient evaluation, especially when trying to differentiate Charcot arthropathy from musculoskeletal infections in the foot and ankle. The radiographic work-up should begin with all patients undergoing plain weight-bearing films of the foot and ankle, if possible. These radiographs commonly display moderate to advanced bony disorganization related to the degree of neuroarthropathy. Two common radiographic patterns described are: (1) an atrophic pattern with bone resorption and joint disintegration and (2) a hypertrophic pattern with much formation of periarticular bone, osteophytes, collapse of joints, and incomplete bone bridging of fractures throughout the affected area [9] (Fig. 5.1a, b). However, plain

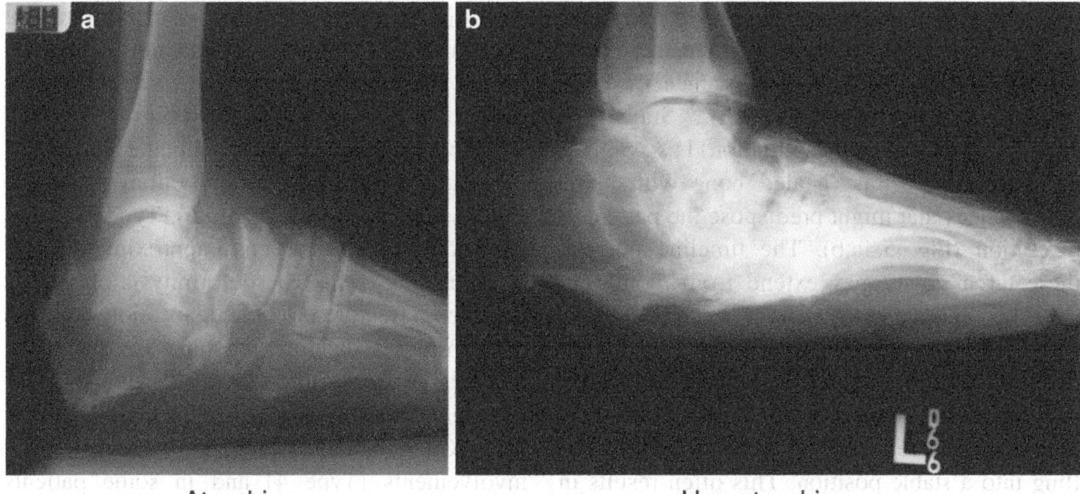

Fig. 5.1 (a, b) Radiographic patterns of neuroarthropathy

radiograph sensitivity in diagnosing osteomyelitis is poor. If concern for infection exists, magnetic resonance imaging (MRI) should be ordered. Despite its wide variation in reported sensitivity and specificity, it is presently considered the gold standard for diagnosing osteomyelitis. Although an MRI helps to identify the presence or absence of abscess cavities and deep soft tissue infection, its primary disadvantage is its inability to differentiate between arthropathy and osteomyelitis, since both are associated with bone edema [10]. When plain films and an MRI makes the diagnosis of an infection uncertain, the use of a simultaneous Indium-labeled white blood cell and technetium-labeled phosphate bone scans has been shown to be helpful in diagnosing osteomyelitis [7] (Table 1, see Appendix).

The diagnostic work-up should continue by evaluating the patient's laboratory values including a complete blood count (CBC), their chemistry profile, including an evaluation of their hemoglobin A1c, and, if infection is suspected, evaluating the erythrocyte sedimentation rate (ESR) and C-Reactive protein (CRP) levels. In the absence of a fever, along with normal white counts, ESR, and blood glucose levels one can nearly eliminate the diagnosis of infection. However, a leukocytosis greater than 11×10^9/L associated with a fever greater than 100.5° has been associated with an increased risk of amputation [11, 12]. A simple test to help determine whether or not the patient has an infection is with a trial of 2 h of bed rest of the elevated foot. If the swelling and erythema resolve it usually indicates that there is no infection; however, these physical findings will persist in the presence of infection [2]. In patients presenting with an ulcer, worsening control of glycemic levels can be an early and reliable indicator of a foot infection. Although ESR and CRP are sensitive for inflammation and infection, they are not specific to delineate between colonization, local infection, and osteomyelitis [8]. In fact, a CRP can be normal in the diabetic patient with deep infection [13]. In patients with suspected deep infections or osteomyelitis deep tissue swabs and bone biopsies remain the gold standard to identify an infection.

Staging and Classification

In 1966, Eichenholtz [9] developed a classification system describing three different stages that occur with Charcot arthropathy. Stage I (Development and Fragmentation) is described with physical signs of erythema, warmth, and swelling and radiographically with periarticular bony debris, subchondral fragmentation, fractures, subluxations, and dislocations (Fig. 5.2a,b).

Stage II (Coalescence) also has warmth, erythema, and swelling and demonstrates new bone formation, sclerosis, and coalescence of large bony fragments (Fig. 5.3a,b). Stage III (Reconstruction and Consolidation) has swelling but may demonstrate healed bone with some prominences that might predispose the patient to ulceration (Fig. 5.4a,b). The timeline through these three stages may extend from months to several years and if the patient is provided with sufficient off-loading devices, a functional position and adequate healing can occur. However, weight-bearing stresses can overpower the healing process preventing the foot or ankle from settling into a stable position. This often results in predictable deformities [10].

When describing the location of the Charcot arthropathy one classification that is commonly used divides the foot and ankle into four regions [11]. Type 1 occurs in the tarsometatarsal region and is seen in almost to 60 % of Charcot arthrop-

athies [12]. It can result in rocker bottom foot deformity, along with displacement of the metatarsals and cuneiforms (Fig. 5.5). Type 2 is the second most common location, occurs in up to 35 % of cases, and affects the subtalar and transverse tarsal joints. A rocker bottom deformity can also be seen [14] (Fig. 5.6). Type 3 affects the ankle joint and is seen in approximately 9 % of cases (Fig. 5.7). The deformity is often preceded by a fracture or ankle dislocation, can lead to deformities that prevent nonoperative brace management, and may lead to the development of ulcers on the medial or lateral malleoli [15]. Some Charcot arthropathies have multiple joint involvements (Type 4) and in some patients (Type 5) only the forefoot is involved. This can result in plantar ulceration of the metatarsophalangeal joints which may result in osteomyelitis. Further discussions can be found in the chapter on the Classification of the Charcot foot and Ankle.

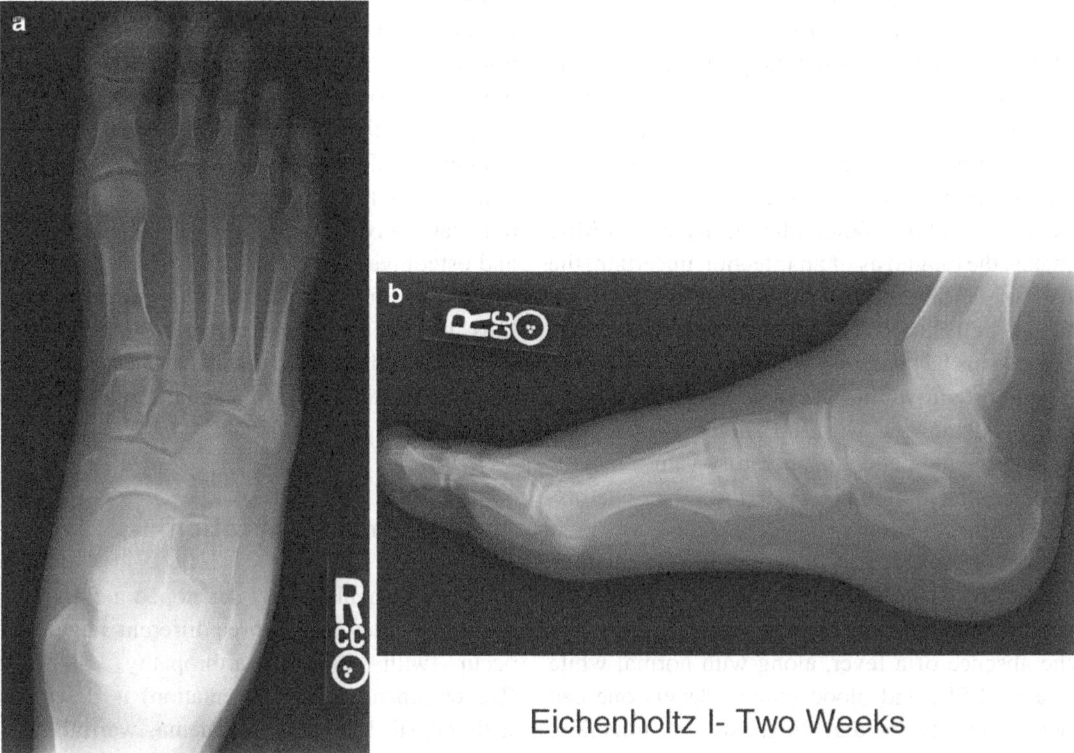

Fig. 5.2 (a, b) AP and lateral radiographs of early 1st TMT disruption

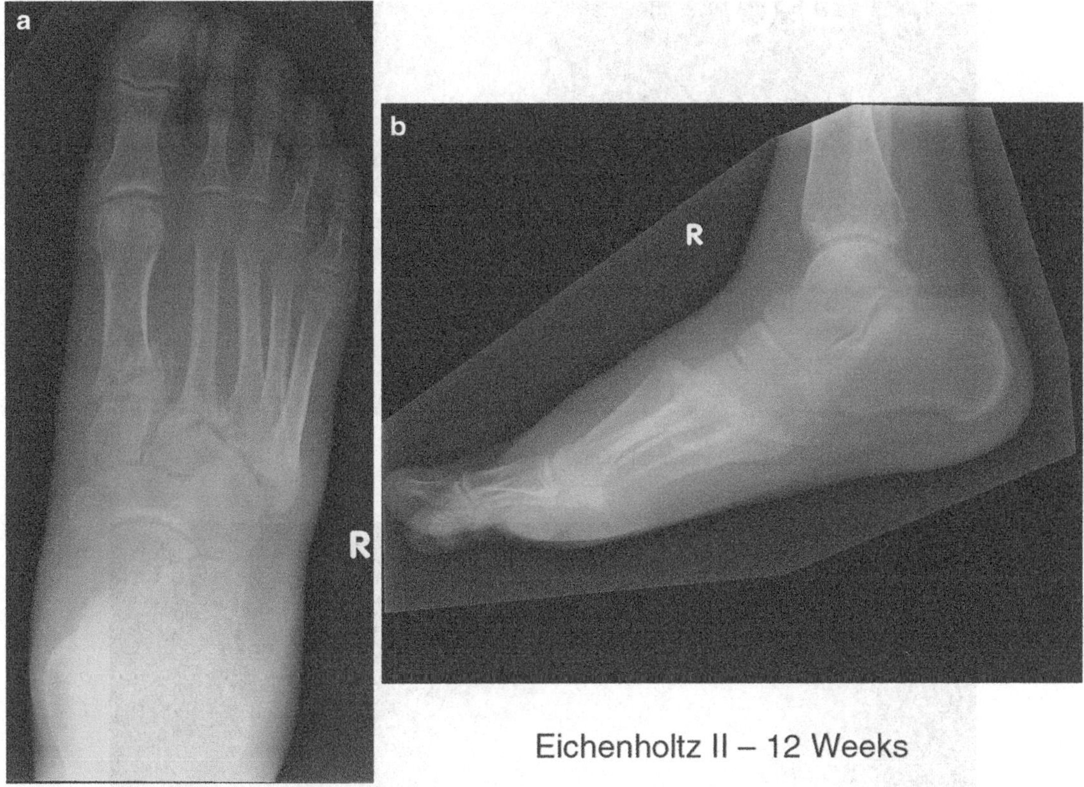

Fig. 5.3 (**a**, **b**) AP and lateral radiographs of progressive medial and lateral column TMT collapse

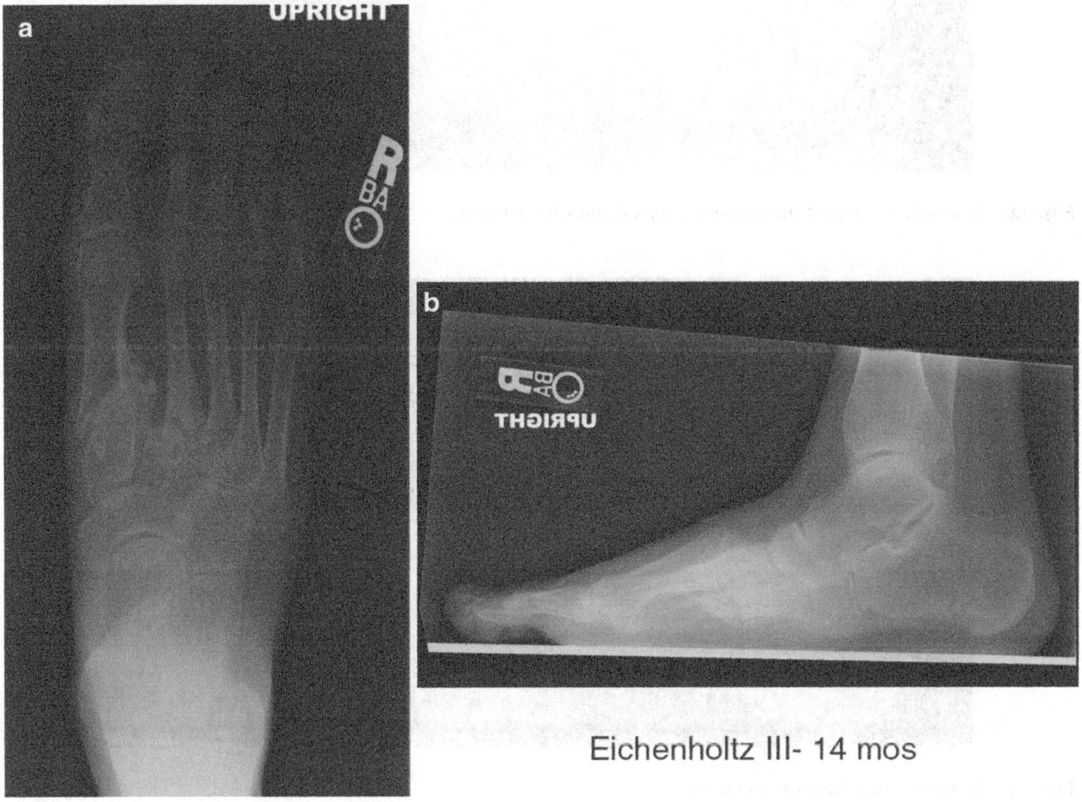

Fig. 5.4 (**a**, **b**) Natural history: tarsometatarsal fracture-dislocation—Eichenholtz III

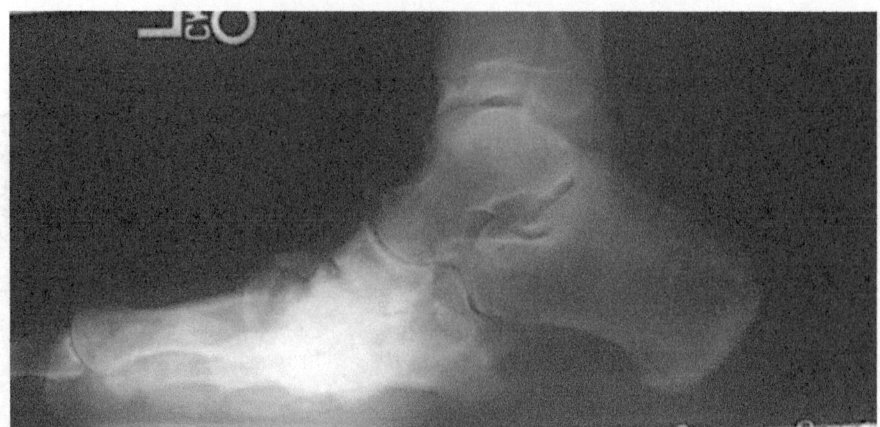

Fig. 5.5 Anatomic classification: tarsometatarsal joints

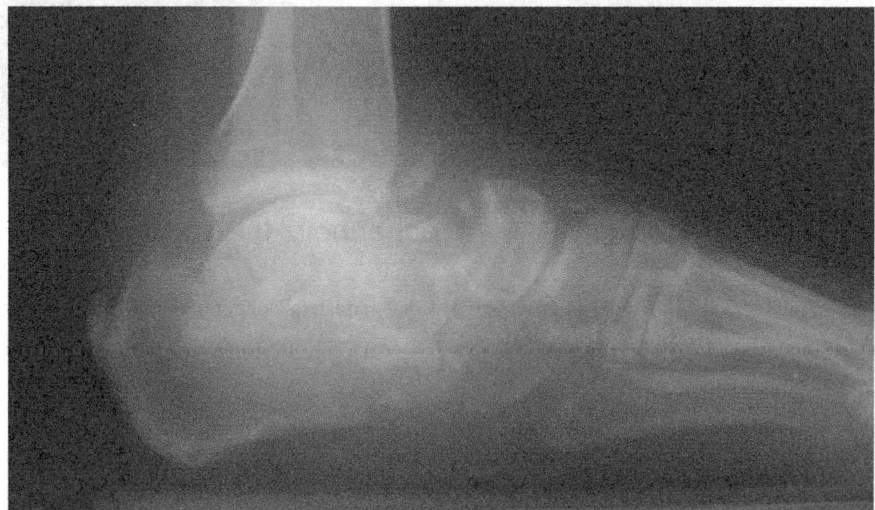

Fig. 5.6 Anatomic classification: transverse tarsal and subtalar joints

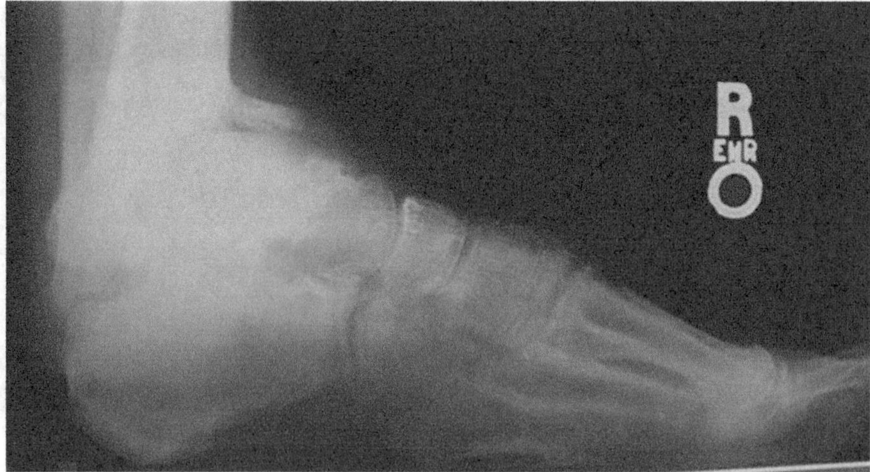

Fig. 5.7 Anatomic classification: ankle joint

Nonoperative Foot Care

The goals for the nonoperative management of the diabetic foot and ankle are to obtain a stable and plantigrade foot, to avoid abnormal plantar pressures in feet with bony deformities, to prevent ulcers from developing or reoccurring, and to allow the patient to ambulate using a combination of footwear and orthoses [15]. By the time a patient is referred to the specialist, a prior foot care program may have been established by another physician. Their program must be reviewed to learn whether the patient has been instructed to perform daily, routine inspection of the foot, does not surgically trim their own calluses, applies skin moisturizer to the foot daily and wears well-fitting footwear. An optimal function can be anticipated with this type of instruction.

Patients may be immediately classified for nonoperative treatment based on a history of ulceration, current deformity, a previous amputation, absence of pulses, and loss of sensation [7]. Categories for failure of nonoperative care are graded 0–3 and are based on the risk of developing a complication. A category-0 patient presents with normal appearing feet and normal sensation. The patient is instructed on basic diabetic foot care, returns at yearly intervals for an examination of the foot and ankle, and can wear normal footwear. The category-1 patient presents with only sensory loss. They are instructed to perform a daily foot examination and are recommended to wear extra-depth shoes or possibly total contact orthoses.

Category-2 patients have no history of ulceration but presents with moderate claw or hammer toe deformities. There is evidence of plantar callosities and possible lesser digit or ray amputations. The patient is instructed to perform daily foot examinations, prescribed extra-depth shoes, custom molded foot orthoses, rocker bottom sole modifications, and is advised to return for an evaluation every 4–6 months.

Category-3 patients present with numerous risk factors including a history of ulceration, presence of a deformity, previous ablation procedure(s), possible loss of distal pulses, and advanced sensory neuroarthropathy. These patients are to be prescribed custom, total contact boot wear. Close evaluation of any new skin or nail problems must be addressed prior to routine weight-bearing, and subsequent bimonthly evaluation is recommended by an orthopaedic foot and ankle surgeon to maintain the optimum status of the foot and ankle and avoid problems.

Skin and Nails

Nonoperative care begins with routine care of the skin and nails. Patients need to understand that this is an important part of treatment, which can help avoid developing ulcerations and infections about the foot and ankle. They should be educated about calluses and corns often developing due to routine pressure phenomenon but also informed that these can be treated with regular use of a pumice stone, along with appropriate orthotic and shoewear. If this fails to resolve their calluses, the use of high speed abraider and scalpel by the treating physician are often necessary, in order to avoid the development of hyperkeratotic calluses. However, they should also be told that the diabetic foot with advanced plantar medial or lateral column prominence may not be effectively managed nonoperatively and may warrant surgical realignment of the bony geometry.

Routine toenail care is also important to maintain a healthy foot and requires trimming nails transversely and maintaining the medial and lateral margins distal to the nail fold, to minimize the risk of an ingrown toenail. Any infection due to an ingrown toenail must be treated by culture-guided antibiotics and may subsequently require a partial or complete matrixectomy of the nail. Topically applied antifungal agents (miconazole, griseofulvin) have shown lower cure rates than oral medications (griseofulvin, itraconazole) but the oral medicines must be monitored for toxicity to the liver and heart [7]. At times the treatment of nail fungal infections may require a dermatologic consultation.

Shoewear

Proper footwear is an important part of the overall treatment program, especially for those patients in the earliest stages of the disease, those with a lack of sensation, or in patients presenting with any kind of neuropathy. That is because excessive pressure and friction that can occur from the wrong kind or poorly fitting shoe can lead to blisters, calluses, and ulcers, and potentially lead to an amputation.

The orthopaedic surgeon should develop a relationship with a certified pedorthist, who gets to know the surgeon's foot and ankle practice. This relationship allows the physician to monitor the quality of products made and make adjustments to a patient's custom product, which ultimately improves patient compliance. The proper footwear for diabetics should achieve the following objectives:

- **Relieve areas of excessive pressure**. Footwear should relieve areas with excessive pressure on the foot that can lead to skin breakdown or ulcers, which can also lead to other problems.
- **Reduce shock and shear**. The footwear should reduce the amount of vertical pressure or shock to the bottom of the foot, as well as to decrease horizontal (shear) movement of the foot within the shoe.
- **Accommodate, stabilize, and support deformities**. Deformities resulting from conditions such as Charcot arthropathy, loss of plantar fatty tissue, the development of hammer toes, and any amputations must be accommodated. Many deformities need stabilization to relieve pain and avoid further problems. In addition, some deformities may need to be controlled or supported to decrease progression of the deformity.
- **Limit motion of joints**. Limiting the motion of certain joints can often decrease inflammation, relieve pain, and result in a more stable and functional foot. The width of the shoe is just as important as the length. The proper width of a shoe is determined when the widest part of the patient's foot, across the base of the toes, is also the widest part of the shoe. The proper length of a shoe should be 3/8- to 1/2-in. longer than the distal tip of the longest toe. The shoe should also come with laces or wide Velcro straps to provide adjustability that is needed to accommodate for swelling or other local deformities. When the shoe fits properly it should not slip off the foot when walking.

Prescription Footwear

- **Healing shoes**. Most often used following surgical reconstruction or ulcer treatment. A healing shoe may be necessary before a regular or custom shoe can be worn. These include custom sandals (open toe), heat-moldable healing shoes (closed toe), and postoperative shoes (Fig. 5.8a,b).
- **In-depth shoes**. The in-depth shoe is the basis for most footwear prescriptions. This is an oxford-type or athletic shoe that is made with an additional 1/4- to 1/2-in. of depth throughout the shoe. This allows extra volume for the inserts or orthoses, as well as to accommodate for any deformity associated with the diabetic foot. In-depth shoes also tend to be light in weight, have shock-absorbing soles, and come in a wide range of shapes and sizes (Fig. 5.9).
- **External shoe modifications**. This modifies the outside of the shoe, such as a rocker bottom sole modification, or by adding shock-absorbing or stabilizing materials to the shoe (Fig. 5.10).
- **Orthosis(es) or Inserts**. An orthosis is a removable insole that provides pressure relief and shock absorption to the foot. It can be a pre-made or custom-made (from a cast model of the foot) insert and is commonly prescribed for diabetic patients, including a special total contact orthosis, which offers a high level of comfort and pressure relief (Fig. 5.11).
- **Custom-made shoes**. Used when severe deformities are present. It is constructed after a cast model of the patient's foot is made. With extensive modifications of in-depth shoes, even the most severe deformities can usually be accommodated (Fig. 5.12a, b).

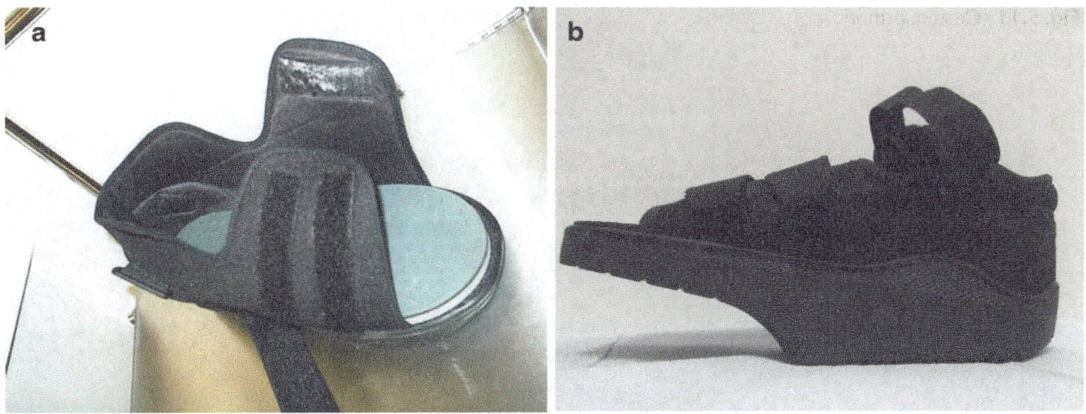

Fig. 5.8 (**a**, **b**) Footwear: (**a**) Post-Op (**b**) Forefoot Unloader Post-Op Shoe

Fig. 5.9 Footwear: in-depth shoe with custom orthotic

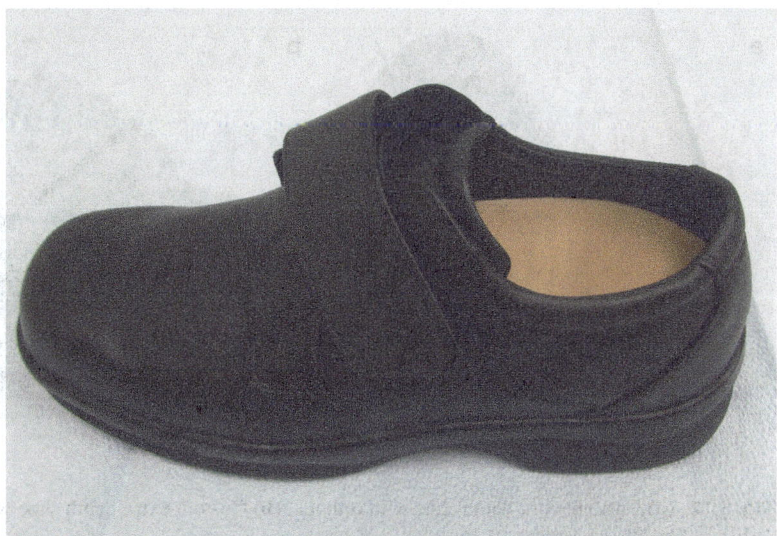

Fig. 5.10 Rocker bottom sole modification

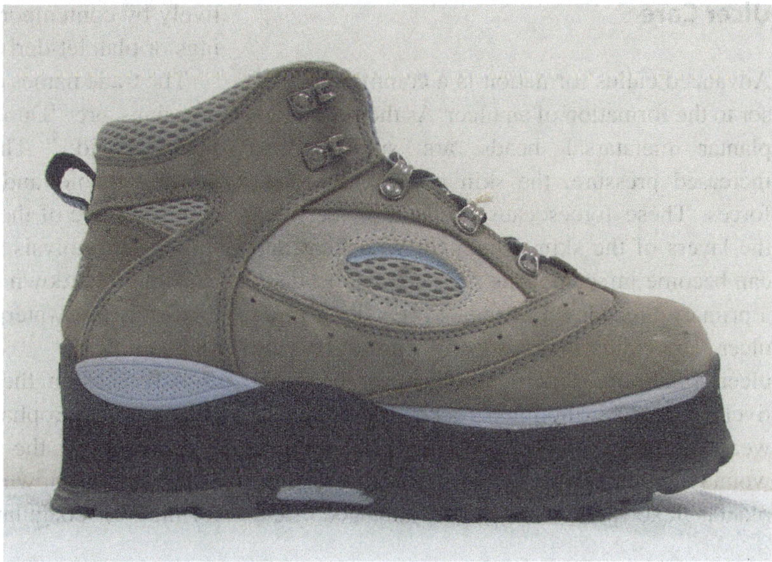

Fig. 5.11 Custom orthotic

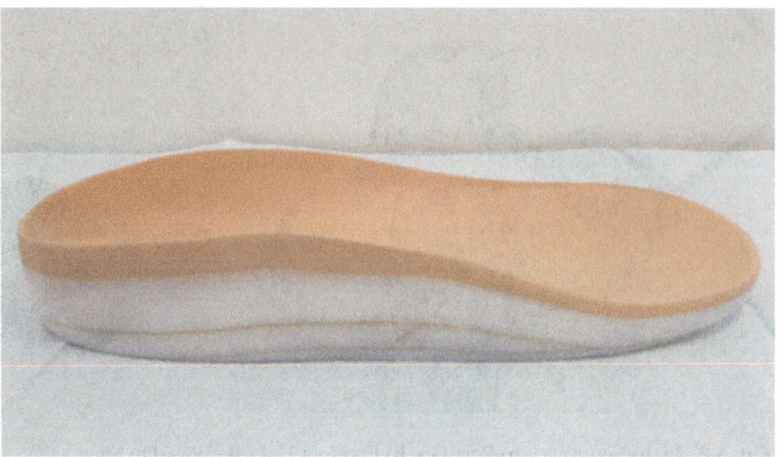

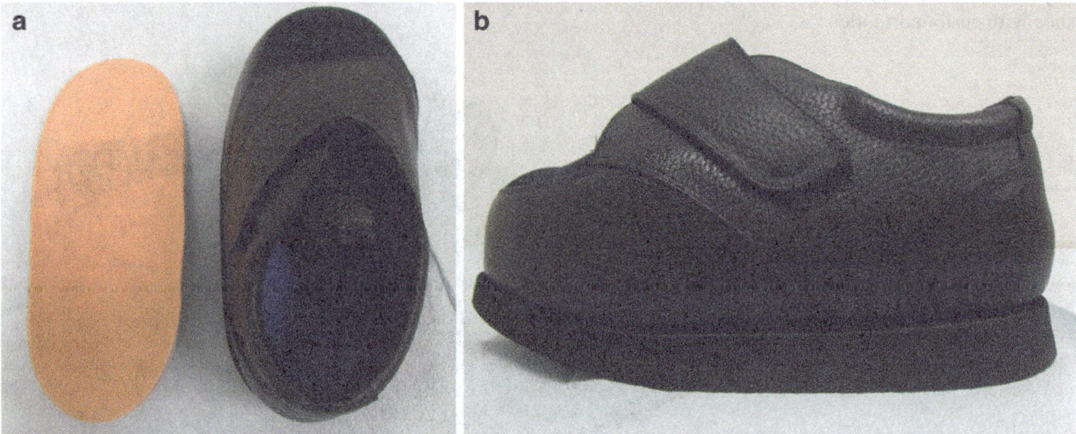

Fig. 5.12 (**a**) Custom extra-depth shoe with orthotic. (**b**) Custom extra-depth shoe with rocker bottom sole

Ulcer Care

Advanced callus formation is a common precursor to the formation of an ulcer. As the prominent plantar metatarsal heads are subjected to increased pressure, the skin experiences shear forces. These forces cause separation between the layers of the skin, which fill with fluid and can become infected. This pressure also leads to a primary breakdown of the skin resulting in an ulcer. The callus may also cover an underlying ulcer. Small, dry, superficial ulcers can be effectively treated by modified rocker bottom shoewear with pressure dissipating insoles. The wound healing of larger ulcers, superficial to plantar flexor paratenon, can be managed effec-

tively by contemporary hydrocolloid type dressings or platelet-derived wound healing factors.

The trade names of two common hydrocolloid dressings are "Duoderm®" and "3M Tegaderm Hydrocolloid®." The hydrocolloid dressing is non-breathable and adheres to the skin. The active surface of the dressing on the wound promotes fibrinolysis and angiogenesis without causing breakdown of tissue. Most hydrocolloid dressings are waterproof, allowing for washing and bathing.

Advances in the biology of wound healing show that macrophages and platelets are the primary cells in the repair process of wounds. Platelets are known for their role in hemostasis forming a coagulant surface which leads to thrombin generation and fibrin formation. A commercial topical platelet derived grown factor approved by the FDA to treat diabetic foot and leg ulcers is "Regranex®."

Antibiotic ointments and topical medications do little to stimulate granulation tissue. As ulcers superficial to flexor tendon paratenon get larger, the dressings tend to become more bulky and complicated for the patient to apply for themselves [3]. At this point Total Contact cast application is recommended. If the ulcer reveals direct communication to bone, one can be suspicious for the presence of osteomyelitis. This may warrant a more aggressive treatment, including surgical debridement and antibiotic control, prior to total contact cast treatment.

Total Contact Casting

Currently total contact casting remains the gold standard for the treatment of diabetic foot ulceration. Conventional short leg cast application can be used successfully to heal neuropathic ulcers [16], but the cast padding may slip in a short time and, with associated pistoning of the foot and ankle inside the cast, may cause the ulcer to progress. The minimal use of cast padding during the application of a total contact cast allows for more precise contouring of the cast mold, which reduces vertical pressures and soft tissue shear forces. The practical problems with total contact casts are fluid shifts, associated with edema, obesity and poor balance. The contraindications to total contact casting include deep infection, extensive drainage from the ulcer, poor skin about the entire foot, advanced arterial insufficiency, and poor patient compliance [17].

The benefits of the total contact cast are its ability to increase the weight-bearing surface area and reduce pressure by distributing it over a larger area. The immobilization can reduce edema and improve circulation, which enhances the healing of the ulcer. The time required to heal ulcers is largely correlated with the ulcer size. Studies routinely show healing of ulcers from 70 to 90 % of cases in one to six weeks [18]. Recurrent ulceration is known to be the most common complication of total contact casting, occurring in up to 40 % of patients within the first 2 years of treatment [19, 20]. The technique is labor intensive and requires that the cast be changed every 1–2 weeks. The cast allows for weight-bearing during the healing period of the ulcer.

Application of the total contact cast may be performed with the patient in either the supine or prone position with the ankle always in a neutral position.

The goal of the cast is to achieve an intimate fit to the foot and leg by safely padding all bony prominences and subsequently performing meticulous contouring of the foot, ankle, and leg using plaster of Paris. To begin, apply gauze or lambs wool in between toes to prevent maceration. The ulcer is covered with a sterile nonadherent dressing. Following, a single layer of stockinette from toes to knee without creases is applied covering the toes. The forefoot is covered with adherent foam padding. Felt pads are carefully applied to the tibial crest, and malleoli and secured with paper tape.

With patient lying supine or prone, ankle in neutral position, a single roll of 6″ webril followed by a thin (single roll) of 6″ plaster of Paris is applied covering the entire cast. Plaster is carefully molded to leg, ankle, and foot. A thin layer of fiberglass casting rolls is applied from the tibial tubercle to enclose the foot distally. The completed cast encloses the entire foot and leg. A rocker bottom sole may be designed using fiberglass casting rolls to allow for weight-bearing.

Technique

The following figures demonstrate a step-by-step approach used for the application of a total contact cast (see Figs. 5.13, 5.14a, b, 5.15a, b, 5.16a, b, and 5.17a, b).

Immobilization

Non-weight-bearing has historically been the principle for the initial nonoperative management of the Charcot foot and ankle [10, 12, 15].

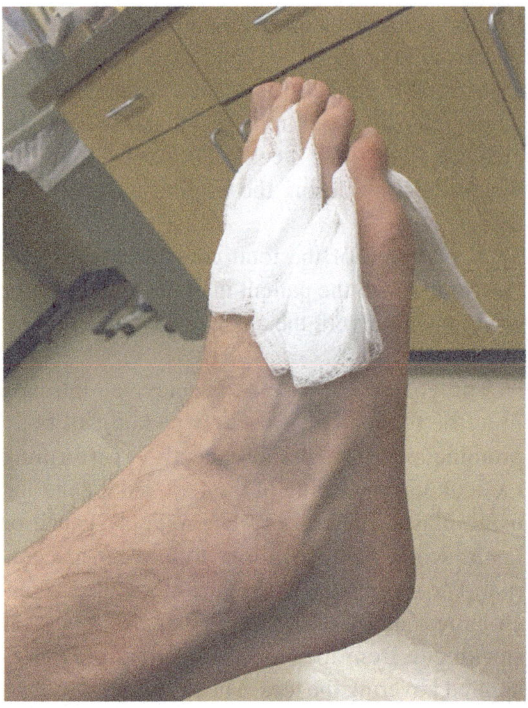

Fig. 5.13 Gauze or lambs wool is applied in between toes to prevent maceration

In the acute stage (Eichenholtz stage I), the goal is to control swelling, provide bony stability, protect soft tissues, and maintain even distribution of weight-bearing surfaces of the foot. In the author's opinion, immediate swelling from a stable, closed fracture of the ankle or midfoot, or well-aligned dislocations of the hindfoot, midtarsal, or tarsometatarsal joints, may be best treated by a well-padded, compressive foot and ankle dressing with posterior splint, elevation, and non-weight-bearing. A displaced, unstable fracture or dislocation, requiring manipulation, is best managed by open reduction with internal fixation.

Once the swelling has resolved, a total contact cast is recommended, whether or not an ulcer is present [5, 21]. An Unna® boot and compression stocking are known to help reduce swelling but require monitoring and offer little stability to the bones and soft tissues by themself [22]. During this early stage of immobilization, other methods such as a well-padded, bivalved cast or prefabricated pneumatic walking boot have been used successfully. However, frequent patient visits are

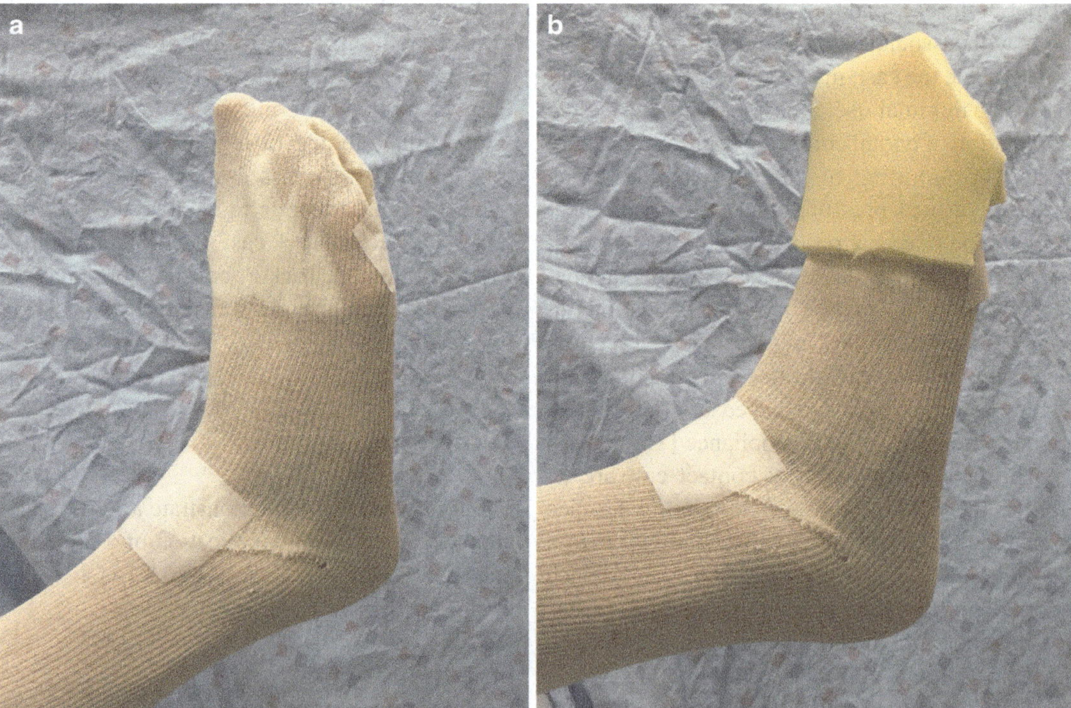

Fig. 5.14 (**a**, **b**) The ulcer is covered with a sterile nonadherent dressing. Following, a single layer of stockinette from toes to knee without creases is applied covering the toes. The forefoot is covered with adherent foam padding

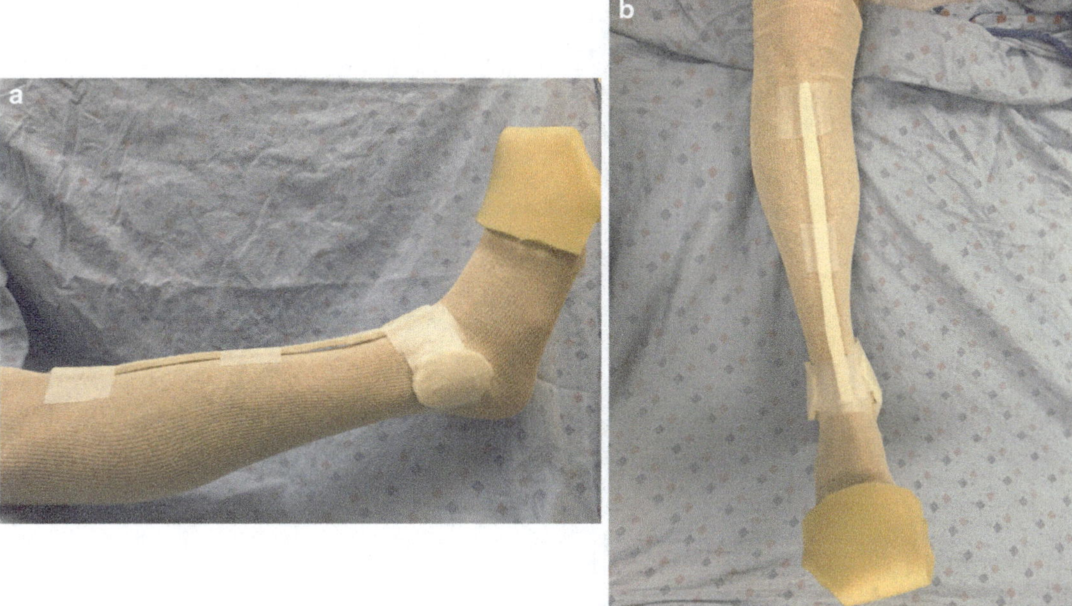

Fig. 5.15 (**a**, **b**) Felt pads are to the tibial crest, and malleoli and secured with paper tape

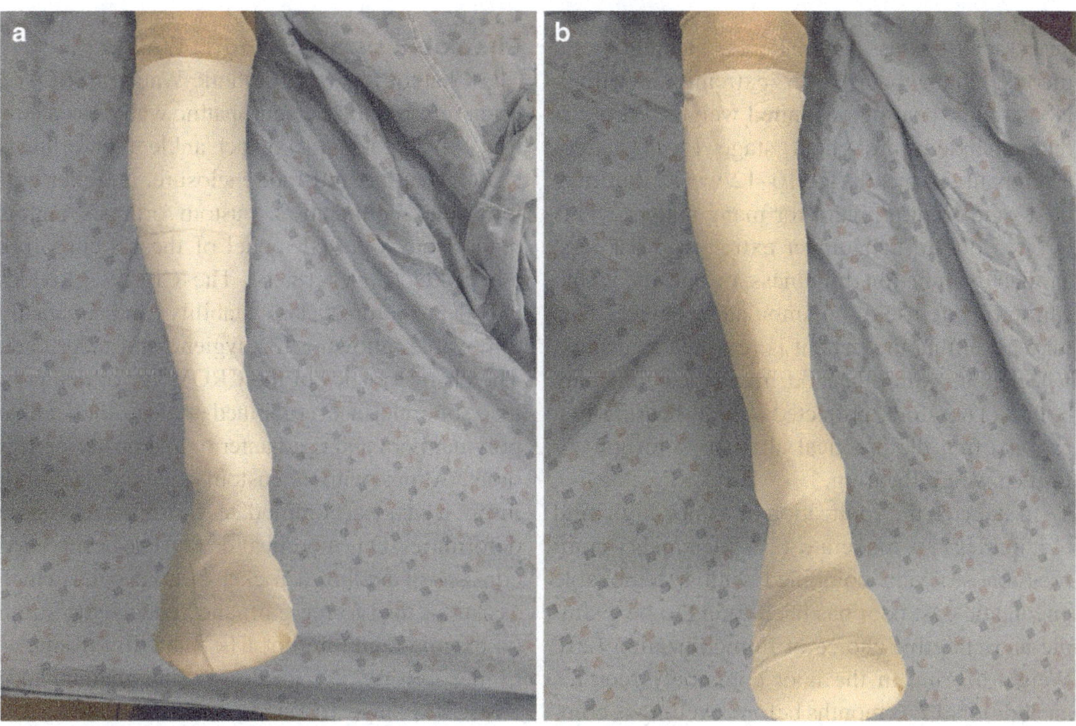

Fig. 5.16 (**a**, **b**) With patient lying supine or prone, ankle in neutral position, a single roll of 6″ webril followed by a thin (single roll) of 6″ plaster of Paris is applied covering the entire cast. Plaster is carefully molded to leg, ankle, and foot

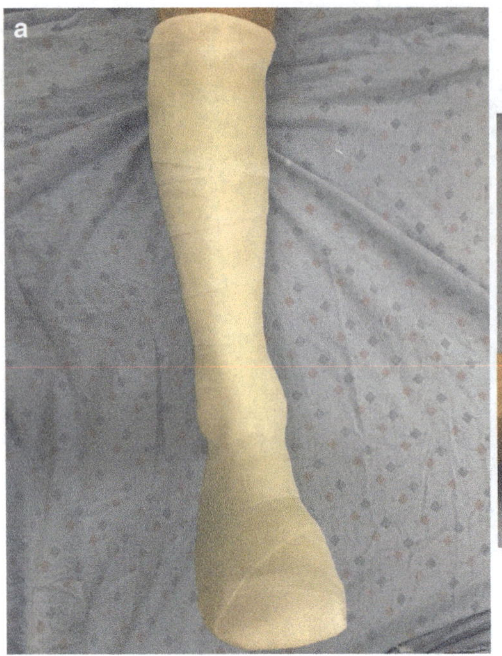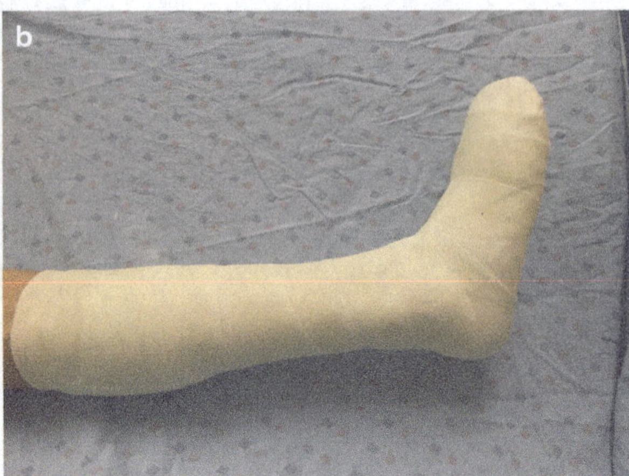

Fig. 5.17 (**a, b**) Fiberglass casting rolls are applied from the tibial tubercle to enclose the foot distally. The completed cast encloses the entire foot and leg. A rocker bottom sole may be designed using fiberglass to allow for weight-bearing

necessary to assess for malleolar ulceration and marked changes in lower extremity swelling. Non-weight-bearing or limited weight-bearing is recommended throughout stage I of Charcot arthropathy, typically for 10–12 weeks, but may be a significant problem for many patients. This is often due to their upper extremity weakness, cardiac dysfunction, blindness, or obesity, which can limit safe use of an ambulatory device. This may mean that the patient is resigned to using a wheelchair, which can be impractical in many homes. Therefore, protected weight-bearing in a cast is often the practical alternative to non- or limited weight-bearing.

In stage II, the application of a knee-high mild (15 mmHg) to moderate (20–30 mmHg) compression stocking combined with a removable pneumatic cast boot has been found to be a simple and effective choice of immobilization [23]. Weight-bearing in the boot commonly requires an additional 2–3 months before swelling is completely resolved and stage III consolidation of Charcot neuropathy is achieved.

Charcot Resistant Orthotic Walker

The Charcot Restraint Orthotic Walker (CROW), often referred to as a neuropathic walker, is a custom, bivalved, total contact ankle foot orthosis (AFO) that has full foot enclosure, a rocker bottom sole modification, custom orthosis and is made from a casted model of the patient's foot and ankle (Fig. 5.18a,b). The CROW provides excellent comfort and stability and is easily removable, allowing for hygiene and ulcer care. The characteristics of the CROW are a total contact soft interface combined with a solid ankle polymer boot and rigid anterior and posterior sections. Along with a custom total contact foot insert, it easily accommodates most foot and ankle deformities. One modification that can be included consists of adding a rocker bottom sole, which assists in heel-to-toe gait, and reduces the strain on the mid- and forefoot. The main disadvantages of the CROW are its design and maintenance costs. If a stage III patient's foot and ankle soft tissues are dry and present with an ulcer less than 2 cm, the use of a CROW is recommended. If the

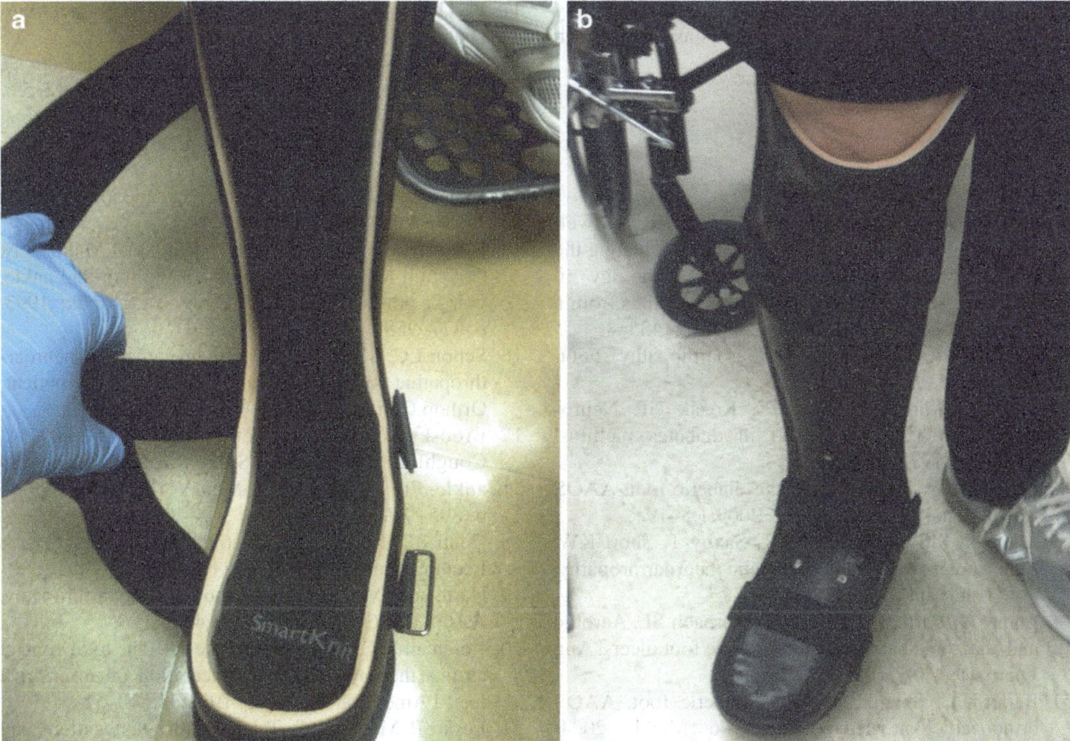

Fig. 5.18 (**a, b**) Charcot restraint orthotic walker

ulcer is moist and is greater than 2 cm in size, particularly with plantar ulceration of the midfoot and malleolar ulceration of the ankle, the decision concerning surgical debridement, ostectomy of bony prominences, and possibly reconstructive foot and ankle surgery must be considered prior to placing the patient in CROW device.

Long-Term Nonoperative Diabetic Foot and Ankle Summary

Diabetic neuroarthropathy is a disabling disease to a patient and a clinical challenge for the treating physician. Often the diagnosis of acute disease is delayed, there is poor patient understanding regarding the significance of their disease process, especially during early neuropathic changes to the foot and ankle, and they may exhibit a certain indifference when it comes to seeking advice about their foot and ankle problems. The use of nonoperative diabetic foot care requires relatively high maintenance from the physician to orchestrate a management team that should include internal medicine, used to manage their diabetes and associated comorbidities, nursing, used to provide instructions for adequate foot and antibiotic care, and routine visitation to the pedorthist to maintain adequate shoewear to allow the patient to have as normal a function and quality of life as possible. The complications associated with nonoperative care include ulceration of the skin, infection, osteomyelitis and the progression of foot deformity associated with diabetic neuropathy [24]. However, nonoperative management with the use of modalities such as the total contact cast and long-term CROW bracing and an AFO has shown to be effective for patient care in up to 75 % of patients initially presenting with stage I and II disease. Because reconstructive surgery is challenging and is not often recommended, unless well planned by an experienced surgeon, the use of nonoperative care should be considered for all patients.

Acknowledgment The author wishes to gratefully acknowledge Luke Brewer, CPO, for his assistance with images provided for this chapter.

References

1. Lavery LA, Armstrong DG, Wunderlich RP, Tredwell J, Boulton AJ. Diabetic foot syndrome: evaluating the prevalence and incidence of foot pathology in Mexican-Americans and non-Hispanic whites from a diabetic cohort. Diabetes Care. 2003;26:1435–8.
2. Marks RM, Myerson MS. Neuroarthopathy. Foot. 1995;5:185–93.
3. Sinha S, Munichoodappa CS, Kozak GP. Neuro-arthropathy (Charcot joints) in diabetes mellitus. Medicine. 1972;51:191–210.
4. Brodsky JW. Evaluation of the diabetic foot. AAOS Instructional Course Lectures. 2009;1:5–19.
5. Myerson MS, Henderson MR, Saxby T, Short KW. Management of midfoot diabetic neuroarthropathy. Foot Ankle Int. 1994;15:233–41.
6. Louie TJ, Bartlett JG, Tally FP, Gorbach SL. Aerobic and anaerobic bacteria in the diabetic foot ulcers. Ann Intern Med. 1976;85:461–3.
7. Berlet GC, Shields NN. The diabetic foot. AAOS orthopaedic knowledge update. Foot Ankle. 2004; 3(12):123–34.
8. Chantelau E, Ma XY, Hernberger S, Dohmen C, Trappe P, Babba T. Effect of medial arterial calcification of O_2 supply to exercising diabetic feet. Diabetes. 1990;39:938–41.
9. Eichenholtz SN. Charcot joints. Springfield: Charles C Thomas; 1966.
10. Trepman E, Nihal A, Pinzer MS. Charcot neuroarthropathy of the foot and ankle. Foot Ankle Int. 2005; 26(1):46–63.
11. Frykberg RG, Veves A. Diabetic foot infections. Diabetes Metab Rev. 1996;12:255–70.
12. Saltzman CL, Pedowitz WJ. Diabetic foot infections. AAOS Instructional Course Lectures. 2009;4:47–59.
13. Williams DT, Hilton JR, Harding KG. Diagnosing foot infections in diabetes. Clin Infect Dis. 2004;39(2): 583–6.
14. Johnson JTH. Neuropathic fractures and joint injuries. J Bone Joint Surg. 1967;49-A:1–30.
15. Brodsky JW. The diabetic foot. In: Mann RA, Coughlin MJ, editors. Surgery of the foot and ankle, vol. 2. 6th ed. St. Louis: Mosby-Year Book; 1993. p. 877–958.
16. Schon LC, Marks RM. The management of neuroarthropathic fracture-dislocations in the diabetic patient. Orthop Clin North Am. 1995;26:375–92.
17. Brodsky JW. The diabetic foot. In: Mann RA, Coughlin MJ, editors. Surgery of the foot and ankle. 7th ed. St. Louis: Mosby-Year Book; 1999. p. 895–969.
18. Conti SF. Total contact casting. AAOS Instr Course Lectures. Foot Ankle. 2009;11:35–50.
19. Harrelson JM. The diabetic foot: Charcot arthropathy. AAOS Inst Course Lect. 1993;42:141–6.
20. Coleman WC, Brand PW, Birke JA. The total contact cast: a therapy for plantar ulceration on insensitive feet. J Amer Podiatr Assoc. 1984;74:548–52.
21. Lesko P, Maurer RC. Talonavicular dislocations and midfoot arthropathy in neuropathic diabetic feet. Clin Orthop. 1989;240:226–31.
22. Conti SF. Total contact casting. AAOS Instr Course Lect. 1999;48:305–15.
23. Helm PA, Walker SC, Pullium GF. Total contact casting in diabetic patients with neuropathic foot ulcerations. Arch Phys Med Rehabil. 1991;72:967–70.
24. Huband MS, Carr JB. A simplified method of total contact casting for diabetic foot ulcers. Contemp Orthop. 1993;26(2):143–7.

Michael S. Pinzur

Diabetic foot ulcers and infections are the precursors to over 65,000 lower extremity amputations performed yearly in the United States. The United States Centers for Disease Control estimates that the total cost to our society, in both direct medical and indirect costs, is over $174 billion annually [1]. In addition to consuming a great deal of medical resources, the negative effect, on health-related quality of life, appears to be similar to that of a major lower extremity amputation [2–5].

The clinical presentation of diabetic individuals with a foot infection generally includes an open wound(s) and clinical signs of sepsis. A careful examination should be performed in patients without obvious open wounds, as an infected ingrown toenail or skin cracks between the toes can serve as the portals for entry of the bacteria that initiate infection. Erythema, warmth, and swelling in the absence of a wound or clinical signs of sepsis, should alert the clinician to the possibility of Charcot Foot arthropathy as an alternative diagnosis. Many patients have unneeded surgical biopsies and contamination of noninfected inflammatory bone when Charcot Foot arthropathy is incorrectly diagnosed as infection [6].

M.S. Pinzur, M.D. (⊠)
Department of Orthopaedic Surgery, Loyola
University Health System, 2160 South First Avenue,
Maywood, IL 60153, USA
e-mail: mpinzu1@lumc.edu

Risk Factors/Pathophysiology of Diabetic Foot Ulcers and Infection

The most important risk factor, for individuals who are *at-risk* for the development of diabetes-associated foot ulcers, foot infection, or Charcot Foot arthropathy, is peripheral neuropathy. Almost half of diagnosed diabetics have electrical evidence of peripheral neuropathy. However, insensitivity to 10 g of pressure, applied with the Semmes-Weinstein 5.07 monofilament, is the clinical threshold that identifies an eightfold increase for the likelihood of developing diabetic foot-associated morbidity [5, 7, 8] (Fig. 6.1). This loss of protective sensation is present in one of four adult diabetics. The presence of peripheral neuropathy appears to be significantly more predictive for the development of diabetic foot-associated morbidity than the presence of peripheral vascular disease as defined by the absence of palpable pedal pulses [5, 7–9].

Most physicians understand and accept the role of loss of protective sensation. What they do not appreciate is the concomitant motor and vasomotor consequences of peripheral neuropathy. The neuropathy affects small nerves, i.e., small muscles, before affecting larger muscles, leading to a motor imbalance between the stronger plantar flexors and the

© Springer International Publishing Switzerland 2016
D. Herscovici, Jr. (ed.), *The Surgical Management of the Diabetic Foot and Ankle*,
DOI 10.1007/978-3-319-27623-6_6

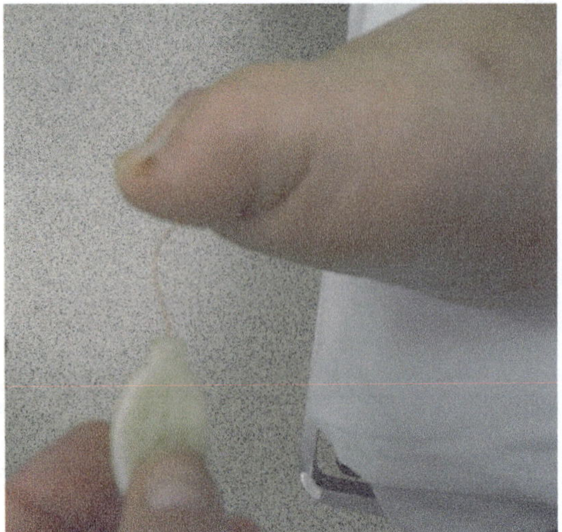

Fig. 6.1 The Semmes-Weinstein 5.07 (10 g) monofilament imparts ten grams of pressure when applied to the pulp of the toes. This amount of pressure has been demonstrated to be the clinical threshold of peripheral neuropathy designating patients *at* risk for developing diabetes-associated foot morbidity <6,14,16>

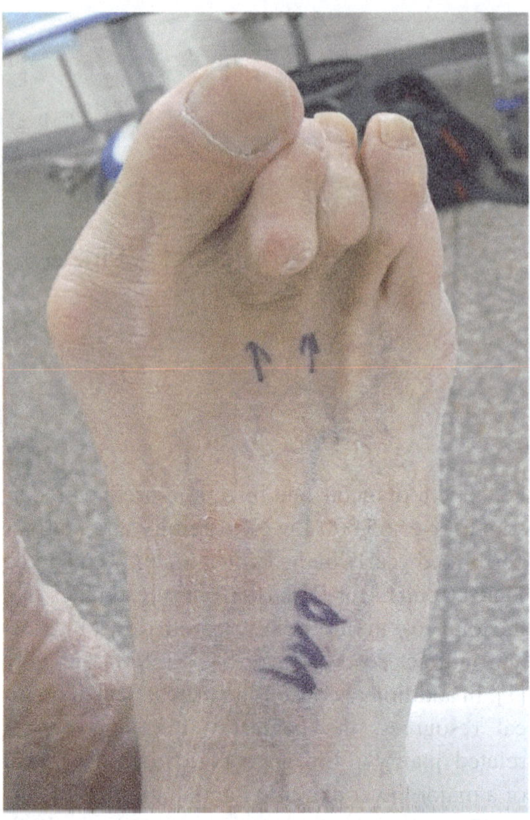

Fig. 6.2 Example of diabetic foot with hallux valgus and hammertoes. Diabetic patients develop foot ulcers from shearing forces applied to skin overlying bony deformities. The most common locations for the development of diabetic foot ulcers are under the metatarsal heads, overlying hammertoe or hallux valgus deformity or under the heel

weaker dorsiflexors. This can lead to tissue breakdown and usually occurs due to shearing forces over bony prominences. This results in foot wounds that occur medially with a hallux valgus deformity, over the dorsal prominence or distal tip abnormality associated with hammertoes or clawtoes, over prominent plantar metatarsal heads, with an "uncovered" talar head that is associated with adult-acquired flatfoot, or in bony deformities associated with Charcot Foot arthropathy (Fig. 6.2). The vasomotor component of peripheral neuropathy leads to venous swelling, increasing the potential for tissue breakdown due to increased pressure or shear [8, 10].

Other key risk factors associated with the development of ulcers or infections include: (1) absent dorsalis pedis and posterior tibial arterial pulses, (2) one absent pedal pulse and three advanced trophic skin changes, including decreased hair growth, abnormal toe nails, discoloration, or atrophy of the skin, (3) history of claudication with walking, (4) venous insufficiency, especially in morbidly obese patients, (5) nontraumatic partial or whole foot amputation, (6) presence or history of a foot ulcer and (7)

bony deformity including hammertoes, clawtoes or severe hallux valgus (Fig. 6.2). Systemic risk factors consist of morbid obesity, poor diabetic control as measured by Hemoglobin A1C values >8 %, clinical immune deficiency, or the immune deficiency associated with longstanding diabetes [7–9, 11]. The relative grading of risk factors can be appreciated on a spectrum and is dependent on a variety of clinical findings.

Clinicians are often lulled into thinking that these individuals develop infections or ulcers due to poor health choices, because they are in denial, or because they are noncompliant. In actuality, diabetic patients often have cognitive and judgment deficits, secondary to their central neuropathy. A constant re-enforcement of foot care guidelines is necessary to avoid preventable

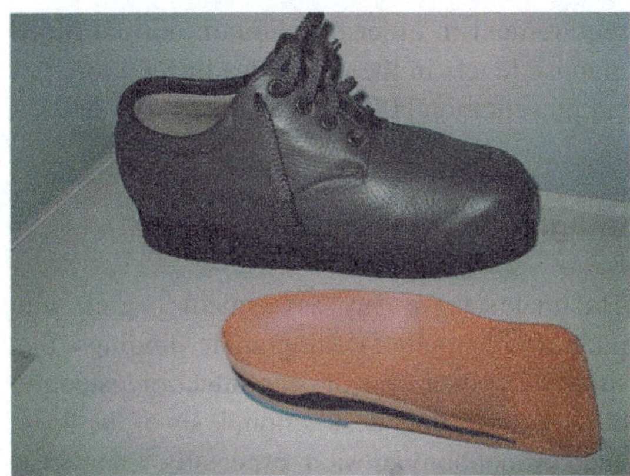

Fig. 6.3 Commercially available therapeutic footwear. The shoes are constructed with oxford style to accommodate swelling, inlay-depth to accommodate foot orthoses and have a high toe box to accommodate forefoot deformities. The leather is soft and the soles are cushioned to absorb shock at impact. The custom accommodative foot orthoses dissipate weight-bearing forces over an enlarged surface area

foot morbidity, due to their central neurologic-associated poor judgment. In addition, therapeutic footwear is an essential component of preventive care, especially for those individuals presenting with an inadequate protective plantar soft-tissue envelope, prominent metatarsal heads, bony deformity or hammertoes [5, 7, 8] (Fig. 6.3). Surgical correction of these deformities can be avoided when accommodative therapeutic footwear is utilized.

Evaluation of Diabetic Foot Infections

Clinical Presentation and Physical Examination

Diabetic foot infections typically develop within preexisting wounds in diabetics with peripheral neuropathy. The wounds can be neuropathic, ischemic, secondary to venous disease or traumatic in origin. Wounds inevitably become colonized by multiple bacteria. Superficial swab cultures should be avoided, as the results are often misleading. Wounds present for greater than 30 days are more likely to transition from colonized to infected. Controversy exists whether the virulence of the colonizing bacteria, the

impaired immune defense of the host or a combination of these factors allow progression from colonization to clinical infection, tissue destruction, bacteremia, and systemic sepsis.

Historically, patients with infection will often report a feeling of malaise, describe increasing blood glucose levels or an increased insulin need, in order to maintain normal glucose levels, which is not common in those with Charcot foot arthropathy. On clinical presentation, the infected diabetic foot wound is characterized by swelling of the foot and involved leg, warmth, erythema surrounding the wound(s), pain and tenderness. The transition from a colonized to an infected wound is generally characterized by a change in the character of the drainage from serous and clear to purulent and malodorous. In contrast, erythema, warmth, and swelling, in the absence of a wound, should alert the clinician to the possibility of Charcot foot arthropathy as an alternative diagnosis. The erythema is frequently decreased with elevation in Charcot Foot arthropathy, which is not the case for infection [12]. In addition, patients with Charcot arthropathy will often remember an incident of trauma, often trivial, just prior to the onset of swelling. Pain can be present with either condition (See Appendix, Table 1).

The "probe-to-bone" test should be performed on every diabetic foot wound (Fig. 6.4). When the applicator or culture swab directly contacts bone, there is a very high probability that the bone is infected. To the contrary, a negative "probe-to-bone" test should not give the examiner confidence to suggest that the bone is not infected [8, 9, 11, 13]. Superficial swab cultures, while tempting, should be avoided due to the presence of contaminants. Empiric treatment with a first generation cephalosporin can be initiated pending obtaining tissue following a surgical preparation of the wound.

A careful assessment for both arterial and venous disease is also essential. Noninvasive vascular laboratory assessment is advised whenever the dorsalis pedis and posterior tibial pulses are not fully normal (Fig. 6.5). In addition, patients should also be assessed for any venous insufficiency. This is a known risk factor for the development of a diabetic foot infection, especially in

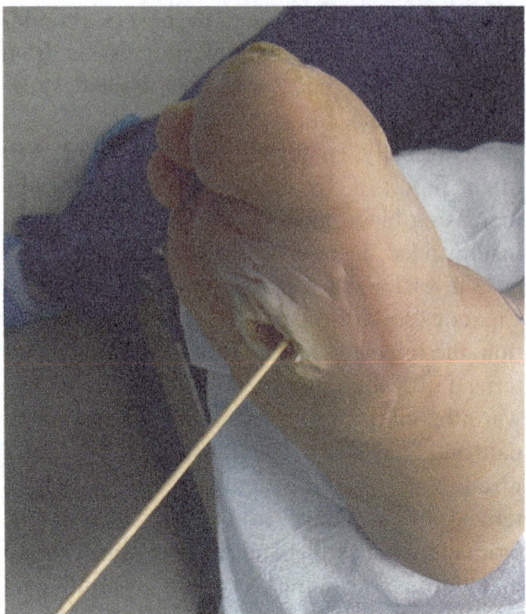

Fig. 6.4 The *probe-to-bone* test is a valuable clinical test. Every foot wound or ulcer should be probed with an applicator stick or culturette. If the applicator tip, i.e., probe, contacts the bone, there is a high likelihood for the presence of bony infection. A negative test is <u>not</u> predictive of absence of infection

morbidly obese patients, and can lead to chronic swelling of dependant lower extremities. Swollen tissues are less tolerant to the shear forces that initiate diabetic foot ulcers, making affected individuals more prone to develop ulcers and deep infection.

Laboratory Evaluation

The initial laboratory assessment of a suspected foot infection should start with a complete blood cell count (CBC). A leukocytosis (with a left-shifted differential) along with elevated erythrocyte sedimentation rate (ESR) and C-reactive protein (CRP) levels support the clinical diagnosis of infection. However, this is not always the case, due to the immunodeficiency and dysfunction of circulating white blood cells observed in this patient population. A valuable observation, as previously stated, is that patients with infection frequently describe increasing blood glucose levels or an increasing insulin

requirement in order to maintain normal blood glucose levels in the period leading up to clinical presentation [14, 15].

Imaging Studies

The mainstay of any assessment begins with plain radiography. Radiographic findings that support the diagnosis of deep infection/osteomyelitis include bony destruction, lysis of the bone, and cortical bony erosion, especially when these findings are in direct contact with a wound. The mere presence of osteopenia and small lytic areas that do not violate bony cortices may simply be suggestive of the osteoporosis associated with disuse as opposed to infection [16].

Magnetic Resonance Imaging (MRI) is helpful, especially a when soft-tissue abscess is suspected. Bony destruction is most suggestive of abscess/infection when it is associated with an open wound. Bony destruction without infection or abscess formation is often observed in patients with active Charcot Foot arthropathy [16–19]. Gadolinium is not necessary to make the diagnosis [20]. Nuclear medicine scans, especially labeled leukocyte scans, have demonstrated sensitivity for an infection, but unfortunately, are not very specific [21].

Vascular Assessment

Lower extremity amputations, in the diabetic patient, are generally classified into those resulting from infection and those due to peripheral arterial disease. While the rate of lower extremity amputations, secondary to infection, has not changed recently, the rate of amputation due to peripheral arterial disease has dropped tenfold in the United States over the past 10 years [22]. This is likely due to the emergence of endovascular surgical techniques that allow arterial inflow surgery to be expanded distally, with less peritreatment morbidity.

All patients with calf pain at rest, exertional leg pain, (i.e., claudication), or patients with less than normal palpable dorsalis pedis or posterior

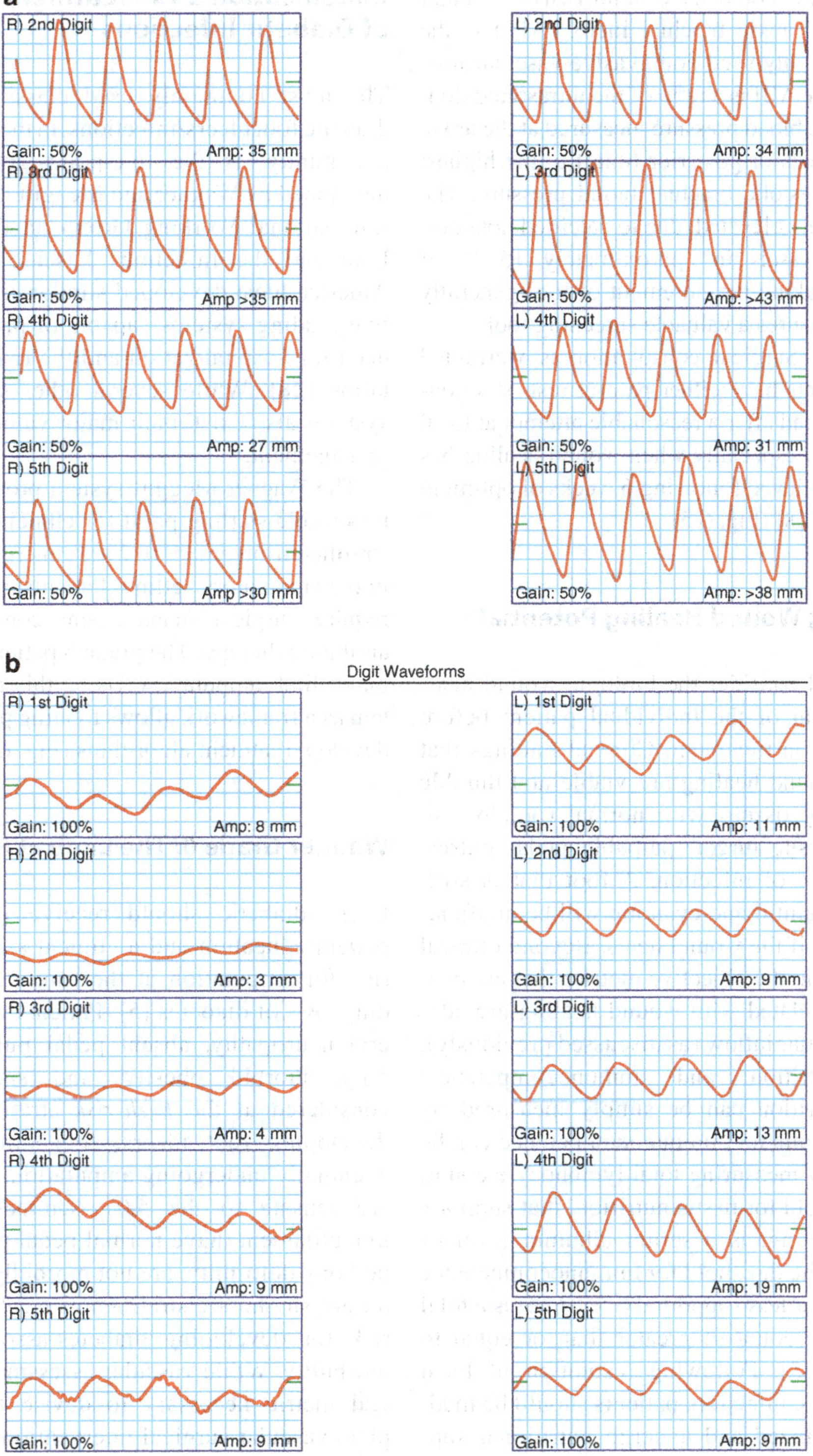

Fig. 6.5 Noninvasive vascular laboratory studies will provide arterial inflow information based on arterial pressure or estimated blood velocity at various levels

tibial pulses, should have noninvasive vascular testing. The ankle brachial index (ABI) is the most commonly used noninvasive vascular testing tool. The ABI is a ratio of the ultrasound doppler systolic blood pressure measured at the ankle (dorsalis pedis or posterior tibial) to the highest measured systolic brachial blood pressure. The ABI is falsely elevated, due to calcified noncompressible vessels in approximately 15 % of patients, making measurement of toe (generally hallux) pressures a valuable screening tool.

Vascular Surgical consultation is warranted when patients have either pain at rest or a nonhealing wound after a reasonable attempt at local wound care, especially when wound healing has not been achieved following 6 weeks of optimum wound care [8] (Fig. 6.5).

Assessing Wound Healing Potential

One should consider the biologic wound healing potential of the individual patient before embarking on treatment. Clinical findings that support wound healing are viable and durable surrounding tissues with normal (or close to normal) tissue turgor, palpable pedal pulses, and absence of infection. A foot that is stiff, atrophic, painful and cyanotic will be nonfunctional even if the wound heals. Beyond clinical examination, the objective metrics that are positively correlated with wound healing are adequate vascular inflow (as discussed previously), tissue nutrition, and immunocompetence. Tissue nutrition can be simply measured by serum albumin and immunocompetence can be assessed by measuring total lymphocyte count. The threshold for tissue nutrition, that supports wound healing, is a serum albumin level of 3.0 g/dL. The threshold for immunocompetence (although far less supported over time) is a total lymphocyte count of greater than or equal to 1500 [23–25]. Following resolution of local and systemic infection, patients should be medically optimized and undergo nutritional support before performing definitive surgical reconstruction.

Classification and Treatment of Diabetic Infections

The most commonly used classification, for diabetic foot ulcers/infections, in the Orthopedic community, is the five-point grading scale developed by Wagner and Meggitt [26, 27]. The International Working Group on the Diabetic Foot and the Infectious Disease Society of America have developed similar semiquantitative grading systems capable of predicting the need for hospitalization and the risk for amputation [28]. While several other stratification systems also exist, their major value is for data management.

The Wagner-Meggitt system provides a very reasonable starting point for clinicians. Patients stratified from grades 0–2 are generally managed in the ambulatory setting. Patients graded 3 or 4 require surgical management combined with antibiotic therapy. The grade 5 patient requires a major limb amputation. Using this grading system as a framework allows treating physicians to develop treatment algorithms (Fig. 6.6).

Wagner Grade 0: The Limb at Risk

Every diabetic should receive foot-specific patient education and a clinical assessment of risk for amputation at the time of the initial diagnosis of diabetes [5]. Patients with peripheral neuropathy, absent pedal pulses, deformity, morbid obesity, and smoking are considered at the *high-risk* stratification for developing foot ulcers, foot infection, and eventually undergoing amputation. Those who are sensate to the 5.07 Semmes-Weinstein monofilament, have normal pedal pulses, have no bony deformity, are not morbidly obese and do not smoke are stratified as a relatively low risk for developing diabetes-associated foot morbidity. While vascular assessment is a crucial metric necessary to devise a treatment plan, vascular surgical intervention is not warranted until the patient has either pain at rest or a nonhealing wound. For the at-risk patient there are no practical preventive measures,

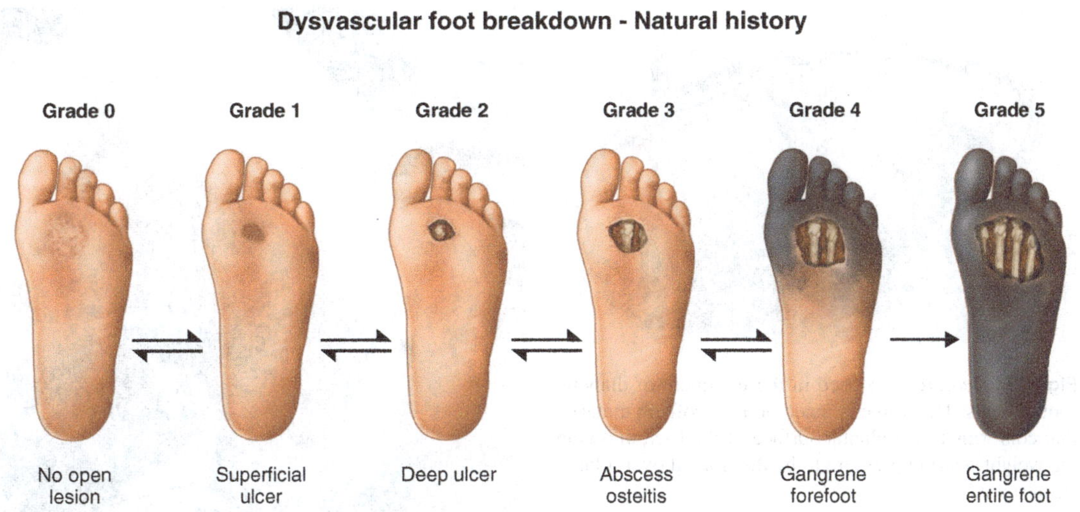

Dysvascular foot breakdown - Natural history

Fig. 6.6 Wagner-Meggitt Classification System for Diabetic Foot wounds. Reproduced, with permission from Wagner FW Jr. The dysvascular foot: a system for diagnosis and treatment. Foot Ankle 1981; 2:64–122

short of exercise, that can be employed proactively in order to avoid developing a foot infection. However, patients with peripheral neuropathy and deformity can decrease their risk for developing foot ulcers or infection with a combination of foot-specific patient education and therapeutic footwear (Fig. 6.3).

Wagner Grade I: Superficial Ulcer

Partial thickness superficial foot ulcers, in the diabetic, represent tissue breakdown due to shear or pressure of the tissues overlying bony prominences. When accompanied by surrounding cellulitis, empiric treatment with an oral first generation cephalosporin antibiotic is warranted until the localized cellulitis/erythema resolves. If the cellulitis does not resolve, once should consider the possibility of deep infection. Transitioning to a second antibiotic should be based on the results of surgically obtained tissue-infected tissue culture, generally from the involved infected bone [9].

Treatment of superficial ulcers should involve sharp debridement of surrounding non-vascular callus, in order to provide a healthy vascularized wound bed. This can be repeated at 5- to 7-day intervals, if the quality of the granulation tissue does not convert to healthy appearing tissue. If a bony deformity is responsible for the plantar ulcer, a consideration for surgical correction can be made following wound healing. Offloading, i.e., distributing the loading forces over a larger surface area, can be accomplished with a total contact cast, commercially available fracture boots or healing shoes (Fig. 6.7). Following wound healing, the patient can be transitioned to custom accommodative foot orthoses and therapeutic footwear [5, 7, 8, 11].

Wagner Grade II: Deep Ulcer/No Bony Involvement

These patients have soft-tissue involvement without extension into the underlying bone. Clinically, these ulcers do not behave like a soft-tissue abscess. Clinical, radiographic, and laboratory investigations should support the diagnosis of soft-tissue loss and/or infection without bony involvement. Cellulitis can be empirically treated with an oral first-generation cephalosporin and can be accomplished in the ambulatory clinic.

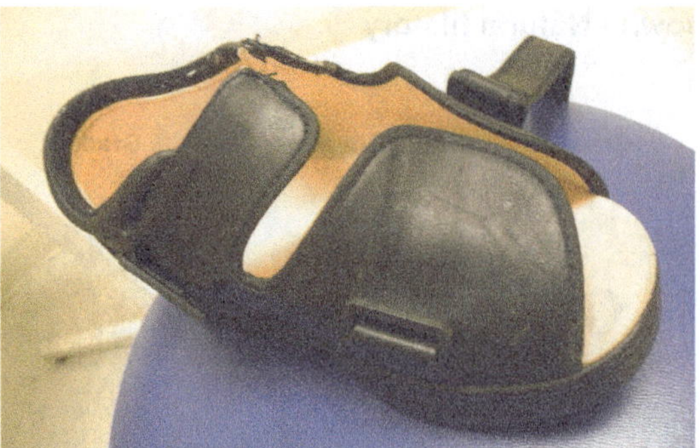

Fig. 6.7 *Healing shoe* used in the treatment of diabetic foot wounds. The insole is made of a microfoam material that conforms to the plantar surface of the foot, allowing the weight-bearing pressure to be distributed over a large surface area

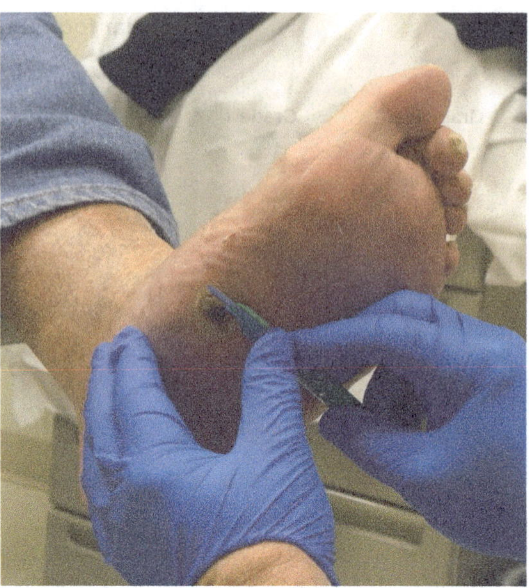

Fig. 6.8 Debridement of callus surrounding ulcer, (**a–c**) This longstanding diabetic had a clinically noninfected plantar ulcer that was receiving serial outpatient debridement. He developed the swelling, erythema, and drainage during the 48 h prior to presentation. He was afebrile and had a white blood cell count of 10,500. His blood sugars were mildly elevated from normal. (**d**) Incisions should be longitudinal and respect vascular angiosomes. (**e, f**) Photos at two weeks following surgery. He had local wound care and culture-specific antibiotic therapy. The lateral wound is healed and the plantar wound will heal by secondary intention. The surrounding dysvascular callus was debrided to allow wound healing

When debridement is necessary, it should remove all infected or devitalized tissues. The wounds are frequently surrounded by a thick build-up of callus. This callus should be sharply resected to produce a smooth contour, to promote healing (Fig. 6.8). Empiric antibiotic therapy can be changed based on deep tissue cultures, which are generally obtained at surgery following antiseptic preparation of the wound. Once the wound is converted from an infected /devitalized ulcer to one that is clean with healthy appearing granulation tissue, the management can be accomplished using a total contact cast, a commercially available fracture boot or a healing shoe, depending on the specific demands of the wound and the patient [5, 7, 8, 11] (Fig. 6.7).

Wagner Grade III: Deep Infection/ Osteitis

Once the patient has developed an abscess with bony involvement, hospitalization, and surgical debridement in the operating room are necessary [9]. Parenteral first-generation cephalosporin antibiotic can be initiated, with definitive antibiotic therapy based on surgically obtained deep tissue cultures. The risk of both medical and surgical complications is increased when operating on patients with increased blood sug-

ars, nonreversed coagulopathy, or an unstable cardiac status [4]. Therefore, preliminary medical optimization, prior to surgical debridement, should be undertaken in patients who are not critically ill.

All incisions should be longitudinal and the approach should consist of an aggressive resection of all infected bone and soft tissues. While sharp dissection is the *gold standard*, there is increasing interest in new technical methods of surgical debridement, which take advantage of pulsed ultrasound lavage. Some suggest that these devices allow for a more precise and consistent debridement of infected and dysvascular wounds, when compared with traditional surgical debridement. Incisions should also respect the tissue angiosomes [29]. Whether pulsed ultrasound or traditional sharp debridement is

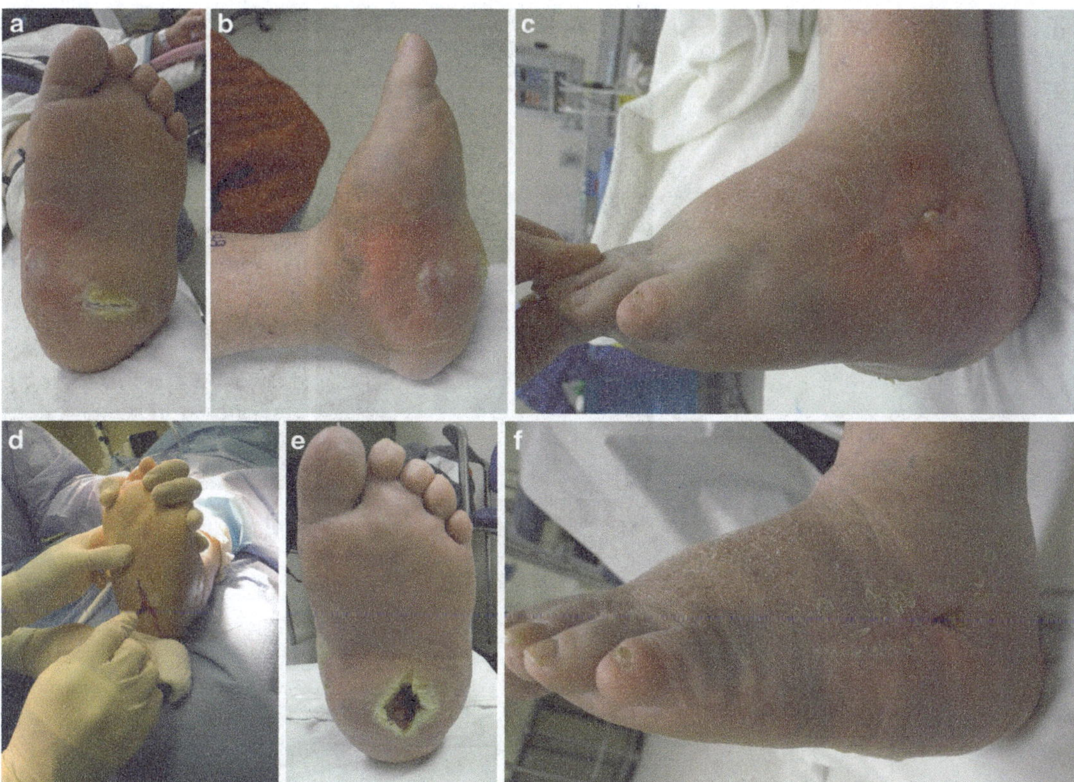

Fig. 6.9 (**a**) This longstanding diabetic had an ulcer under the first metatarsal head for several months prior to becoming acutely ill. An applicator stick probed to bone (see Fig. 6.4). (**b**) Radiographs reveal destruction of the metatarsal phalangeal joint. (**c**). The MRI demonstrates significant signal changes, but is not able to isolate the extent of the disease process. (**d**, **e**) Following thorough debridement, he is well on the way to healing and management longitudinally with therapeutic footwear

employed, the end result should be a clean, vascularized wound without any retained nonviable or infected tissues. Deep tissue cultures should guide parenteral antibiotic therapy. Current evidence would suggest a 6-week course of culture-specific intravenous antibiotic therapy and primary wound closure should be avoided [9]. The most-popular method used for the management of the open wound is a vacuum-assisted wound care (VAC) modality until a healthy noninfected wound bed is obtained.

When the infection has been resolved and a healthy wound granulation base is achieved, wound closure can be accomplished with plastic surgery flap closure, skin grafting, or healing by secondary intention. Several tissue-engineered products are currently available for obtaining expedited wound healing. None of these appear to be sufficiently durable to advise routine use. Lessons learned from the management of trauma would suggest that attempting wound closure or reconstruction within the zone of injury risks wound failure. Wound healing is an interim goal in providing a clinically plantigrade foot capable of bearing weight with commercially available therapeutic footwear (Figs. 6.9 and 6.10).

Wagner Grade III: Forefoot Amputations

The forefoot acts as a lever arm during terminal stance phase of gait. A stable foot allows the quadriceps muscle to extend the knee and propel the foot forward. Loss of length or stability within the forefoot impedes propulsion.

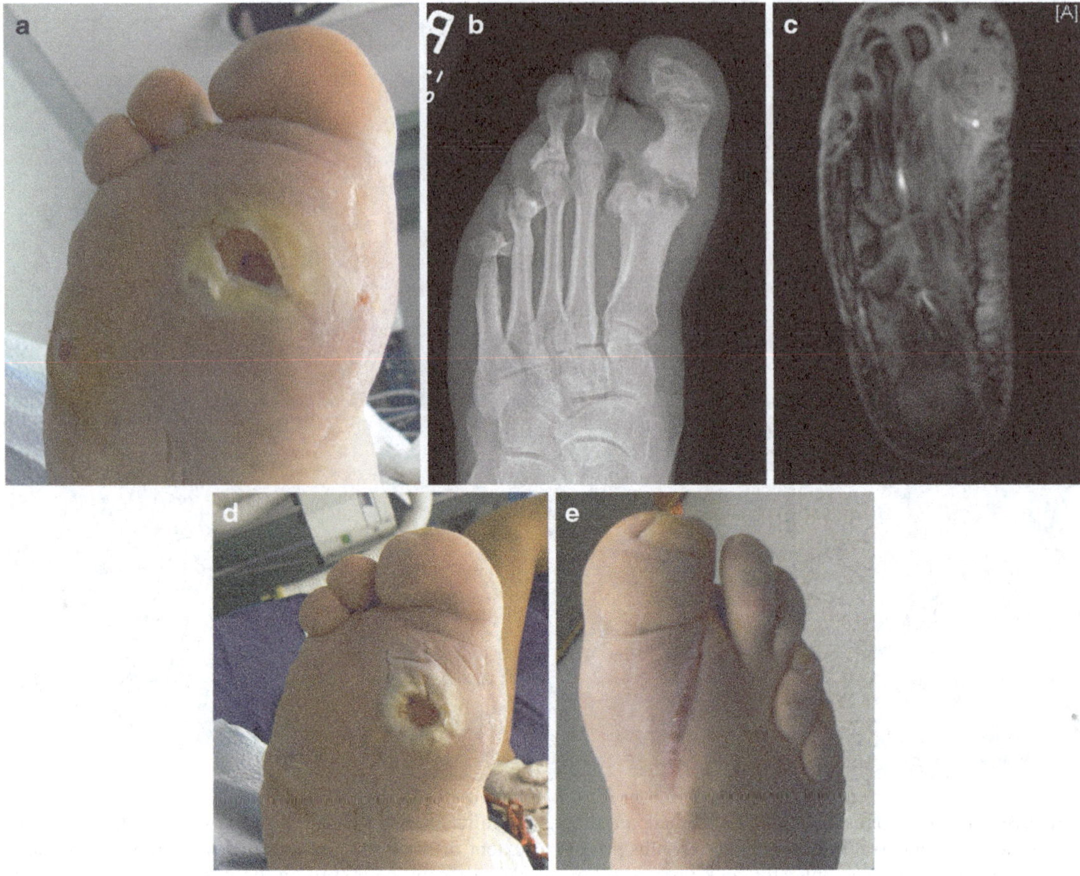

Fig. 6.10 (**a**) Osteomyelitis of the interphalangeal joint of the hallux. (**b**, **c**) The proximal metaphysis of the proximal phalanx was retained to maintain medial column stability

Attention should be directed towards maintaining length and durable plantar tissue, to retain surface area, to preserve stability, and sustain a lever arm for push-off during gait. At times resolution of an infection is best resolved with a resection of all infected or nonfunctional tissue, i.e., amputation and reconstruction with a functional residual limb. When considering an amputation one should be cognizant that skin flaps used for bony coverage are based on the availability of local viable tissue.

Hallux Amputation

A crucial component of stability of the medial column of the foot is achieved, during terminal stance phase of gait, by the action of the flexor hallucis longus and brevis tendons. Relative stability can be maintained by retaining the proximal metaphysis of the proximal phalanx, which preserves the stabilizing function of the flexor hallucis brevis. When the entire hallux and/or the distal metatarsal are resected, it disengages the hallux flexors and significantly impairs medial column stability during terminal stance phase of gait. This leads to a relatively propulsive gait pattern (Fig. 6.11).

Lesser Toe Amputation

The critical component for any lesser toe amputation is to maintain the parabola (curvature) appearance of the forefoot. Leaving prominent individual toes can lead to areas that can produce pressure concentration resulting in late tissue breakdown. When a resection of the entire second toe is performed it can lead to a severe hallux valgus deformity and tissue breakdown overlying the prominent medial eminence deformity. Retention of the proximal metaphysis of the second toe proximal phalanx can prevent this late complication (Fig. 6.12).

Metatarsal heads can be removed, when prominent, to enhance wound healing.

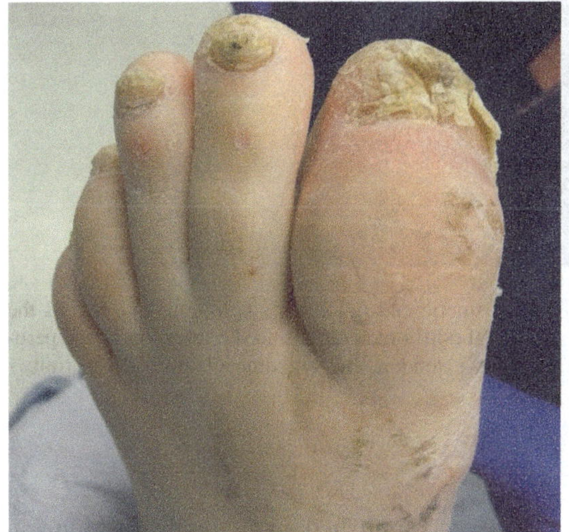

Fig. 6.11 Amputation of the entire second toe allows shoes to create a severe hallux valgus deformity with a very prominent medial eminence

Ray Resection

Resection of a single medial or lateral outer ray is easily accommodated with therapeutic footwear. When possible, the proximal metaphysics of the first metatarsal can be retained. The amputation of the metatarsal should be contoured from medial to lateral to avoid a bony prominence. Resection of the first ray leads to a relatively propulsive gait pattern due to the functional loss of the flexor hallucis longus and brevis at terminal stance. This is a reasonable option for an older, more sedentary patient, but can be very disabling in a younger patient. When an infection necessitates a resection of the entire fifth metatarsal, it often leads to a late dynamic varus deformity. This can be avoided by retaining the base of the fifth metatarsal, which preserves the muscle balancing capacity of the peroneus brevis. The contour of the retained fifth metatarsal should be from lateral to medial to again avoid a bony prominence. If late dynamic varus does occur it can be addressed with either fractional muscle lengthening of the posterior tibialis or lateral transfer of the tibialis anterior tendon [30] (Fig. 6.13). A single central ray resection is generally performed during the initial stage of the infectious debridement and is often combined with open wound management. Vacuum-assisted wound care followed by either secondary wound healing or dorsal wound skin grafting is generally required. Even a single central ray resection can

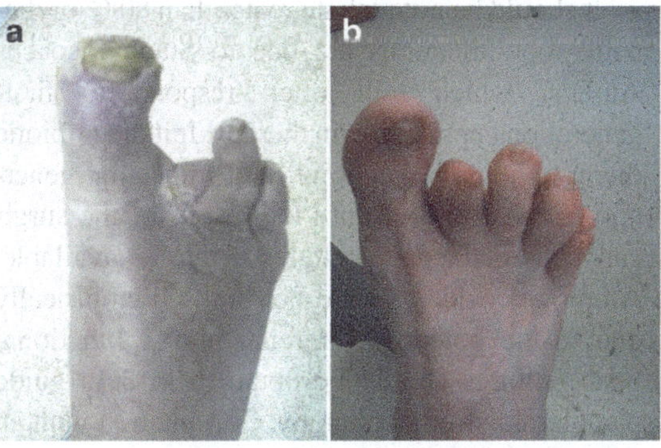
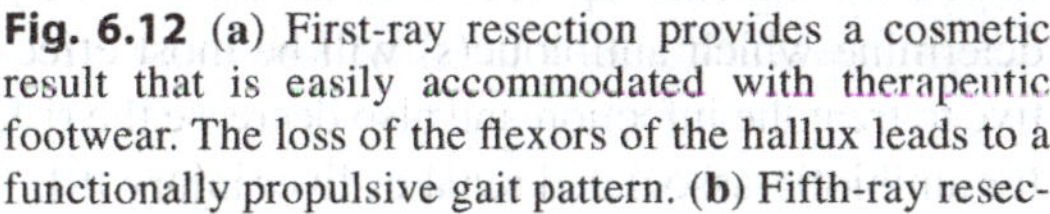
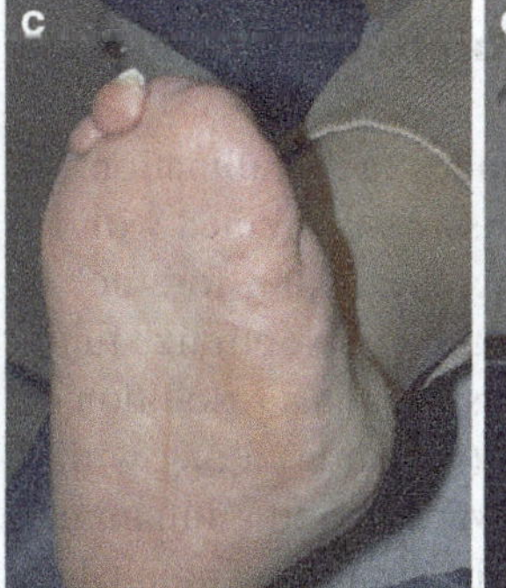
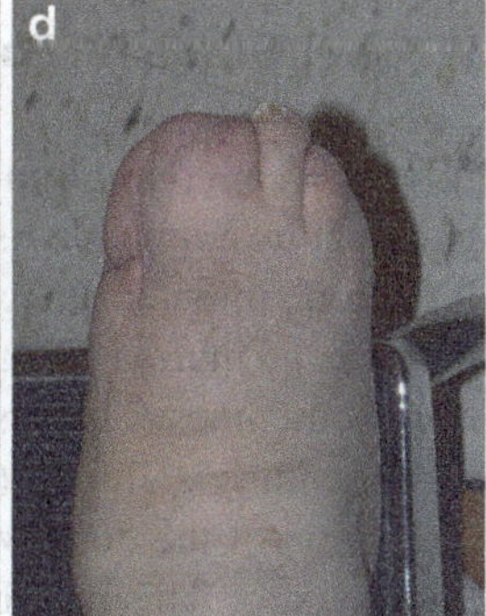

Fig. 6.12 (**a**) First-ray resection provides a cosmetic result that is easily accommodated with therapeutic footwear. The loss of the flexors of the hallux leads to a functionally propulsive gait pattern. (**b**) Fifth-ray resection is both cosmetic and functional, as long as one retains the base of the fifth metatarsal and the insertion of the peroneus brevis tendon, thus avoiding a late varus deformity

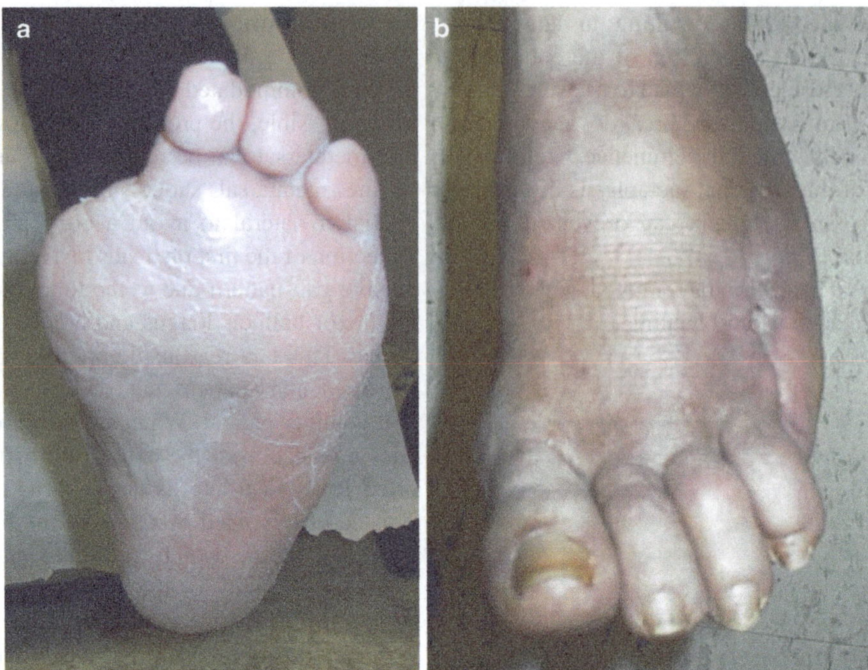

Fig. 6.13 (a) First-ray resection provides a cosmetic result that is easily accommodated with therapeutic footwear. The loss of the flexors of the hallux leads to a functionally propulsive gait pattern. b. Fifth-ray resection is both cosmetic and functional, as long as one retains the base of the fifth metatarsal and the insertion of the peroneus brevis tendon, thus avoiding a late varus deformity

lead to a challenging secondary wound closure due to the loss of structural stability. Involvement of more than one metatarsal shaft generally requires a more proximal amputation level to create a residual limb capable of bearing weight.

Wagner Grade IV: Forefoot Gangrene

Infected gangrene implies a combination of gangrenous nonviable tissues combined with an infection. Infected gangrene of the forefoot is best treated in a staged fashion to optimize functional outcomes. The first step is a resolution of the ascending cellulitis (infection) along with a correction of the downward trending inflammatory markers. This may be simply accomplished using parenteral first-generation antibiotic therapy. Beginning treatment in this manner allows clinical optimization of the patient prior to subjecting them to the risks of surgery. If this can-

not be accomplished in a timely fashion, an urgent resection of all infected tissues, combined with antibiotic therapy, is required. Resection of all gangrenous nonviable and infected tissue is necessary prior to considering any sort of reconstruction.

It should be noted that greater than 80 % of diabetic foot infections are due to Staphylococcus Aureus, which will often respond to first-generation cephalosporin therapy. Initial antibiotic therapy should be accomplished with a first-generation cephalosporin until the results of the surgically obtained cultures are available. Aminoglycosides should not be used empirically due to the potential for renal injury. Junctional bone cultures should be obtained to help guide parenteral antibiotic therapy. Consultation with an Infectious Disease specialist is advised to help determine which antibiotic(s) will be most effective to treat the infection and also decrease the risk for antibiotic-associated renal or liver injury [9].

Infected wounds are best managed with open wound therapy and/or the use of vacuum-assisted wound closure ± secondary dorsal skin grafting. The initial use of vacuum-assisted wound treatment allows an excellent method of retaining healthy tissue to be available for creation of a terminal organ of weight bearing. During treatment it is important to remember that infection depletes protein stores, often making the post-infection diabetic malnourished, i.e., protein deficient [23]. Following the resolution of clinical sepsis, attention should be directed to systemic medical optimization of diabetic and cardiopulmonary markers. Consultation with specialist from the appropriate medical disciplines is crucial in managing this highly complex, comorbid patient population.

The first goal of treatment is the resection of all infected and nonviable tissue. This task may require serial debridements at 5- to 7-day intervals. Once all infected tissue has been resected, reconstruction of the available tissue to create a terminal organ of weight-bearing is the next consideration. Therefore, the reconstruction in a patient with a Wagner grade IV wound will be, at a minimum, a Syme's ankle disarticulation. Proximal amputation should always be considered in patients where a more proximal amputation level will provide a more functional weight-bearing organ.

Midfoot Amputation

Both transmetatarsal and tarsal–metatarsal (Lisfranc) amputation levels function equally well in older patients [23]. In spite of the loss of lever arm, these levels are valuable function-sparing levels in older dysvascular patients, since they do not require a prosthesis for walking. While multiple orthotic designs have been described, these patients fare well with a simple toe-filler. In younger patients, who wish to return to heavy lifting and running, the surgeon should consider Syme's ankle disarticulation, which will allow the use of a dynamic elastic response prosthetic foot [31]. Plantar-based myocutaneous flaps are best, but dorsal skin may be necessary, depending on the available viable tissue. Distal metatarsal levels retain a more efficient lever arm, but are prone to re-

ulcerate under the ends of the retained metatarsal shafts. This can be avoided by performing the amputation at the level of the proximal metaphysis, again at the relative loss of lever arm. Retention of the peroneus brevis insertion on the base of the fifth metatarsal decreases the risk for a late varus deformity. The late development of equinus, noted with an amputation with either level, can be avoided by performing a percutaneous triple hemisection Achilles tendon lengthening or a gastrocnemius ("Strayer") muscle lengthening at the time of amputation. Postoperatively, patients are best managed with a weight-bearing short leg cast for 4 weeks following the surgery.

Hindfoot Amputation

An amputation at the transverse tarsal joint should be avoided for several reasons. These patients have a high potential for the development of a severe late equinus deformity that does not allow plantigrade weight-bearing. Rarely successful, even with a tibias anterior tendon transfer to counteract the strong equines-producing gastrocnemius, the weight-bearing platform is so small that it does not allow the use of standard footwear.

In the author's opinion, the Syme's ankle disarticulation amputation is an underutilized, function-sparing end-bearing amputation level. It can be performed in a single stage, by resecting the malleoli and metaphyseal flares of the tibia and fibula, and it retains the weight-bearing surface of the distal tibia. Heel pad migration is avoided by suturing the heel pad via drill holes to the anterior corner of the residual distal tibia (Fig. 6.14). The major contraindication to this durable amputation level is the loss of the durable fibrous septae connective tissue and overlying skin.

Wagner Grade V

The Wagner V infection implies infection combined with gangrene. This makes limb salvage virtually impossible. Limb salvage in this popu-

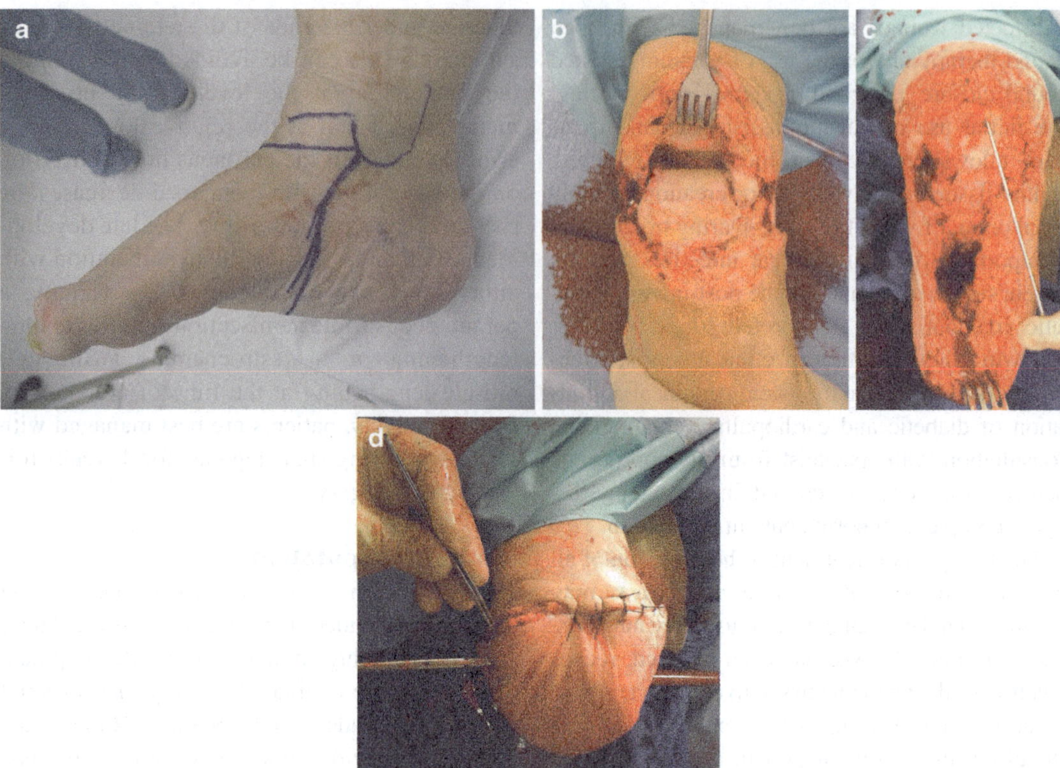

Fig. 6.14 Symes amputation performed in a one-stage surgery. (**a**) Incision. (**b**) The incision is taken directly to bone circumferentially. Care is taken to dissect from the talus and calcaneus, maintaining the blood supply to the heel pad flap, which is based on the posterior tibial artery. This photo is looking into the ankle joint during dissection. (**c**) The heel pad is below in this photo. Nonabsorbable sutures attach the heel pad to the tibia through drill holes in the anterior distal corner of the tibia. (**d**) Anterior view during wound closure

lation can only be achieved with staged resection of all infected tissue, followed by revascularization and reconstruction of a functional partial or complete foot amputation.

Treatment of Necrotizing Fasciitis and Sepsis

Necrotizing fasciitis is a life-threatening disease that requires emergent treatment. Classically, patients present with severe leukocytosis. The presence of hypotension implies imminent cardiopulmonary collapse and death. Blood sugars in the 400+ range are not uncommon. Unfortunately, the immune systems of many diabetics are over- whelmed by sepsis and patients will not be capable of mounting an immune response.

Prompt surgical resection of all infected tissue is necessary in order to avoid a full-blown sepsis and cardiopulmonary failure (Fig. 6.15). Excision of single compartment contents is adequate when the infection is confined to a single compartment. When the infection involves more than one compartment, an open amputation and a secondary closure is required. Open ankle disarticulations or a distal tibial guillotine amputation, combined with longitudinal appropriate compartment incisions, is a simple and expedient option when the purulence tracks into proximal compartments and the necrosis is confined to the foot. One should plan for the eventual

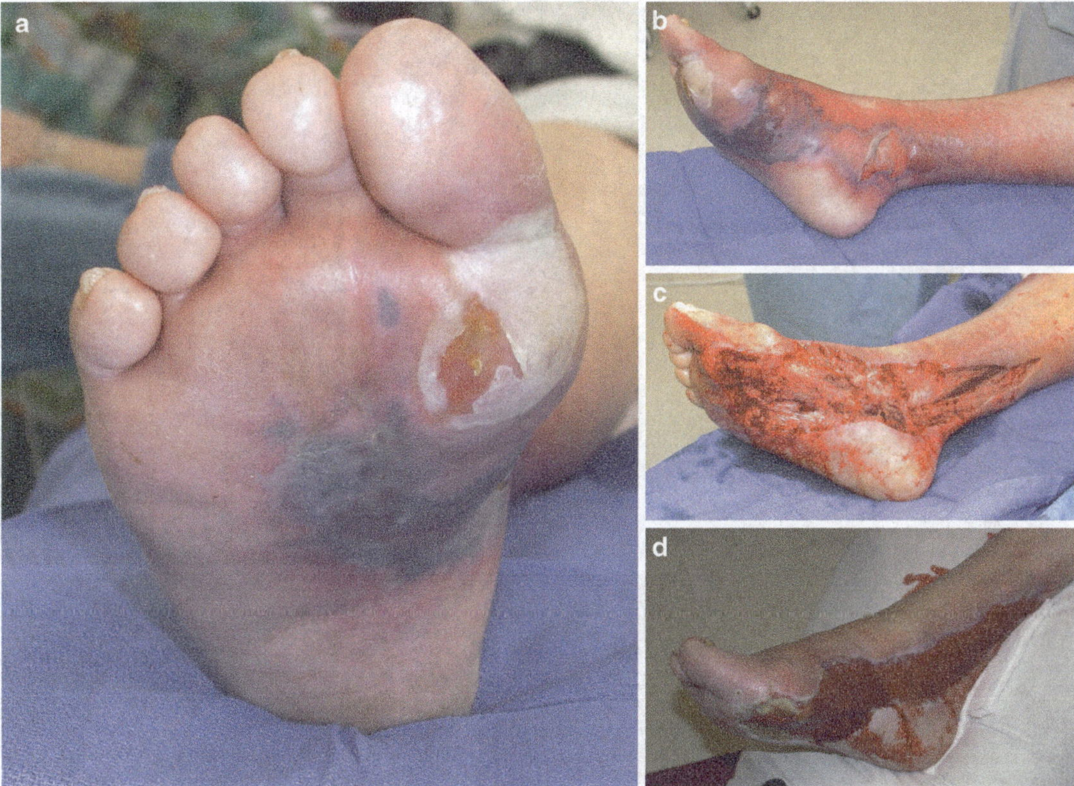

Fig. 6.15 (**a**, **b**) Long plantar flap for midfoot amputation. This durable flap provides the best protection for the residual foot longitudinally. When there is an insufficient amount of plantar tissue, a fish-mouth or increased dorsal flap is a second choice. (**c**) Appearance of the long plantar flap at follow-up

reconstructive amputation level at the time of initial surgery, by retaining any viable tissue, which can be used for the creation of an amputation flap. It should again be stressed that reconstruction, i.e., wound closure, is not accomplished until all infected, nonviable tissue has been resected, a task that occasionally takes repeated debridements.

Treatment of the Charcot Foot with Infection

Historically, the deformity occurring from diabetes-associated Charcot Foot arthropathy has been treated with accommodative bracing. Ulcers and underlying osteomyelitis, from direct pressure overlying the bony deformity, was treated with surgical debridement and localized wound care. Correction of deformity was only attempted as an alternative to amputation, when the deformity could not be accommodated with custom orthoses [32]. The current trend in management is resection of the infection, followed by correction of the bony deformity. This can either be accomplished in a staged fashion with internal fixation to maintain the correction. Most experts now recommend resection of the infection and correction of the deformity with a circular external fixator [33, 34] (Fig. 6.16).

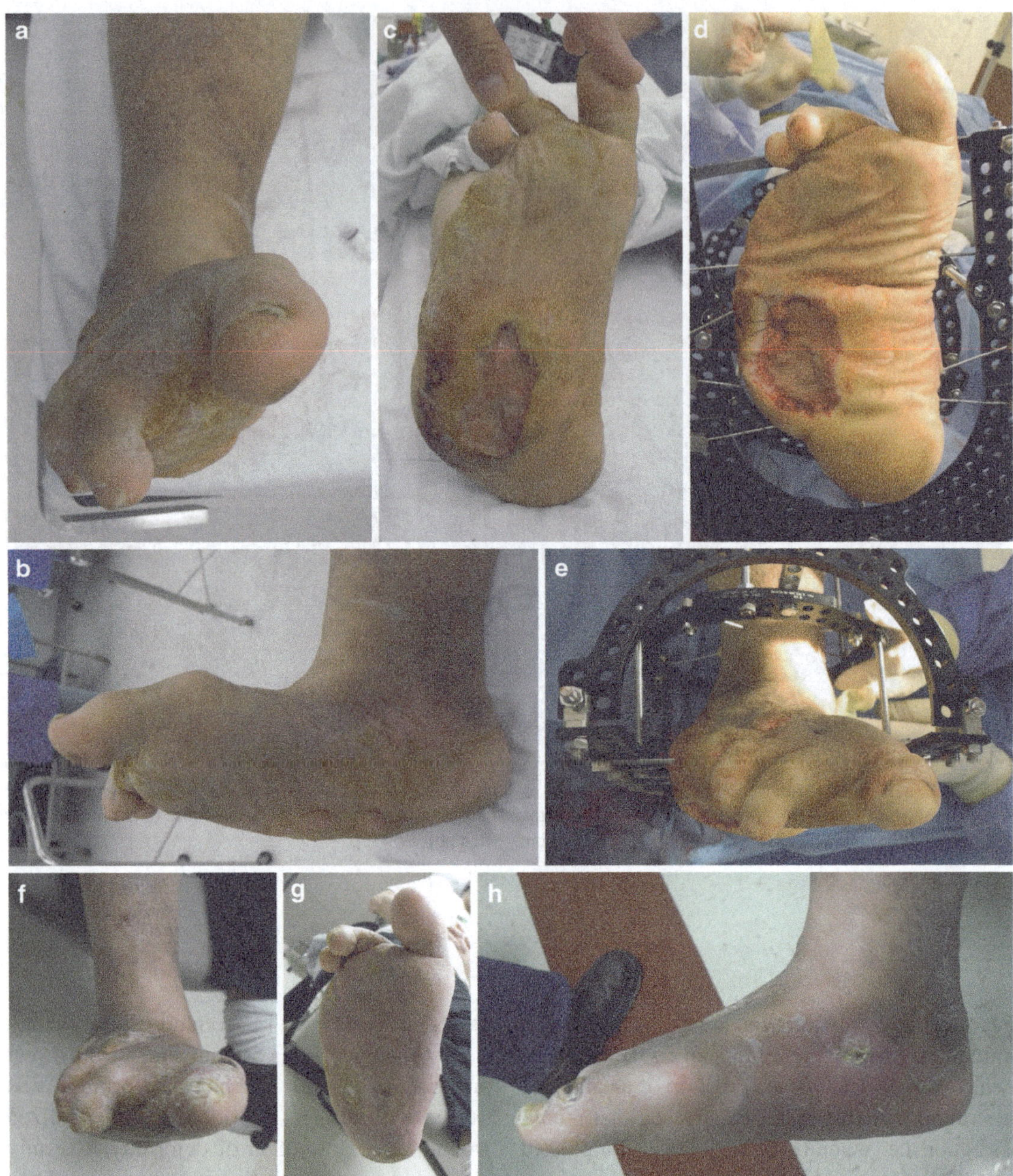

Fig. 6.16 (**a–c**) A sixty-year-old diabetic male with Charcot deformity following fifth-ray resection. Note the rotational deformity of the foot and the wound that has not resolved with treatment. (**d, e**) He underwent posterior tib-ial tendon lengthening, resection of chronic osteomyelitis underlying the wound, correction of the bony deformity, and maintenance of the correction with a static circular external fixator. (**f–h**) 1 year following surgical correction

Summary

The diabetic patient who develops foot ulcers and foot infection is complicated by having concomitant cardiac and renal disease vascular insufficiency and a significant impairment in both immunocompetence and wound healing potential. These patients are often prone to develop sepsis with rapid medical deterioration and death. When present, infections should be addressed aggressively. Resection of deep infection is required prior to a consideration of surgical reconstruction. Surgical reconstruction should be devised to create a durable terminal organ of weight-bearing that will not be prone to repeat infection and periods of morbidity.

References

1. National Diabetes Fact Sheet 2011. http://www.cdc.gov/diabetes/pubs/pdf/ndfs_2011.pdf. Accessed 16 Oct 2013.
2. Willrich A, Pinzur MS, McNeill M, Juknelis D, Lavery LA. Health related quality of life, cognitive function, and depression in diabetic patients with foot ulcer or amputation. A Pilot Study. Foot Ank Int. 2005;26:128–34.
3. Evans AE, Pinzur MS. Health-related quality of life of patients with diabetes and foot ulcers. Foot Ank Int. 2005;26:32–7.
4. Wukich DK, Lowery NJ, McMillen RL, Frykberg RG. Postoperative infection rates in foot and ankle surgery: a comparison of patients with and without diabetes mellitus. J Bone Joint Surg. 2010;92A:287–95.
5. http://ndep.nih.gov/publications/PublicationDetail.aspx?PubId=116. Accessed 12 Feb 2013.
6. Rogers LC, Frykberg RG, Armstrong DG, Boulton AJM, Edmonds M, Van Ha G, Hartemann A, Game F, Jeffcoate W, Jirkovska A, Jude E, Morbach S, Morrison W, Pinzur M, Pitocco D, Sanders L, Wukich DK, Uccioli L. The diabetic Charcot foot syndrome: a report of the joint task force on the Charcot foot by the American Diabetes Association and the American Podiatric Medical Association. Diabetes Care. 2011;34:2123–9.
7. Pinzur MS, Slovenkai MP, Trepman E. American orthopaedic foot & ankle society guidelines for diabetic foot care. Foot Ankle Int. 1999;20:695–702.
8. http://iwgdf.org/. Accessed 12 Feb 2013.
9. Lipsky BA, Berendt AR, Cornia P, Pile J, Armstrong DG, Deery HG, Embil JM, Joseph WS, Karchmer AW, LeFrock JL, Peters EJG, Pinzur MS, Senneville E. 2012 infectious diseases society of America Clinical Practice guidelines for the diagnosis and treatment of diabetic foot infections. Clin Infect Dis. 2012;54:132–73.
10. http://ndep.nih.gov/publications/PublicationDetail.aspx?PubId=116. Accessed 12 Feb 2013.
11. http://pcs.isiknowledge.com/. Accessed 12 Feb 2013.
12. Berendt AR, Lipsky B. Is this bone infected or not? Differentiating neuro-osteoarthropathy from osteomyelitis in the diabetic foot. Curr Diab Rep. 2004;4:424–9.
13. Lavery LA, Armstrong DG, Wunderlich RP, Mohler MJ, Wendel CS, Lipsky BA. Risk factors for foot infections in individuals with diabetes. Diabetes Care. 2006;29:1288–93.
14. Lipsky BA, Polis AB, Lantz KC, Norquist JM, Abramson MA. The value of a wound score for diabetic foot infections in predicting treatment outcome: a prospective analysis from the SIDESTEP trial. Wound Repair Regen. 2009;17:671–7.
15. Lipsky BA, Berendt AR, Deery HG, et al. Diagnosis and treatment of diabetic foot infections. Clin Infect Dis. 2004;39:885–910.
16. Dinh MT, Abad CL, Safdar N. Diagnostic accuracy of the physical examination and imaging tests for osteomyelitis underlying diabetic foot ulcers: meta-analysis. Clin Infect Dis. 2008;47:519–27.
17. Kapoor A, Page S, Lavalley M, Gale DR, Felson DT. Magnetic resonance imaging for diagnosing foot osteomyelitis: a meta-analysis. Arch Intern Med. 2007;167:125–32.
18. Ledermann HP, Morrison WB, Schweitzer ME. Pedal abscesses in patients suspected of having pedal osteomyelitis: analysis with MR imaging. Radiology. 2002;224:649–55.
19. Armstrong DG, Harkless LB. Outcomes of preventative care in a diabetic foot specialty clinic. J Foot Ankle Surg. 1998;37:460–6.
20. Tan PL, Teh J. MRI of the diabetic foot: differentiation of infection from neuropathic change. Br J Radiol. 2007;80:939–48.
21. Schweitzer ME, Daffner RH, Weissman BN, et al. ACR Appropriateness criteria on suspected osteomyelitis in patients with diabetes mellitus. J Am Coll Radiol. 2008;5:881–6.
22. Jing W, Geiss LS, Cheng YJ, Li YF, Gregg EW. Differential trends for ischemic and neuropathic lower extremity amputation rates, United States, 1998–2010. Roger Pecoraro Award lecture. 73rd Scientific Session. Chicago, 2013.
23. Pinzur MS, Kaminsky M, Sage R, Cronin R, Osterman H. Amputation at the middle level of the foot. J Bone Joint Surg. 1986;68:1061–4.
24. Pinzur MS. New concepts in lower-limb amputation and prosthetic management: amputation level selection and immediate post-surgical prosthetic limb fitting. In: Instructional Course Lectures, editor. The American Academy of orthopaedic surgeons, vol. 39. Park Ridge: Instructional Course Lectures; 1990. p. 361–6.
25. Pinzur MS, Stuck R, Sage R, Hunt N, Rabinovich Z. Syme's ankle disarticulation in patients with diabetes. J Bone Joint Surg. 2003;85A:1667–72.
26. Meggitt B. Surgical management of the diabetic foot. Br J Hosp Med. 1976;16:227–332.

27. Wagner Jr FW. The dysvascular foot: a system for diagnosis and treatment. Foot Ankle. 1981;2:64–122.
28. Lavery LA, Armstrong DG, Murdoch DP, Peters EJ, Lipsky BA. Validation of the infectious diseases society of America's diabetic foot infection classification system. Clin Infect Dis. 2007;44:562–5.
29. Attinger CE, Evans KK, Bulan E, Blume P, Cooper P. Angiosomes of the foot and ankle and clinical implications for limb salvage: reconstruction, incisions, and revascularization. Plast Reconstr Surg. 2006;117(7 Suppl):261S–93.
30. Sage R, Pinzur MS, Cronin R, Preuss HF, Osterman H. Complications following mid-foot amputation in neuropathic and dysvascular feet. J Am Podiatr Med Assoc. 1989;79:277–80.
31. Pinzur MS, Wolf B, Havey RM. Walking pattern of midfoot and ankle disarticulation amputees. Foot Ankle Int. 1997;18:635–8.
32. Pinzur MS, Sage R, Stuck R, Kaminsky S, Zmuda A. A treatment algorithm for neuropathic (Charcot) midfoot deformity. Foot Ankle. 1993;14:189–97.
33. Pinzur MS, Sammarco VJ, Wukich DK, Charcot foot: a surgical algorithm. Instructional course lectures of the American Academy of Orthopaedic Surgeons. 2012;61: 423–40.
34. Pinzur MS, Gil J, Belmares J. Treatment of osteomyelitis in Charcot foot with single stage resection of infection, correction of deformity and maintenance with ring fixation. Foot Ank Int. 2012;33: 1069–74.

Management of Acute Hindfoot Fractures in Diabetics

Stefan Rammelt

Introduction

Acute fractures of the hindfoot (talus and calcaneus) are among the most challenging injuries to the orthopedic and trauma surgeon. The ultimate goal for these fractures is to obtain an anatomic reconstruction of any joint incongruity and attain an axial realignment in order to obtain a stable, plantigrade foot with near normal joint function [1–3]. Due to the tenuous soft-tissue coverage surrounding the talus and calcaneus, the direct damage to the soft tissues resulting from the injury, indirect damage that occurs through the pressure of displaced bony fragments, and through the use of extensile approaches that are routinely employed for reductions and fixations, one can see why the management of these fractures is prone to minor and major complications [2, 4]. Any malunion, non-union, or postoperative complication leading to a bone infection or resulting in a compromise of the soft-tissue envelope, can lead to severe restrictions of hindfoot function due to joint incongruities, axial mal-alignment, alteration of hindfoot shape, and soft-tissue impingement [5, 6]. Therefore, a balanced approach is needed for patients with relevant comorbidities.

S. Rammelt, M.D., Ph.D. (✉)
University Center of Orthopaedics and Traumatology, Technische Universität Dresden, Fetscherstrasse 74, Dresden 01307, Germany
e-mail: stefan.rammelt@uniklinikum-dresden.de

Acute talar and calcaneal fractures have to be differentiated from pathological fractures, especially those due to diabetes mellitus that often present with an associated polyneuropathy. As a general rule, the suspicion of a neuropathic fracture should be considered in patients presenting with atypical fracture patterns, a history of low-energy trauma, the presence of edema and mild or diffuse pain, and for any patient who presents more than 24–48 h after their initial injury [7]. The associated neuropathy frequently produces an altered pain perception leading to a delay in the diagnosis and treatment, resulting in a progressive destruction of the bone ultimately producing significant instability and dislocations of adjacent joints [8]. At this point, a diagnosis of a Charcot neuroarthropathy (CN, Charcot foot) is often made. The CN most commonly results from diabetes mellitus, in western civilizations, but can also occur due to other etiologies [9, 10]. Although the specific cause is not completely understood, important causative factors have included repetitive overloading due to unrecognized trauma, poor bone quality due to metabolic changes, and local inflammatory changes with dysfunctional bone formation and resorption [9, 11, 12]. Additionally, acute fractures treated in a delayed manner can also trigger the onset of CN [13].

Sanders and Frykberg [14], observed a forefoot pattern in about 80 % of their patients, but recent studies have discussed a shift towards the ankle and hindfoot [15, 16]. This results in a high

© Springer International Publishing Switzerland 2016
D. Herscovici, Jr. (ed.), *The Surgical Management of the Diabetic Foot and Ankle*,
DOI 10.1007/978-3-319-27623-6_7

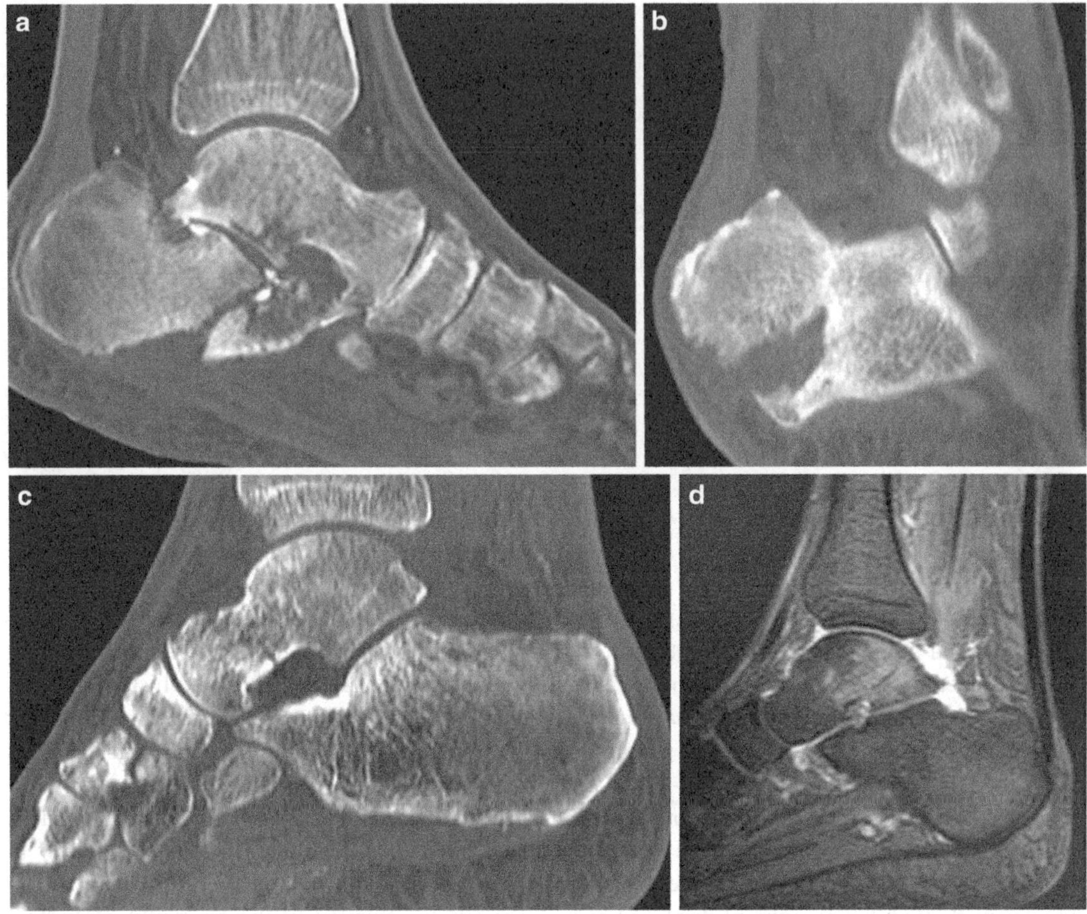

Fig. 7.1 Typical pathologic calcaneal and talar fracture patterns in diabetic patients: (**a**) Reverse oblique fracture through the anterior calcaneal process, (**b**) "beak" fracture of the calcaneal tuberosity. By definition, the subtalar joint is not involved. (**c**) Talar neck stress fracture in a diabetic patient with (**d**) massive edema. (from Zwipp H, Rammelt S. Tscherne Unfallchirurgie: Fuss. Berlin/Heidelberg/New York, Springer, 2014)

degree of instability that is difficult to manage with a cast or brace. These patients often have a dramatic decrease in quality of life and are at considerable risk for an amputation [10, 14]. Isolated, extra-articular calcaneal fractures are seen in only about 1–2 % of patients with diabetic arthropathy [16]. Acute fractures occur as one of three patterns: a fracture through the anterior calcaneal process, one that presents as a reverse oblique fracture through the tuberosity exiting anterior to the sinus tarsi, and a more frequent pattern that presents as a displaced avulsion fracture off of the superior portion of the tuberosity ("beak" fractures, Fig. 7.1) due to the pull of the Achilles tendon [17]. The latter fracture pattern is frequently associated with an increased risk of skin breakdown over the displaced fragment that can lead to a subsequent ulceration and the development of an infection [18].

Studies have shown that the presence of diabetes mellitus is a risk factor for the development of wound complications and infection in acute hindfoot fractures (Fig. 7.2). Folk et al. [19] found a 2.8-fold increased infection rate in diabetic patients with acute calcaneal fractures. More recently, Ding et al. [20] calculated an odds ratio of 6.23 for diabetes mellitus as a risk factor for postoperative wound complications while Wukich et al. [21] found a fivefold increase in postoperative infection rates in persons with

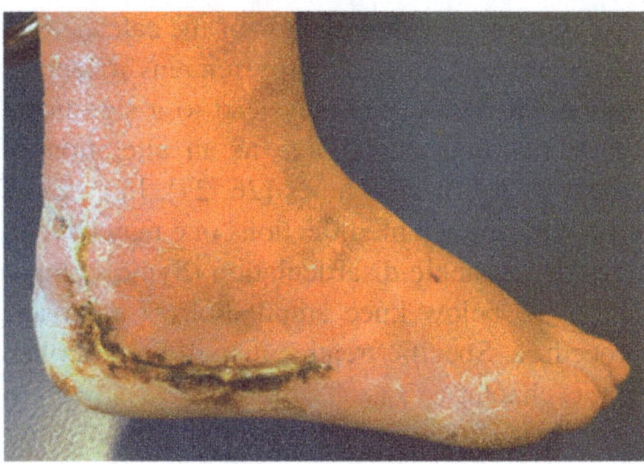

Fig. 7.2 Extensive wound edge necrosis after plate fixation via an extensile lateral approach for a displaced intra-articular calcaneal fracture in a 72-year-old patient with insulin-dependent diabetes mellitus

diabetes compared to non-diabetics. In the latter study, the presence of complicated diabetes increased the risk of postoperative infection by a factor of ten, compared with non-diabetics, and by a risk factor of six when compared to patients with uncomplicated diabetes. Interestingly, there was not much difference of developing a postoperative infection when non-diabetics were compared to patients with uncomplicated diabetes.

Another complication associated with diabetes is that the time to fracture healing is often prolonged, especially with poorly controlled diabetes [22]. However, in the absence of manifest neuropathy, vasculopathy or nephropathy, similar results as in non-diabetic patients can be expected after internal fixation, provided that the patients' blood glucose levels are well controlled and that prolonged offloading can be ensured in compliant patients [7, 13]. Lastly, bony issues have also been noted after performing primary or secondary fusions of the hindfoot. As noted with fracture healing, in the presence of abnormally high glucose levels, and despite adequate surgical technique, patients will demonstrate increased rates of delayed and non-union of the fusion mass [23]. Acute fractures of the talus or CN involving the talus and peritalar joints can also occur producing significant instability of Chopart's, the subtalar and the tibiotalar joints. Further information regarding classifications can be obtained in Chap. 4.

Treatment Recommendations

The goals for the management of these patients, is to protect the foot, minimize soft-tissue breakdown and ulcerations, and to keep the patient as normally ambulatory as possible. However, the literature on the management of acute hindfoot fractures in diabetic patients is scarce and no controlled studies are available. From the available previously cited sources, discussions with colleagues and the author's own experience [7] some guidelines can be offered when considering the surgical management of these injuries.

In compliant patients with well-controlled diabetes (HbA$_{1C}$ < 6.5), and without neuropathy, angiopathy, or nephropathy, a standard open reduction and internal fixation may be carried out. Due to potential healing problems, it is recommended that blood glucose levels be kept within normal limits throughout the time of healing.

In patients with poorly controlled diabetes (HbA$_{1C}$ > 6.5), poor or non-compliance, along with manifest complications of neuropathy, angiopathy, or nephropathy, no extensile approaches should be used due to a compromised immune system along with an impaired wound and bone healing. Patients presenting with open fractures should still undergo an urgent irrigation and debridement. In the presence of grossly displaced fractures and fracture-dislocations, the author's recommendation is to use minimal incisions that allow fixation to be performed either percutaneously or augmented with external fixation. Once healing has occurred, the presence of any symptomatic arthritis can be managed electively with an arthrodesis, without the need for an extensile approach.

Patients presenting with acute neuropathic talus or calcaneus fractures, impeding CN, or an unstable hindfoot should not be managed with standard internal fixation since it will invariably fail because of poor bone quality, impaired healing potential, impaired proprioception and loss of sensation that makes offloading of the foot by the patient unpredictable. For most neuropathic fractures, immobilization and offloading in a well-padded cast is the first line of treatment.

This treatment might even lead to a full restitution in case of early neuropathic changes, i.e., stress fractures that are detected as bone marrow edema on the MRI [7, 8, 16]. Any grossly displaced or unstable hindfoot fractures or fracture-dislocations (combination of Sanders Frykberg Types IV and V) that are not amenable to bracing should be treated with a hindfoot fusion using internal and/or external fixation. In these highly unstable conditions, an acute fusion at the time of presentation, which usually is not the time of injury, will also help transforming them into a more stable Eichenholtz stage while bracing will only maintain the vicious circle of chronic instability and thus progression of the disease [7, 24, 25].

Chronic ulcerations and bony prominences leading to skin necrosis also have to be debrided according to the individual pattern of deformity. Isolated exostectomy and ulcer debridement with primary or secondary wound healing will only be successful in cases of minor deformities. When associated with major deformities and/or gross instabilities, only surgical treatment of these underlying pathologies will eventually result in ulcer healing. In recalcitrant or chronic ulcerations that fail conservative approaches and are associated with osteomyelitis of the calcaneus, a partial or total calcanectomy remains a salvage option. However, this may lead to a significant functional impairment due to an alteration of the overall foot mechanics [26, 27]. In cases of otherwise intractable infections one may have to consider an ankle disarticulation (Syme's amputation) or below knee amputation as a salvage procedure. Specific treatments will be described in this chapter.

Non-Operative Treatment

The use of non-operative management for talar and calcaneal fractures should be considered in all patients who present with non-displaced fractures. Additionally, any patient presenting with poorly controlled diabetes ($HbA_{1C} < 6.5$), poor compliance, neuropathy, angiopathy, or nephropathy, or fractures that will have a stable collapse (i.e., do not produce any bony prominence on the plantar surface of the foot) can be considered candidates for non-operative care in order to avoid the potential risks of surgery (Fig. 7.3). Minimally or non-displaced fractures of the calcaneus (Sanders Frykberg Type V) may be treated

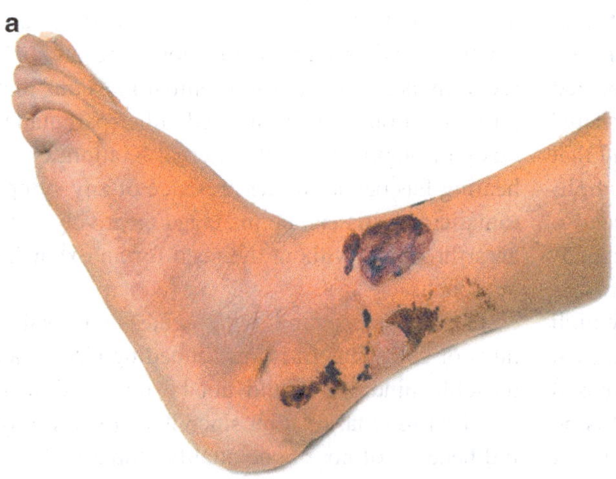
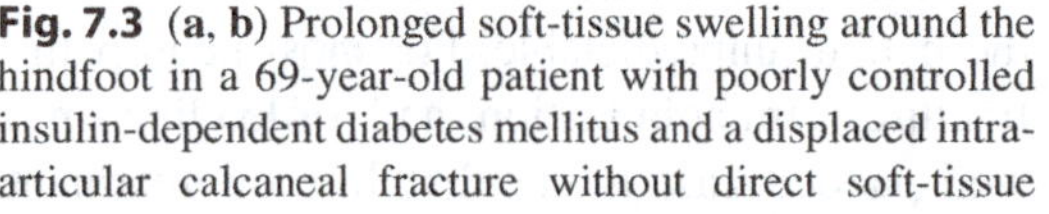
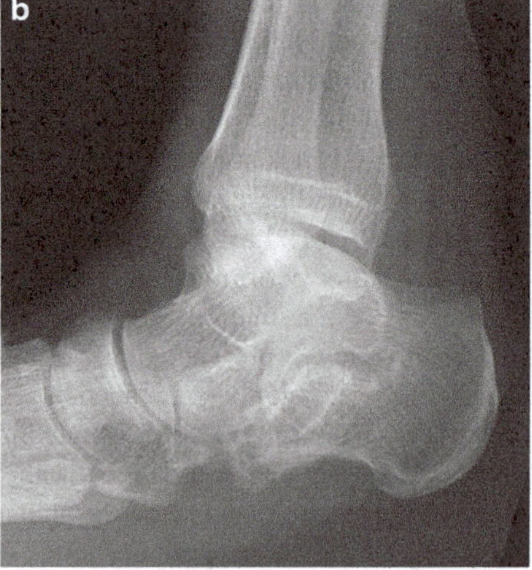

Fig. 7.3 (a, b) Prolonged soft-tissue swelling around the hindfoot in a 69-year-old patient with poorly controlled insulin-dependent diabetes mellitus and a displaced intra-articular calcaneal fracture without direct soft-tissue compromise. The skin blistures healed at 2 weeks. Non-operative treatment was initiated because of the significantly increased perioperative risk

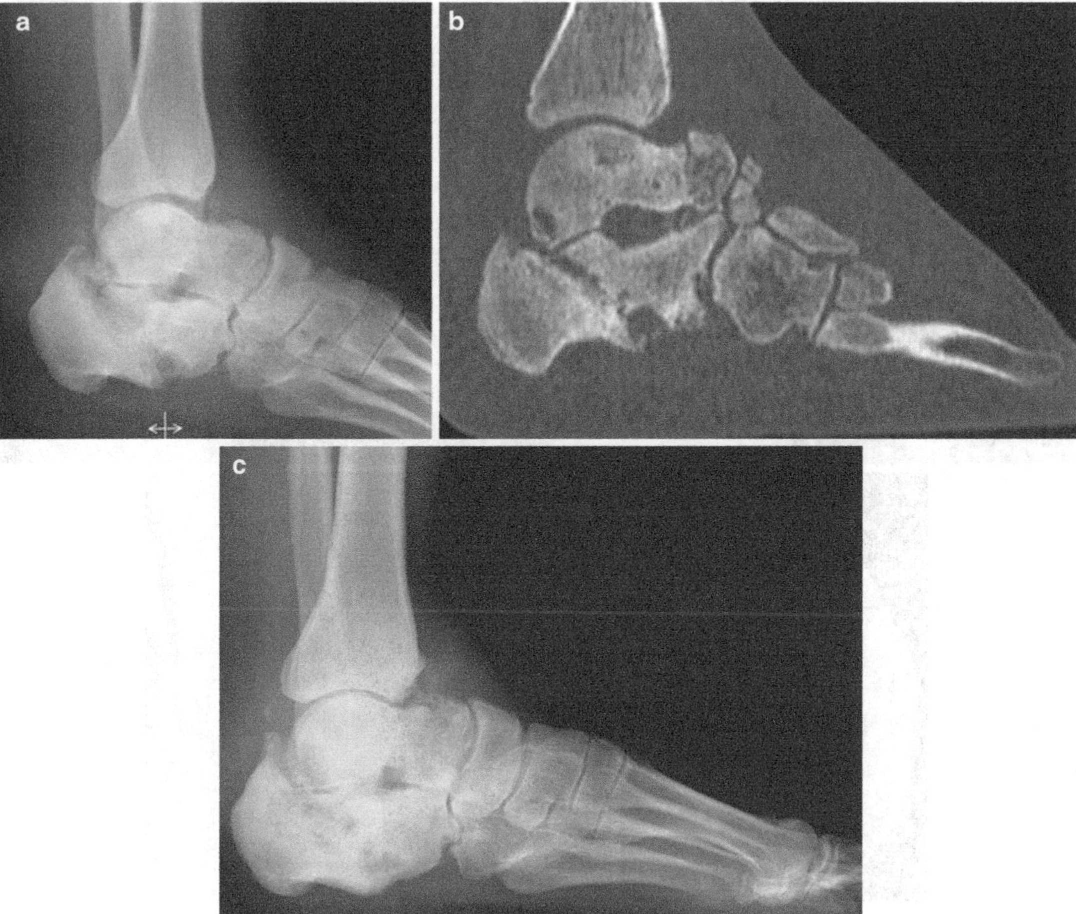

Fig. 7.4 Acute neuropathic fracture of the calcaneus and talar head without gross displacement or soft tissue compromise in a 34-year-old female with severe, poorly controlled insulin-dependent diabetes. (**a, b**) The patient reported increasing pain and swelling over the heel after a misstep on a stair. The calcaneal fracture displays an oblique course with only marginal involvement of the subtalar joint, compatible with a Sanders/Frykberg Type V fracture pattern. Treatment consisted in offloading in a walker. After 3 months (**c**) the fracture has consolidated and soft-tissue swelling has subsided. (from Zwipp H, Rammelt S. Tscherne Unfallchirurgie: Fuss. Berlin/ Heidelberg/New York, Springer, 2014)

with offloading in a cast or a cam walker boot for 6–12 weeks. In the author's experience, neuropathic talar fractures present either as stress fractures (see Figs. 7.1 and 7.4) or as progressive necrosis with gradual dissolution until there is a complete collapse ("disappearing talus," see Fig. 7.5). Patients with minimally or non-displaced fractures are restricted to non-weight-bearing in a well-padded below-knee cast until solid a fracture union is noted. Weight-bearing is then gradually increased after radiographic evidence of bone healing, usually beginning after 6–12 weeks. Alternatively, in compliant patients which adhere to non-weight-bearing, an orthotics cam walker boot may be used.

It is important that a coordinated team approach be used to manage these patients. This includes obtaining or continuing the medical treatment of their diabetes. Patients should also be informed that special foot care is mandatory in order to avoid deleterious complications, not only from the acute fracture but also from the sequelae of diabetes. Foot care should include special individually fitted shoewear with soft insoles.

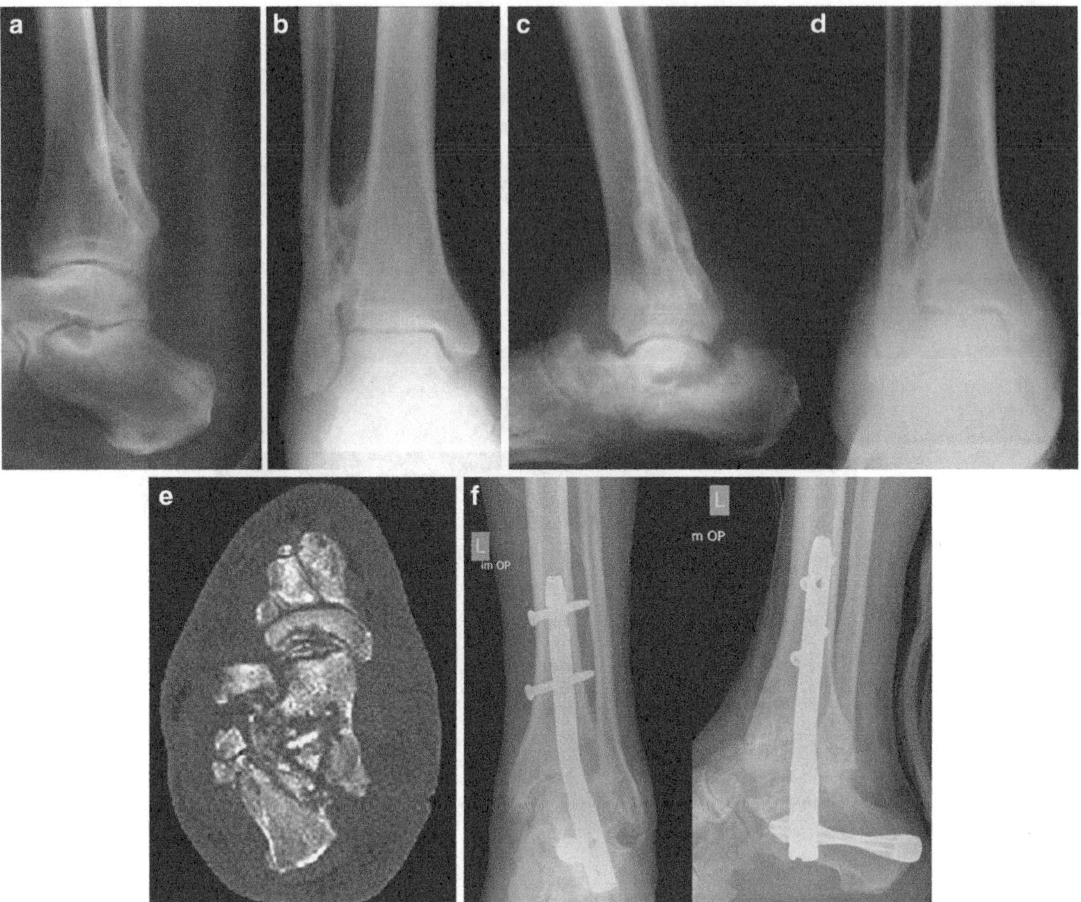

Fig. 7.5 A 50-year-old male with insulin-dependent diabetes mellitus underwent hardware removal for residual pain 9 months after an acute ankle fracture that had healed with prolonged immobilization. (**a**, **b**) He presented 6 months later with increasing pain and deformity. (**c**, **d**) Radiographs and CT scans revealed a CN with destruction of the subtalar joint. (**e**) Because of the high degree of instability, the hindfoot was stabilized with a curved retrograde nail (**f**)

Standard Operative Treatment

Any patient presenting with an open fracture should be managed the same as any non-diabetic patient presenting with an open fracture. This includes emergent or urgent debridement and irrigation, repeated every 48–72 h as needed, the early use of broad spectrum intravenous antibiotics, dispensing tetanus prophylaxis and closure of the wound or providing coverage as soon as possible. Grossly displaced closed fractures and fracture-dislocations that threaten the skin should be reduced as soon as possible using minimal incisions and fixed either percutaneously with screws and/or with the use of an external fixator. Pinning with K-wires is not encouraged as they do not provide adequate stability and constitute a potential source of infection. Definitive fixation is performed in a staged manner after soft-tissue consolidation. As previously stated, a standard open reduction and internal fixation without crossing any joint can be considered for compliant patients who present with acute talar and calcaneal fractures that have an HbA_{1c} less than 6.5, are able to sense a 5.07 or smaller Semmes-Weinstein monofilament, have palpable foot pulses, do not have osteoporotic bone, and are without any manifestations of autonomic dysfunction.

If these criteria are met, displaced talar fractures should be reduced and fixed with screws and/or small plates using the classical two-incision approach, with or without the addition of a posterior approach, depending on the individual fracture anatomy as evaluated by preoperative CT scans [1, 7]. Postoperatively, the patients are restricted to partial weight-bearing with 20 kg or less, which is equivalent to the foot just touching the ground without loading, in a cast or walker for 10–12 weeks until bony union.

Displaced, intra-articular calcaneal fractures are usually treated according to the individual fracture pattern using either locking plate fixation via an extended lateral approach (Fig. 7.6) or, if possible, screw fixation via a minimally invasive approach [2, 3, 28]. The latter is often a good option for simple fracture patterns like tongue-type fractures with large or easily accessible articular fragments (Fig. 7.7). Meticulous handling of the soft tissues is of utmost importance in these cases. Additionally, patients have to be told about the possibility of increased risk of infection and increased time to union. The postoperative regimen has to be tailored to the individual course, with repeated clinical follow-up. The author's preference is to mobilize patients into their own shoe with weight-bearing restricted to a maximum of 20 kg until radiographic evidence of bone healing, usually identified after 8–10 weeks. Over the whole course of treatment the serum glucose levels have to be controlled tightly and kept within normal limits in order to avoid complications. With careful soft-tissue handling, anatomic fracture reduction, and adequate follow-up, similar results can be expected as seen in non-diabetic patients.

Late Arthrodesis

Regardless of whether patients are treated operatively or non-operatively, the sequelae of posttraumatic arthritis may develop. However, prior to undertaking any arthrodesis, any patient presenting with a chronic infection should first undergo serial debridements and then be managed by external fixation or staged internal fixation, and intravenous or oral antibiotics, until they appear clinically clean.

In the presence of symptomatic arthritis, an arthrodesis may be carried out on consolidated fractures via less extensile approaches. With poor skin conditions, percutaneous, arthroscopically assisted arthrodesis techniques may be employed both at the ankle and subtalar joint as they have similar fusion rates as open techniques [29]. Compression may also be obtained using a hybrid wire, hexapod, or Charnley external fixation frame. If an external device is employed it is important that the pin sites be cleaned on a regular basis and the fixators inspected for pin track infections. If a pin tract infection develops either new and separate pins and site are exchanged or the entire frame has to be removed and treatment continues in a cast. If the need arises for an ankle fusion, this can be preformed either with screws alone or in combination with plates while retrograde nailing may offer the best stability for a tibiotalocalcaneal fusion [24, 25, 30].

For malunited calcaneal fractures with posttraumatic subtalar arthritis, the author's preferred approach is a subtalar fusion performed with the patient placed into a prone position using a straight posterolateral approach [5]. This approach is much less prone to complications than a standard extensile lateral approach to the calcaneus. It furthermore allows adequate visualization and lengthening of the collapsed heel with a bone block distraction arthrodesis in patients with good bone stock (Fig. 7.8). Diabetic patients who present with malunited talar fractures or patients who develop avascular necrosis of the talar body with subsequent collapse often require a tibiotalocalcaneal fusion for a salvage of the hindfoot [5, 30, 31].

Patients undergoing an arthrodesis must be followed closely with radiographic examinations every 6 weeks. It has to be borne in mind that in the presence of diabetes, prolonged times to bone healing have to be expected not only for acute fractures but also for fusions about the foot and ankle [22, 23]. There is poor evidence for the efficacy of additional measures like the use of a

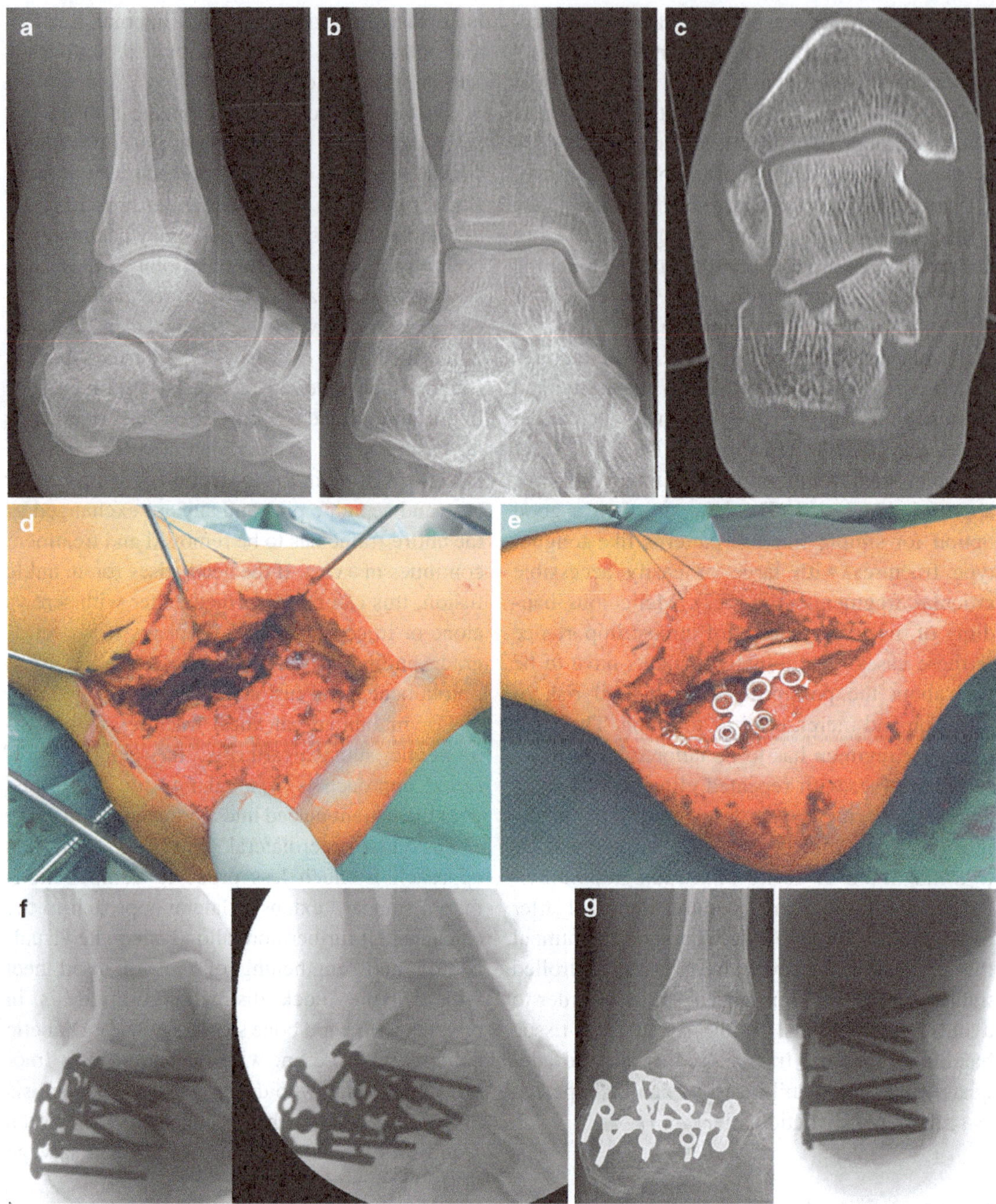

Fig. 7.6 (**a–c**) Displaced intra-articular calcaneal fracture with excessive broadening of the heel, peroneal tendon dislocation (note the bony avulsion of the superior peroneal retinacle) and two displaced fracture lines in the subtalar joint (Sanders type III) in a 53-year-old male patient with well-controlled diabetes. (**d, e**) Treatment consisted of a standard open reduction and internal fixation, via an extensile lateral approach, with reconstruction of the joint and the calcaneus. The epiperiosteal full-thickness soft-tissue flap is held by a suture and gently retracted with K-wires placed into the lateral talar process. No sharp retractors were employed. The peroneal tendons were reduced after fixation of the calcaneus with the torn retinaculum reattached to the tip of the fibula. (**f, g**) Intraoperative fluoroscopic images and postoperative radiographs showing anatomical reduction of the joint and the calcaneal shape. The soft tissues healed uneventfully

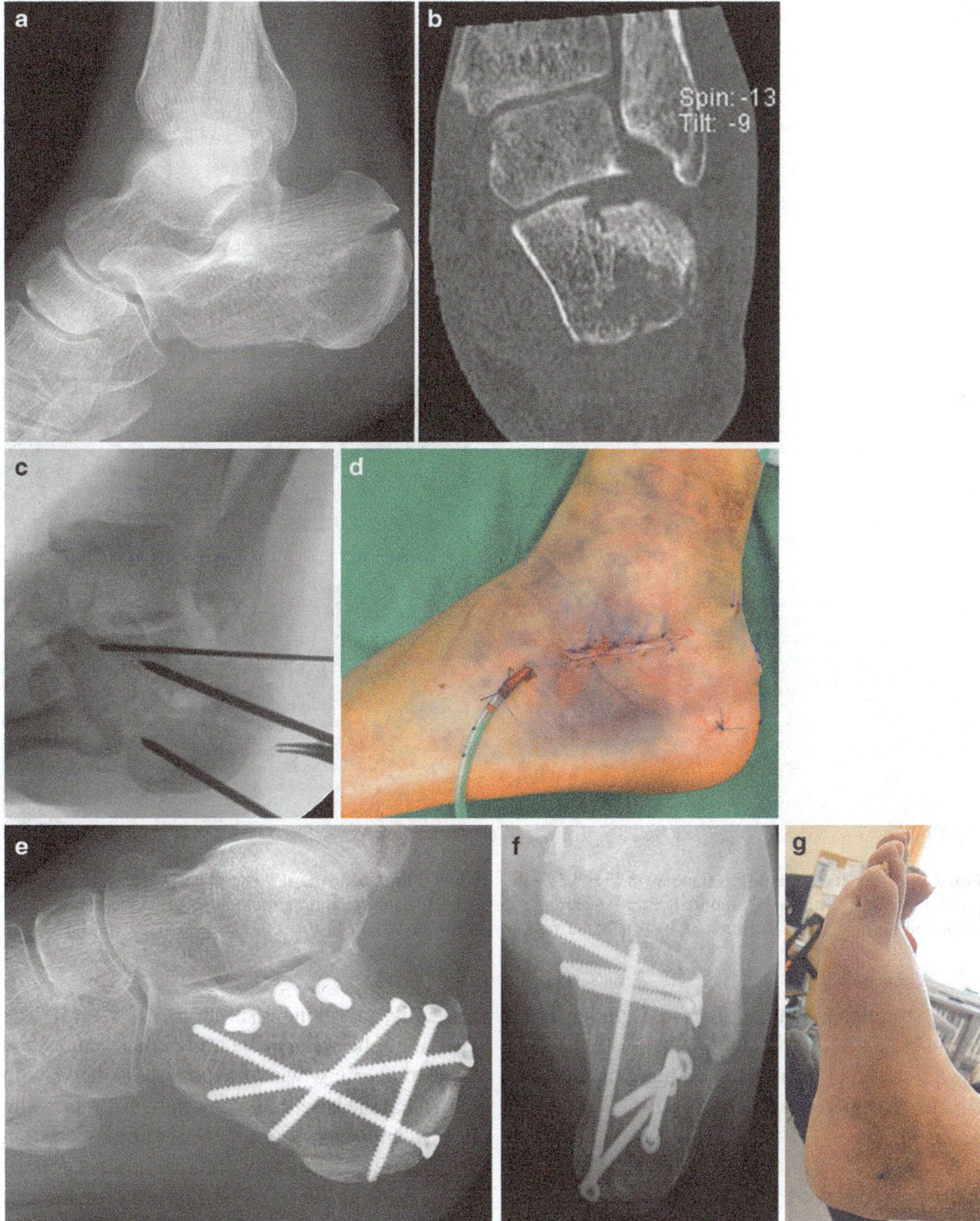

Fig. 7.7 (a–c) Minimally invasive fixation of an acute calcaneal fracture with a single displaced lateral fragment in the posterior facet of a 72-year-old patient with well-controlled diabetes mellitus. Anatomic reduction of the joint is verified with fluoroscopy using a small sinus tarsi approach. (d–f) Screws were introduced through small incisions or percutaneously. (g) Six weeks after the surgery, the soft tissues have healed uneventfully

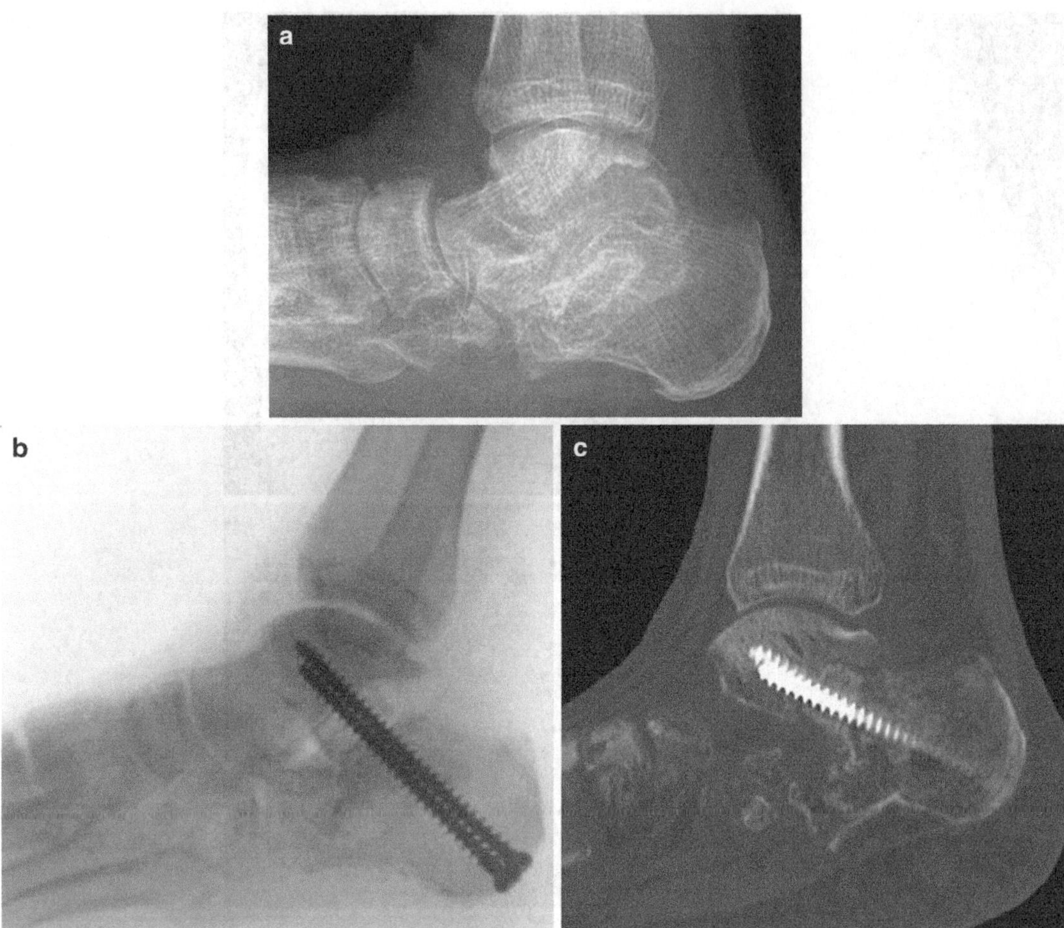

Fig. 7.8 A diabetic patient (the same as in Fig. 7.3) with painful subtalar arthritis 3 months after sustaining a displaced intra-articular fracture. (**a, b**) A subtalar fusion was performed using a posterolateral (Gallie) approach. (**c**) CT scanning at 6 months shows good incorporation of the bone block. The soft tissues healed uneventfully

bone stimulator. Rather, in these patients the blood glucose levels should be controlled and in the presence of manifest osteoporosis, specific treatment should be used [9, 21, 23].

Management of Neuropathic (Charcot) Fractures

Treatment of diabetic CN of the hindfoot is directed towards achieving a stable plantigrade foot that is free of infection or ulceration and allows the patient to ambulate in an orthopedic shoe [7, 10]. Realignment and stable fixation is important in order to break the vicious circle of instability and bone resorption [12, 32, 33]. The distinction between acute traumatic fractures and those presenting with fractures associated with CN is that the latter often present with neuropathy (i.e., inability to sense a 5.07 Semmes-Weinstein monofilament), no history of trauma, have noticed more swelling of the foot than usual making it difficult to place their foot into a shoe, possess signs of autonomic dysfunction (dry, scaled, and reddened skin with diffuse edema of the extremity), have unusual fracture patterns, may or may not have pain, and often have late rather than acute presentations. However, is important to remember, that an acute fracture can also trigger the onset of CN of the hindfoot (Fig. 7.5).

Traditionally, these patients are managed non-operatively with prolonged offloading and immobilization of the affected foot in a total contact cast (TCC). The cast is applied and patients are completely offloaded for a minimum of 6 weeks or until radiographic signs of bony consolidation are seen. Patients are then placed into a special boot or walker (like an ankle foot orthosis, AFO, or a Charcot restraint orthotic walker, CROW). Patients are instructed that they will require individually fitted orthopedic shoes and regular foot care for the rest of their lives in order to avoid deleterious consequences like gross instability, undetected lesions, plantar ulcerations, and subsequent infections with the potential need for amputation.

Surgery is usually reserved for highly unstable, non-braceable deformities and in patients with non-healing ulcers or deep infections [14, 34]. Unfortunately, CN of the ankle/hindfoot type regularly results in severe deformity and instability that does not respond well to casting [7, 16]. Moreover, non-operative treatment in a cast often requires long periods of immobilization and failure rates approach 40 % even in the best of hands [35, 36]. In addition, patients with CN frequently have a poor compliance and difficulties controlling the amount of weight-bearing because of altered pain perception, proprioceptive difficulties and gait disturbance resulting from systemic neuropathy [11]. Consequently, implants have to withstand high loads which may cause implant failure.

Several classifications exist for the lesions at the foot and ankle in CN [10, 15, 16]. The classification most often used by the author is described by Sanders and Frykberg [14] and refers to the anatomical site of the arthropathy. Type I describes a lesion at the forefoot, type II at the tarsometatarsal joint, type III at the mid-tarsal joint, type IV at the hindfoot, i.e., ankle and subtalar joint, and type V extra-articular lesions at the calcaneus. However, neuropathic deformities can occur at several sites at once, therefore combinations of these types are frequently seen. This chapter deals specifically with hindfoot fractures, i.e., Sanders/Frykberg types IV and V.

Sanders/Frykberg Type IV Pattern (Ankle/Hindfoot)

Grossly displaced and unstable hindfoot fracture-dislocations (Sanders Frykberg type IV) that are not amenable to bracing should be treated with a hindfoot fusion technique using internal or external fixation. Advantages of using an external fixation are the low amount of implant mass within the bone, the ability to avoid any medullary reaming, the use of small incisions, and the possibility of stepwise reduction of gross deformities. Disadvantages are high rates of pin track infections and the relatively low biomechanical stability compared to internal fixation methods [25, 35].

Biomechanically, retrograde intramedullary nailing (Fig. 7.5) provides the most stable fixation available [30]. The complication rates following hindfoot fusion with retrograde nailing are significantly higher in patients with CN than for patients presenting with hindfoot arthritis or deformities of other origins [24]. The reported rates of limb salvage range between 86.7 and 100 %, and fusion rates between 77 and 95 % [24, 37, 38]. The use of curved nails provides more bony purchase within the calcaneus [30, 38]. Stability can be further enhanced with the use of a spiral blade within the calcaneus (see Fig. 7.5) and multiple locking screws within the nail.

Sanders/Frykberg Type V Pattern (Calcaneus)

Rarely, does CN develop in the hindfoot as an isolated entity. It is estimated that approximately 1 % of all CN fractures occur in the calcaneus (Sanders Frykberg Type V). By definition, these do not involve the subtalar joint (Figs. 7.1 and 7.6). The majority of these fractures may be treated with offloading in a cast or walker for 6–12 weeks (Fig. 7.4). Chronic ulcerations and bony prominences leading to skin necrosis have to be debrided according to the individual pattern of deformity. Of particular challenge is an acute calcaneal fracture that presents with an ulceration of the heel. However, good outcomes can be obtained with complete healing of both the fracture and ulceration after serial deep debridements and a prolonged course of offloading in a TCC has been used (Fig. 7.9). Patients are seen on an outpatient basis at least once a week until complete wound healing. After soft-tissue and bone consolidation, weight-bearing is gradually increased in a special boot or walker, depending on the patient's compliance.

Using conventional internal fixation for the treatment of these patients will invariably be prone to failure. Implants usually fail and lead to further bony and soft-tissue complications (Fig. 7.10). In the author's opinion, in the presence of CN only open calcaneal fractures or grossly displaced fractures with severe deformity of the hindfoot and direct compromise to the soft tissues should be treated operatively. Depending on the size of the fragments fixation may be obtained using combinations of short plates, screws, tension band wiring, or suture anchors [28, 39]. Most fractures are extra-articular, and involve the posterior tuberosity of the calcaneus. This allows fixation to be achieved using minimal incisions or with percutaneously placed screws. Because the Sanders/

Frykberg type V lesions are either completely extra-articular or only marginally involve the subtalar joint, additional joint trans-articular fixation or fusion is usually not needed. Rather, these additional procedures only add to surgical trauma and are prone to complications like infection or nonunion of the attempted arthrodesis [21, 23]. Alternatively, a small or fragile posterior tuberosity fragment may be excised and the Achilles tendon reattached to the calcaneus if it inserted on the fragment. In case of an open fracture, the decision to partially or totally resect a fractured fragment can be made in order to achieve wound closure without any tension on the wound edges.

Amputations

The risk of soft-tissue and bone infection after talar and calcaneal fractures is significantly increased in diabetic patients with poorly controlled blood glucose levels and complications such as neuropathy [19–21, 28]. Chronic osteomyelitis that develops after an acute hindfoot fracture, which does not respond to serial debridements and antibiotic therapy, may require a partial

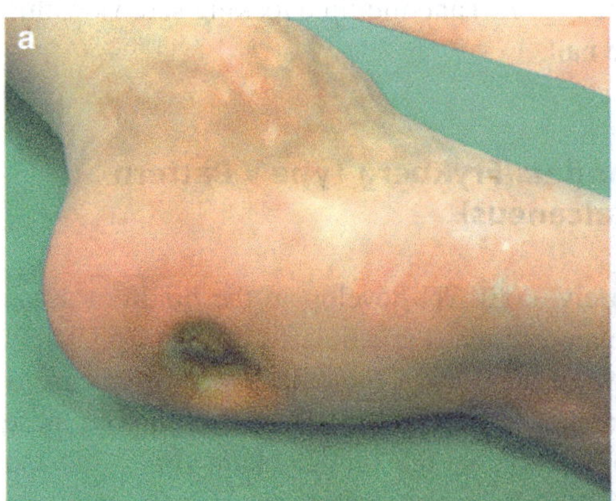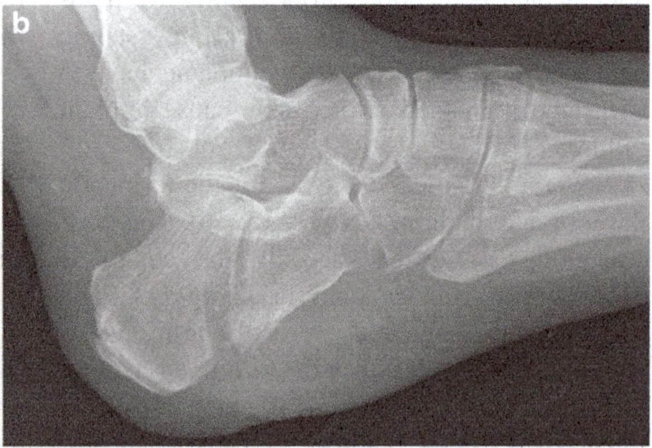

Fig. 7.9 A 65-year-old insensate male presents with acute bleeding from a chronic ulcer below the calcaneal tuberosity. (**a**) He reported hearing a "crack" when standing up in the morning. (**b**) The acute neuropathic fracture displays the typical reverse oblique course without involvement of the subtalar joint but in direct continuity with the heel ulcer. (**c**) Note the air bubbles at the fracture site in the CT scan as a sign for an open fracture. (**d**) An MRI shows the surrounding edema and the absence of diffuse bone infection. (**e**) Treatment consisted of serial local debridements, temporary insertion of an antibiotic bead, and application of antiseptic dressings. (**f, g**) Complete offloading of the heel in a well-padded total contact cast was used for 3 months. (**h, i**) After a prolonged course both the fracture and the ulceration healed completely. Afterwards, the patient was treated with orthopedic shoewear

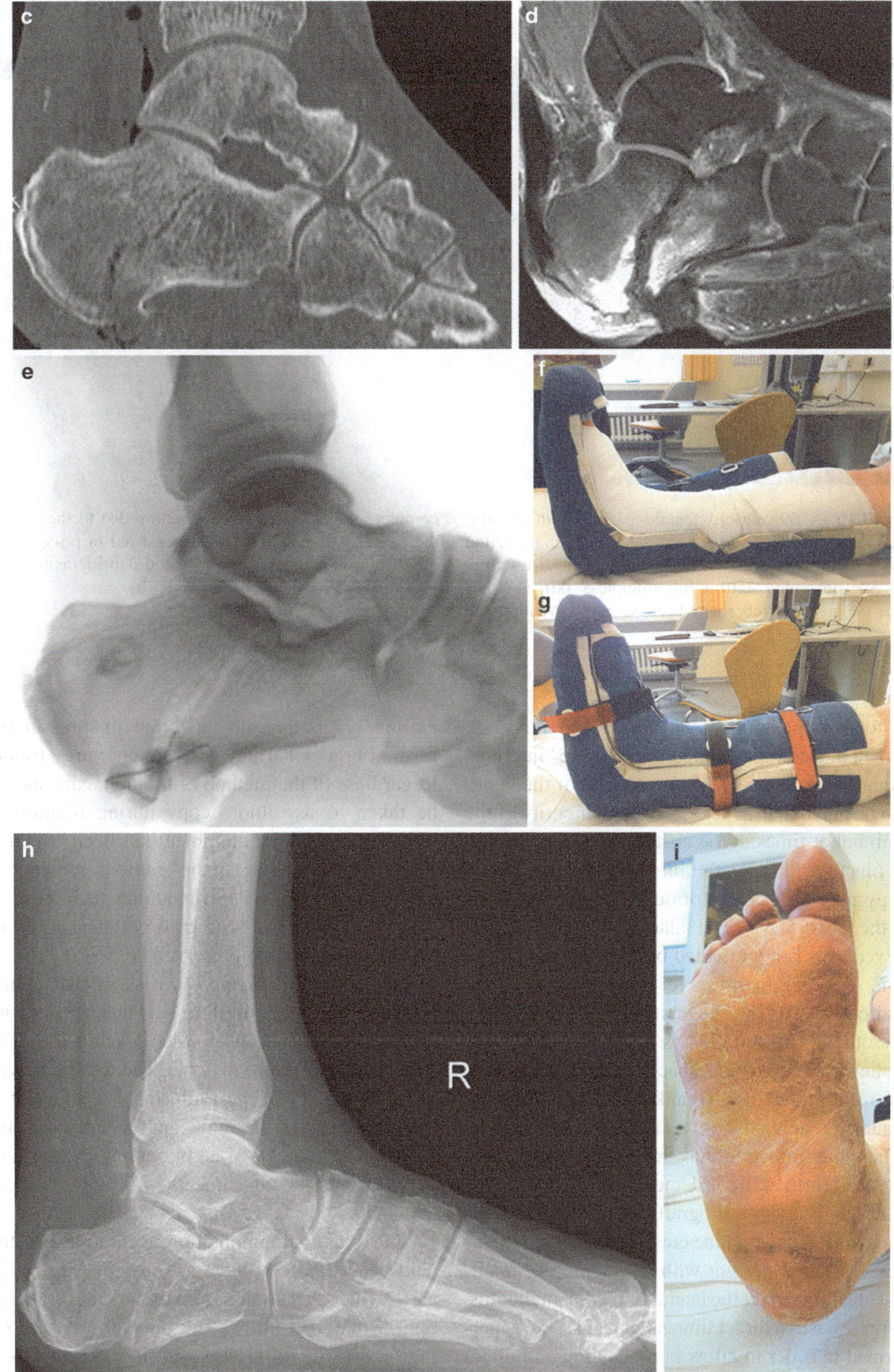

Fig. 7.9 (continued)

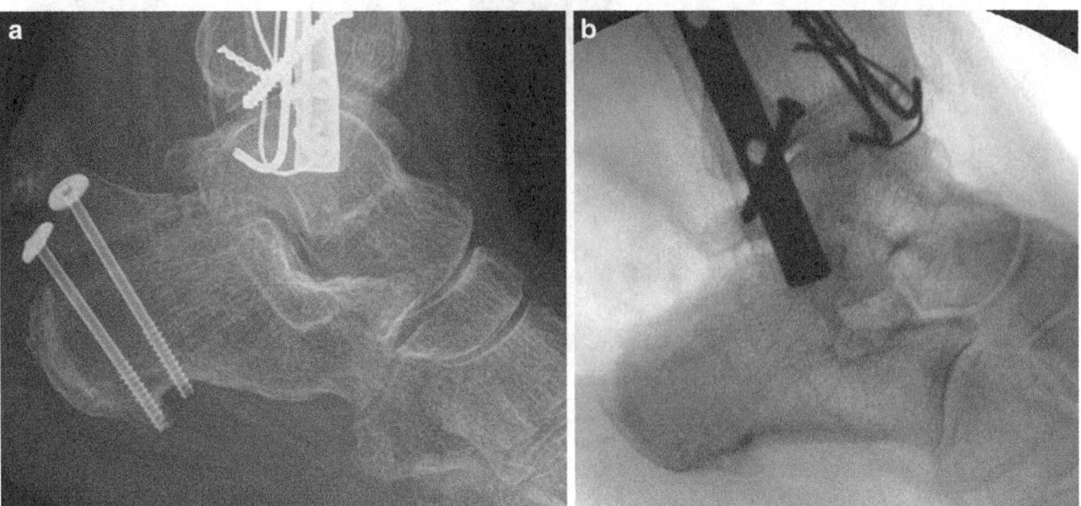

Fig. 7.10 A 59-year-old female patient with insulin-dependent diabetes had been treated with open reduction and screw fixation for a neuropathic calcaneal fracture. (a) She presented with a full thickness skin necrosis over the posterior tuberosity because of a non-union and complete redislocation of the fracture due to the pull of the Achilles tendon. Treatment consisted in resection of the displaced fragment and repeated debridements until soft-tissue closure became possible (**b**)

or total amputation at the ankle and hindfoot. In-lieu of a complete amputation, some "internal" amputations, (i.e., a partial resection of the bone) can be pursued in order to save the integrity of the limb but at times at the cost of considerable loss of function [40]. At the hindfoot, an astragalectomy may also be performed for septic necrosis of the talus [5, 41]. The talar head should be preserved, if it is not affected by necrosis and infection, in order to preserve some motion at the midfoot level [1]. The first step is that all the necrotic or infected bone is resected and an antibiotic bead or cement spacer is introduced into the resulting cavity. An ankle spanning external fixator is applied for temporary stabilization. When the infection has resolved, which may require further debridements, the spacer is replaced by a bulk allograft or corticocancellous bone graft from the iliac crest. Patients with manifest CN often present with threatening or manifest ulceration over the lateral or medial malleolus. In these cases a direct tibiocalcaneal fusion is performed in order to allow bone healing and direct closure of the soft tissues. Fixation is achieved with interlocking plates and screws, intramedullary nailing or compressing external fixation in the form of a Charnley or small wire frame. Regardless of the method of fixation, care should be taken to use fluoroscopy during fixation to note that good axial alignment has been obtained in order to avoid placing the hindfoot into a varus or valgus position The remaining talar head is then attached to the bone graft or anterior part of the tibia if it is being preserved [1, 5].

Partial or total calcanectomy is a salvage option for chronic ulcerations of the heel that present with a diagnosis of calcaneal osteomyelitis [26, 27]. While this procedure may not lead to a perceived loss of integrity of the limb, for the patient it is often associated with significant functional impairment due to the loss of an important lever arm of the heel with the attachments of the Achilles tendon and plantar fascia (Fig. 7.11).

The classical amputation techniques at the ankle and hindfoot, such as Pirogoff (Fig. 7.12) and Syme amputation remain a valid salvage option that still allows the patients to walk on their own sole [40]. However, in cases of otherwise intractable infection, a below-knee amputation is often the best option for these patients.

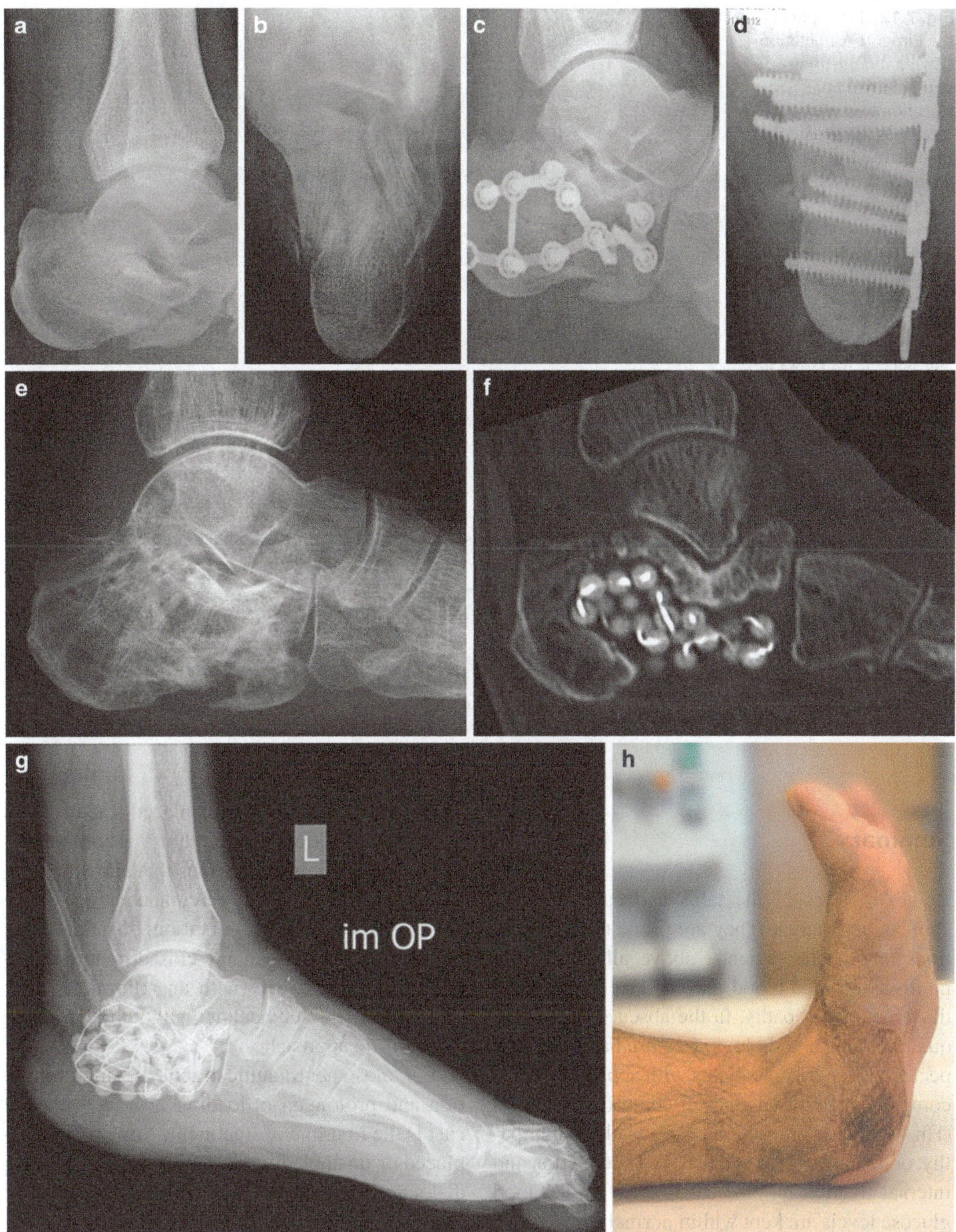

Fig. 7.11 (**a, b**) Lateral and axial views of a 65-year-old diabetic patient with poorly controlled diabetes presenting with a displaced, intr-articular calcaneal fracture. (**c, d**) Initial treatment consisted in lateral plate fixation via an extensile approach. Note the medially and laterally protruding implants and failure to restore calcaneal anatomy. (**e, f**) Despite early implant removal the patient developed chronic osteomyelitis of the calcaneus. Treatment consisted of repeat debridements and implantation of antibiotic beads. (**g, h**) A complete calcanectomy finally lead to a resolution of the infection but with considerable loss of function and shape

Fig. 7.12 Principle of the Pirogoff Amputation (Zwipp modification with minimal bone resection from the calcaneus at the anterior process resulting in only about 2–4 cm limb-length discrepancy). This amputation is useful for septic necrosis of the talus. For patients with CN, a more generous resection of the anterior part of the calcaneus is preferred in order to obtain soft-tissue and bone healing (**a–c**) (from: Rammelt S, Olbrich A, Zwipp H. Hindfoot amputations [German]. Operat Orthop Traumatol. 2011;23(4):265–79)

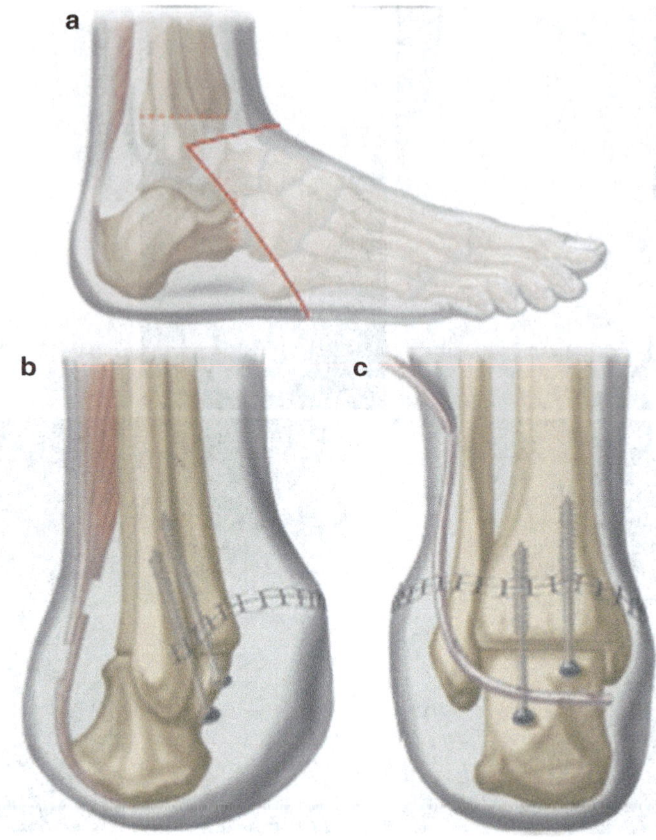

Summary

Acute fractures of the talus and calcaneus are challenging to treat. They are prone to complications in diabetic patients, above all those with poorly controlled blood glucose levels especially those with neuropathy. In the absence of an adequate trauma, a pathologic fracture has to be suspected when seen in patients with apparent CN. In compliant patients with well-controlled diabetes ($HbA_{1C} < 6.5$), and without neuropathy, angiopathy, or nephropathy, a standard open reduction and internal fixation may be carried out while blood glucose levels are kept within normal limits.

In patients with poorly controlled diabetes, poor or non-compliance, along with obvious complications, no extensile approaches should be used and non-operative treatment is preferred. Patients presenting with open fractures should still undergo an urgent irrigation and debridement. In the presence of grossly displaced fractures and fracture-dislocations, the author's recommendation is to use minimal incisions that allow fixation to be performed either percutaneously or augmented with external fixation. Symptomatic arthritis after both open and closed treatment can be managed electively with an arthrodesis after bone and soft-tissue healing, without the need for an extensile approach.

For most neuropathic fractures, immobilization and prolonged offloading in a well-padded cast is the first line of treatment. Any grossly displaced or unstable hindfoot fractures or fracture-dislocations (combination of Sanders Frykberg Types IV and V) that are not amenable to bracing should be treated with a hindfoot fusion using stable internal or external fixation. In cases of otherwise intractable infections one may have to consider a Pirogoff amputation or ankle disarticulation (Syme's amputation) or below-knee amputation as a salvage procedure.

References

1. Rammelt S, Zwipp H. Talar neck and body fractures. Injury. 2009;40(2):120–35.

2. Rammelt S, Zwipp H. Fractures of the calcaneus: current treatment strategies. Acta Chir Orthop Traumatol Cech. 2014;81(3):177–96.

3. Sanders R. Displaced intra-articular fractures of the calcaneus. J Bone Joint Surg Am. 2000;82(2):225–50.

4. Heier KA, Infante AF, Walling AK, Sanders RW. Open fractures of the calcaneus: soft-tissue injury determines outcome. J Bone Joint Surg Am. 2003; 85-A(12):2276–82.

5. Rammelt S, Zwipp H. Corrective arthrodeses and osteotomies for post-traumatic hindfoot malalignment: indications, techniques, results. Int Orthop. 2013;37(9):1707–17.

6. Sangeorzan BJ, Hansen Jr ST. Early and late posttraumatic foot reconstruction. Clin Orthop Relat Res. 1989;243:86–91.

7. Zwipp H, Rammelt S. Tscherne Unfallchirurgie: Fuss. Berlin: Springer; 2014.

8. Wukich DK, Sung W, Wipf SA, Armstrong DG. The consequences of complacency: managing the effects of unrecognized Charcot feet. Diabet Med. 2011; 28(2):195–8.

9. Hofbauer LC, Brueck CC, Singh SK, Dobnig H. Osteoporosis in patients with diabetes mellitus. J Bone Miner Res. 2007;22(9):1317–28.

10. Pinzur MS, Sammarco VJ, Wukich DK. Charcot foot: a surgical algorithm. Instr Course Lect. 2012;61: 423–38.

11. Hamann C, Kirschner S, Gunther KP, Hofbauer LC. Bone, sweet bone—osteoporotic fractures in diabetes mellitus. Nat Rev Endocrinol. 2012;8(5):297–305.

12. Jeffcoate WJ, Game F, Cavanagh PR. The role of proinflammatory cytokines in the cause of neuropathic osteoarthropathy (acute Charcot foot) in diabetes. Lancet. 2005;366(9502):2058–61.

13. Holmes Jr GB, Hill N. Fractures and dislocations of the foot and ankle in diabetics associated with Charcot joint changes. Foot Ankle Int. 1994;15(4):182–5.

14. Sanders LJ, Frykberg RG. Diabetic neuropathic osteoarthropathy: The Charcot foot. In: Frykberg RG, editor. The high risk foot in diabetes mellitus. New York: Livingstone; 1991.

15. Herbst SA, Jones KB, Saltzman CL. Pattern of diabetic neuropathic arthropathy associated with the peripheral bone mineral density. J Bone Joint Surg Br. 2004;86(3):378–83.

16. Mittlmeier T, Klaue K, Haar P, Beck M. Charcot foot. Current situation and outlook [German]. Unfallchirurg. 2008;111(4):218–31.

17. Hedlund LJ, Maki DD, Griffiths HJ. Calcaneal fractures in diabetic patients. J Diabetes Comp. 1998; 12(2):81–7.

18. Athans W, Stephens H. Open calcaneal fractures in diabetic patients with neuropathy: a report of three cases and literature review. Foot Ankle Int. 2008; 29(10):1049–53.

19. Folk JW, Starr AJ, Early JS. Early wound complications of operative treatment of calcaneus fractures: analysis of 190 fractures. J Orthop Trauma. 1999; 13(5):369–72.

20. Ding L, He Z, Xiao H, Chai L, Xue F. Risk factors for postoperative wound complications of calcaneal fractures following plate fixation. Foot Ankle Int. 2013; 34(9):1238–44.

21. Wukich DK, Lowery NJ, McMillen RL, Frykberg RG. Postoperative infection rates in foot and ankle surgery: a comparison of patients with and without diabetes mellitus. J Bone Joint Surg Am. 2010;92(2): 287–95.

22. Follak N, Kloting I, Merk H. Influence of diabetic metabolic state on fracture healing in spontaneously diabetic rats. Diabet Res. 2005;21(3):288–96.

23. Myers TG, Lowery NJ, Frykberg RG, Wukich DK. Ankle and hindfoot fusions: comparison of outcomes in patients with and without diabetes. Foot Ankle Int. 2012;33(1):20–8.

24. Mendicino RW, Catanzariti AR, Saltrick KR, Dombek MF, Tullis BL, Statler TK, et al. Tibiotalocalcaneal arthrodesis with retrograde intramedullary nailing. J Foot Ankle Surg. 2004;43(2):82–6.

25. Chiodo CP, Acevedo JI, Sammarco VJ, Parks BG, Boucher HR, Myerson MS, et al. Intramedullary rod fixation compared with blade-plate-and-screw fixation for tibiotalocalcaneal arthrodesis: a biomechanical investigation. J Bone Joint Surg Am. 2003; 85-A(12):2425–8.

26. Smith DG, Stuck RM, Ketner L, Sage RM, Pinzur MS. Partial calcanectomy for the treatment of large ulcerations of the heel and calcaneal osteomyelitis. An amputation of the back of the foot. J Bone Joint Surg Am. 1992;74(4):571–6.

27. Bollinger M, Thordarson DB. Partial calcanectomy: an alternative to below knee amputation. Foot Ankle Int. 2002;23(10):927–32.

28. Sanders R, Rammelt S. Fractures of the calcaneus. In: Coughlin MJ, Saltzman CR, Anderson JB, editors. Mann's surgery of the foot & ankle. 9th ed. St. Louis: Elsevier; 2013. p. 2041–100.

29. Winson IG, Robinson DE, Allen PE. Arthroscopic ankle arthrodesis. J Bone Joint Surg Br. 2005;87(3): 343–7.

30. Rammelt S, Pyrc J, Agren PH, Hartsock LA, Cronier P, Friscia DA, et al. Tibiotalocalcaneal fusion using the hindfoot arthrodesis nail: a multicenter study. Foot Ankle Int. 2013;34(9):1245–55.

31. Kitaoka HB, Patzer GL. Arthrodesis for the treatment of arthrosis of the ankle and osteonecrosis of the talus. J Bone Joint Surg Am. 1998;80(3):370–9.

32. Mittlmeier T, Klaue K, Haar P, Beck M. Should one consider primary surgical reconstruction in Charcot arthropathy of the feet? Clin Orthop Relat Res. 2010;468(4):1002–11.

33. Papa J, Myerson M, Girard P. Salvage, with arthrodesis, in intractable diabetic neuropathic arthropathy of the foot and ankle. J Bone Joint Surg Am. 1993;75(7): 1056–66.

34. Petrova NL, Edmonds ME. Charcot neuro-osteoarthropathy-current standards. Diabetes Metab Res Rev. 2008;24 Suppl 1:S58–61.
35. Pinzur M. Surgical versus accommodative treatment for Charcot arthropathy of the midfoot. Foot Ankle Int. 2004;25(8):545–9.
36. Saltzman CL, Hagy ML, Zimmerman B, Estin M, Cooper R. How effective is intensive nonoperative initial treatment of patients with diabetes and Charcot arthropathy of the feet? Clin Orthop Relat Res. 2005;435:185–90.
37. Pyrc J, Fuchs A, Zwipp H, Rammelt S. Hindfoot fusion for Charcot osteoarthropathy with a curved retrograde nail [German]. Orthopade. 2015;44(1):58–64.
38. Siebachmeyer M, Boddu K, Bilal A, Hester TW, Hardwick T, Fox TP, et al. Outcome of one-stage correction of deformities of the ankle and hindfoot and fusion in Charcot neuroarthropathy using a retrograde intramedullary hindfoot arthrodesis nail. Bone Joint J. 2015;97-B(1):76–82.
39. Robb CA, Davies MB. A new technique for fixation of calcaneal tuberosity avulsion fractures. Foot Ankle Surg. 2003;9(4):221–4.
40. Rammelt S, Olbrich A, Zwipp H. Hindfoot amputations [German]. Oper Orthop Traumatol. 2011;23(4):265–79.
41. Liener UC, Bauer G, Kinzl L, Suger G. Tibiocalcaneal fusion for the treatment of talar necrosis. An analysis of 21 cases [German]. Unfallchirurg. 1999;102(11): 848–54.

Dolfi Herscovici Jr. and Julia M. Scaduto

Ankle fractures are common skeletal injuries and are one of the most commonly managed joint injuries in orthopedic surgery. Surgical fixation is well-established as the treatment of choice for displaced fractures. This produces an anatomic reduction of the mortise, decreases instability, and lessens the development of posttraumatic arthrosis of the ankle. Although the use of non-operative care for some fractures have demonstrated good outcomes, nonsurgical treatment is currently reserved for patients presenting with non-displaced fractures, those whose medical co-morbidities preclude any surgical intervention, patients who refuse surgery or most often as an intermediate step until the soft-tissue envelope has sufficiently stabilized to allow surgery. These fractures are so routinely treated that there is often a certain disregard for their seriousness and their potential complications, especially in the diabetic patient. At times we fail to remember that the diabetic patient can also present with impaired healing of the wound and bone, along with some vascular insufficiency and neuropathy.

D. Herscovici Jr., D.O. (✉) • J.M. Scaduto, A.R.N.P.
Foot and Ankle/Trauma Service, Tampa General
Hospital, Florida Orthopaedic Institute,
13020 Telecom Parkway, Temple Terrace,
Tampa, FL 33637, USA
e-mail: fixbones@aol.com; juliaarnp@yahoo.com

In the diabetic, chronic hyperglycemia results in high levels of blood viscosity, it impairs the ability of the red blood cell to deliver oxygen, it affects nitric oxide, which functions as an antioxidant and neurotransmitter, and it leads to microvascular compromise. The last of which results in coronary artery disease, stroke, peripheral artery disease and produces nerve ischemia [1, 2]. In addition, hyperglycemia also decreases the ability of immune cells, specifically fibroblasts, from migrating and attaching to wounds ultimately resulting in healing stagnation that may last for up to 8 weeks [3].

In bone physiology, chronic hyperglycemia increases osteoclastic activity, leading to osteoporosis and demineralization, and decreases osteoblastic activity, resulting in a decrease in osteon formation and the ability of the bone to remodel. This impairs proliferation and migration of the osteocytes which results in a decrease in callus formation, tensile strength, and bone stiffness [4]. Ultimately it is a combination of all of these changes that results in a significant delay in bone healing [5], with studies reporting union times increasing to 163 % to that of non-diabetic patients, which is further increased to 187 % of non-diabetics when the fractures are displaced [6, 7]. These bony changes also raise their chances of sustaining a more severe ankle fracture, along with increasing their mortality rates,

© Springer International Publishing Switzerland 2016
D. Herscovici, Jr. (ed.), *The Surgical Management of the Diabetic Foot and Ankle*,
DOI 10.1007/978-3-319-27623-6_8

postoperative complications, lengths of hospital stays and costs, than in the non-diabetic patient [8–11]. It is, perhaps, for all of these reasons that the use of non-operative care is more often considered for management of the diabetic patient who presents with an ankle fracture.

How then, do we manage the acute diabetic ankle fracture? Do we withhold certain treatments because they will be too expensive? Or do we withhold treatments, due to expectations that they will have poorer outcomes than the non-diabetic patient? This comes with the understanding that withholding treatment can produce avoidable complications, result in significant disabilities, and create chronic conditions that can lead to socioeconomic burdens to patients, their families, and to payer systems. The decision driving treatment should be based on the injury pattern and the patient's physiology. If surgery is anticipated a discussion with the patient should include the need for preoperative medical evaluations and whether any adjunctive fixation will be needed to augment the reduction. Additionally, and regardless of whether the patient is treated operatively or non-operatively, a long discussion should be held to discuss prolonged immobilization and non-weight-bearing of the patient. Given the advancements in techniques and implants, this chapter will hopefully provide a rational approach for the physician tasked with managing acute ankle fractures in the diabetic patient.

Epidemiology

The 2014 National Diabetes Statistics reported that 29.1 million people (9.3 % of the US population) have diabetes of which 8.1 million (27.8 % of people) are undiagnosed [12]. Approximately 89 % have one additional co-morbidity and 15 % have four or more [13]. Patients, presenting with neuropathy and at least one other co-morbidity, have higher rates of complications (47 % vs. 14 %) compared to diabetics without neuropathy or another co-morbidity [11]. Although complications are often related to poor glucose control, hypertension, and dyslipidemia, only 36–57 % of patients achieve adequate glycemic or blood pressure levels, while only 13.2 % of all patients achieve all three target levels [14].

The incidence of adult ankle fractures has been shown to be 100.8/100,000/per year. The ratio of men to women is 47:53, with bi- and tri-malleolar fractures increasing in incidence, more so in women, as patients get older [15]. In the United States it has been estimated that approximately 260,000 Americans per year sustain an ankle fracture, with about 25 % undergoing surgical management [9]. Within this population nearly 6 %, or almost 16,000 patients per year, are diabetics who sustain an ankle fracture [8]. If the 25 % needing surgery is extrapolated into the diabetic population, it would mean that one would expect that annually approximately 4000 diabetics sustain an ankle fracture, or less than 2 % of all diabetic ankle fractures in the United States, are going to be managed surgically for their injury.

Preoperative Evaluations

Unless the patient presents with an open fracture or an irreducible dislocation, there is no emergency for surgery. It is important that one understands that both *medical and surgical* treatment will be needed to manage these patients, rather than placing conveniently into the surgical schedule

History

The management begins with a thorough history, specifically asking about the mechanisms and the timing of the injury. Up to 74 % of diabetic patients have scores less than the threshold for osteopenia and 39 % below the threshold for osteoporosis [16]. Therefore, a low (ground level fall) mechanism of energy resulting in a complex fracture pattern may indicate poor bone quality. Additionally, questions about when the injury occurred are also important. Because neuropathy is present in 10 % of diabetics [17] it can be inferred for any patient continuing to ambulate on that extremity and presenting more than 24 h after the injury occurred.

The history should also include questions about the presence of comorbidities since they have been shown to increase the rates of complications [11]. With approximately 89 % of diabetics presenting with one additional comorbidity and 15 % have four or more [2], this means that all medical and vascular evaluations should be performed prior to any surgical intervention. Additional questions should include whether ambulatory aids were used prior to their injury, whether or not they smoke, their use of insulin or other medicines, and whether they have a history of previous ulcers or infections.

Physical Examination

The examination should begin by inspecting the soft-tissue envelope and evaluating the neurovascular structures of the limb. Any wounds or lacerations should be evaluated for an open fracture. Look and palpate for changes in skin color, temperature changes, or any bony prominences, all of which may be an indication of impending skin necrosis. Additionally, fracture blisters or the presence of any tense compartments may indicate that the extremity is not ready for operative fixation.

The neurologic examination should also begin with an observation of the extremity. Motor dysfunction, indicating intrinsic atrophy, is often manifested as clawing of the toes and neuropathic autonomic dysfunction is suspected in patients presenting with dry, cracking, hyperemic skin. Of greatest concern is the loss of protective sensation due to neuropathy. Loss of vibratory sensation, pinprick, sense of position or absence of deep tendon reflexes at the ankle (difficult to perform in the presence of a fracture) may indicate neuropathy but have only a fair agreement amongst evaluators [18]. Although the gold stan-

dard for identifying peripheral neuropathy is a nerve conduction study, the accepted method for detecting the loss of protective sensation is the use of a 5.07 (10-g) Semmes-Weinstein monofilament. This simple exam has a sensitivity and specificity of 91 % and 86 %, respectively [19], which increases with a minimum testing of four plantar sites (great toe, first, third and fifth metatarsals) [18]. Detecting peripheral neuropathy is important since it increases both the risk of noncompliance and postoperative infections by a factor of four [20].

The last part of the physical exam should include a vascular evaluation. This is important since more than 40 % of diabetics present with peripheral arterial disease [21]. The popliteal trifurcation is most often affected however, vessel calcification in the ankle and the foot are suggestive of vascular compromise (Fig. 8.1). Visual signs suggestive of peripheral artery disease include dependant rubor, pallor with elevation of the extremity, dystrophic toenails, and hair loss [22]. The evaluation should continue with an attempt to palpate pulses and comparing it with the contralateral extremity. If pulses are still absent or diminished, after reducing the dislocation or improving the fracture alignment, the aid of Doppler ultrasound can be used to identify the vessels. However, the use of the ankle-brachial (ABI) index is often described as a more sensitive, noninvasive test for evaluating the patient's vascular status. A value of 0.91–1.3 is considered normal. However, in the diabetic, an $ABI \geq 1.1$ can be suggestive of arterial calcinosis and an $ABI > 1.3$ indicates poor compressibility of the vessel [22]. In patients with acute ankle fractures an ABI may be difficult to perform, so for these patients one should pursue additional testing.

Currently, three additional, noninvasive tests are available. The first measures the transcutaneous oxygen pressure (T_cPO_2) of the skin. Pressures >30 mmHg are the minimum value needed to heal surgical wounds [22]. The second test places small blood pressure cuffs around each toe and measures the systolic pressure of

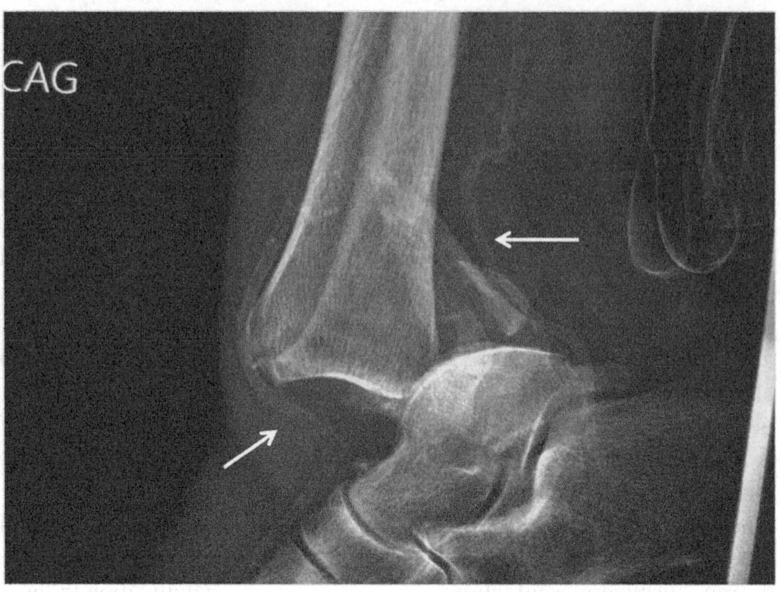

Fig. 8.1 A fracture dislocation sustained in an insulin-dependent diabetic. Note the calcification of the vessels (*arrows*) anteriorly and posteriorly

each toe. A toe pressure >40 mmHg is predictive of good wound healing [22]. If there is any question, however, they should be referred to a vascular surgeon for further work-up. The third test is the toe-brachial index (TBI) and is calculated by dividing the toe pressure by the highest obtained ankle pressure. Currently a value >0.7 has been reported as the cutoff for a normal value [23]. Again, the problem with the TBI is that in the presence of a fracture the patient may not tolerate a cuff placed around the ankle. Currently, the authors' preferred method of evaluation is measuring the patient's toe pressures. Further discussions can be found in the chapter on the Vascular Evaluation and Management of Vascular Disease in the Diabetic Patient.

Laboratory Evaluations

As discussed, uncontrolled hyperglycemia results in pathophysiologic dysfunctions [3, 4, 6–11]. Therefore, in addition to standard preoperative laboratory studies, all patients should also have their hemoglobin A_{1c} (HgA_{1c}) evaluated. Levels >6.5 increase the risk of complications, produce longer hospital stays, and result in poor radiologic outcomes [24]. Those with values >8

have a 2.5 times greater risk of developing an infection [25]. It should be noted that for every 1 % reduction in HgA_{1c}, there is approximately a 25–30 % reduction in the rate of complications [26]. Patients may not necessarily be excluded from surgery, due to an elevated HgA_{1c}, but this information may help manage their diabetes during their postoperative care.

Fracture Management

Whether managed operatively or non-operatively, the goals of treatment are to achieve a stable and congruent joint, restore function, and to prevent complications from occurring. Unfortunately, there is no clear algorithm to guide the treatment, based on fracture displacement, for this population.

Non-operative Treatment

The nonsurgical management can be controversial because of the concern for displacement; however, these patients can be treated to completion successfully. Nonsurgical care is offered to patients presenting with non-displaced fractures, with a good rule of thumb being to double or triple the treatment offered to non-diabetic patients. Therefore, the authors' preferred method for non-operative treatment consists of placing patients into a short leg, non-weight-bearing cast for 10–12 weeks. Weekly or biweekly radiographs and inspection of the soft-tissue envelope should be performed to ensure that there has been no displacement of the mortise and no problems to the soft tissue envelope have developed (Fig. 8.2). After the casting period, patients are placed into a period of protective weight-bearing, using a brace or boot, for an additional 2–3 months.

Very few studies discuss the nonsurgical management of diabetic ankle fractures. Most contain very small numbers of patients and are often discussed as one of the arms of treatment, in-lieu of surgical management [9, 11, 27–29]. The complications reported in these studies have included malunions, due to a loss in the initial reduction; non-unions; the development of Charcot neuroarthropathy; infections; and the development of ulcers. Risk factors for developing a complication include seeing patients infrequently, early weight-bearing or non-compliance, having a long duration of diabetes, the presence of neuropathy, insulin dependence, and those with a history of Charcot neuroarthropathy. Risk factors not associated with complications include age, gender, and type of fracture [9, 11].

Operative Treatment

Preoperative Care and Planning

The indication for surgical management is an unstable ankle fracture. However, before fixation is performed it is important to stabilize the soft-tissue envelope. This includes a prompt reduction and splinting of the extremity, especially if fracture blisters have occurred. Immobilization can be achieved using a well-padded, non-removable splint or with the use of an external fixator, if the reduction cannot be maintained by using the splint alone. The patient is instructed to keep the leg elevated as much as possible and is evaluated at weekly intervals. The ability to wrinkle the skin and a re-epithelialization of the skin, after fracture blisters have resolved, indicates that the soft tissues have stabilized and are ready for surgical management. This may take anywhere between 10 and 21 days and during this period the preoperative evaluations and planning should be performed.

The preoperative planning is undertaken to ensure that all the equipment and implants needed for surgery will be present. This includes small, large, and periarticular bone clamps, extra-long drill bits, extra-long screws, with lengths reaching 90–110 mm in length and in sizes ranging from 2.7 to 4.5 mm, Steinman pins, and extra-long k-wires. In addition, locking mini, small, and large extra-long locking plates, and their corresponding locking screws, should also be readily accessible. A 3.5- or 4.5-mm locking plate, at least ten holes in length, for fixation of the fibula should be utilized while avoiding semi-tubular or easily deformable (malleable) plates. Lamina spreaders or distractors should also be on hand if distraction of the fractures, especially in the fibula, is anticipated. Lastly, an external fixator should also be on hand if the anticipation is that the ankle construct will need to be augmented with external fixation.

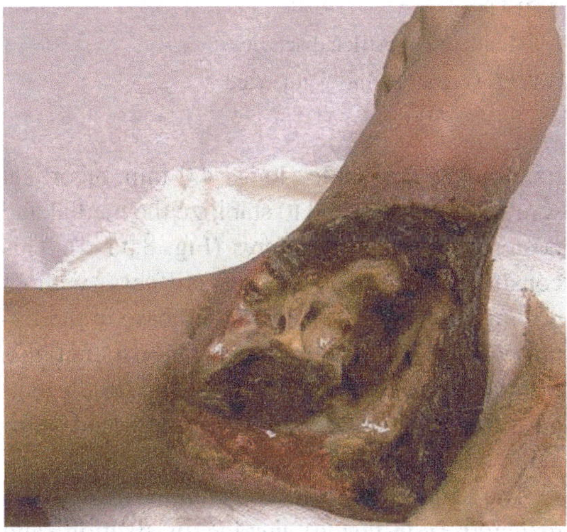

Fig. 8.2 Significant necrosis on the medial surface of the ankle and foot in a neuropathic, non-compliant, type I diabetic treated with a short leg, non-weight-bearing cast for a non-displaced fracture. Patient did not return to clinic for 8 weeks after initial cast application. An amputation was ultimately performed

Operative Management

There are four approaches that can be used to manage the diabetic ankle fracture: standard fixation, trans-syndesmotic, trans-articular, and a combination of these techniques. Standard fixation, with expected good outcomes, can be considered for any patient presenting with an HbA_{1c} less than 7.0, a body-mass index (BMI) less than 25, able to sense a 5.07 or smaller Semmes-Weinstein monofilament, the presence of palpable pulses, non-osteoporotic bone, and those without any manifestations of autonomic dysfunction. Postoperatively, patients can be managed similar to non-diabetic patients.

For patients who do not meet these criteria, three methods of fixation are available. These three techniques are much different than standard methods of ankle fixation but have been developed to maintain an anatomic mortise and decrease the risk that failure of fixation will occur prior to adequate healing. In addition to prolonged immobilization and non-weight bearing, the operative principles for these three techniques include the use of long, rigid, locking fixation, using some kind of adjunctive fixation, considering adding a bone graft, and contemplating the use of a bone stimulator (Table 8.1). Because of the patient's abnormal bony metabolism, the authors' current treatment of choice is to add a bone stimulator to all patients when using one of these three alternative techniques.

The *trans-syndesmotic fixation technique* uses the tibia to help stabilize the fibular fixation. Described using tetracortical screws (crossing four cortices), this method consists of getting the fibula out to length, reducing the fracture, applying at least a 10-hole 3.5 mm or larger locking plate onto the fibula, and then inserting as many locking screws as possible through the fibula and into the tibia [30]. The advantage of using a locking plate is that it provides angular stability, which increases its load-carrying capacity, which allows locking plates to be four times stronger than load-sharing constructs. This means that for failure of fixation to occur it requires that all points of fixation fail as opposed to the loosening of individual screws, as seen with traditional compression plating techniques. To complete the

Table 8.1 Operative principles for non-standard surgical management of ankle fractures

Rigid fixation
Longer and thicker plates (Minimum ten holes)
Locking plate technology
More and longer screws
Tetracortical screws used for trans-syndesmotic fixation
Bicortical screws for medial/posterior malleolar fixation, 4.0 mm or larger
Possible use of an Intramedullary nail
Adjunctive fixation
External fixation
K-wires across ankle joint
Steinman pins across ankle and subtalar joints
Combinations of these techniques
Cement (Calcium Sulfate/Phosphate or polymethyl methacrylate)
Bone graft
Consider using
Bone stimulator
Recommend using these devices
Postoperative care
Week 1: Well-padded postoperative splint
Week 2: Apply short leg non-weight-bearing cast
Week 3: Remove sutures
Week 12: Remove Steinman pins, casting completed
Month 4–5: Boot or brace, therapy, advance to WBAT[a]
Month 6: Unrestricted activity

[a]*WBAT* weight bearing as tolerated

fixation of the ankle, long, 4.0-mm bicortical screws should be used to stabilize the medial and posterior malleolar fractures (Fig. 8.3a–d). This construct improves fixation stiffness without relying solely on the screw's purchase in the fibula. Although there is some concern that this technique may alter the biomechanics of the syndesmosis, this has not been demonstrated clinically. For postoperative care see Table 8.1.

The second alternative technique is a *trans-articular (non-fusion) method* of fixation, and can be approached in one of two ways. The first is to treat the patient using standard reduction techniques, which is then augmented using two or three large, smooth, retrograde tibio-talar-calcaneal Steinmann pins [30] (Fig. 8.4a–c). This produces some stiffness of ankle and the hindfoot but does not rely solely on standard fixation techniques to main the reduction. The second approach is the use of a retrograde tibial-talar-calcaneal intramedullary nail. Although some calcification or arthrodesis of the ankle or subtalar joints is possible, the difference between this method and an arthrodesis technique is that neither the subtalar nor the ankle joint is exposed and prepared as when performing a formal arthrodesis (Fig. 8.5a–c). This approach works well in patients presenting with pilon fractures but can also be used in certain unstable bi- or trimalleolar ankle fractures, especially in patients with morbid obesity. Once the fracture is healed a decision regarding nail removal can be made.

For postoperative care of both approaches see Table 8.1. To complete the discussion of transarticular methods of fixation, immediate arthrodesis of the ankle has been described for non-reconstructable fractures [31] but has rarely been performed for an acute diabetic ankle fracture. However, in the setting of poor bone quality, a poorly controlled diabetic with neuropathy, autonomic changes and poor potential to heal the fracture, an immediate arthrodesis may be considered to improve the outcome of that patient.

The third technique is described as *a combined technique*, with the surgical tactic described in Table 8.2. In this approach the trans-syndesmotic technique is augmented using two or three large, smooth, retrograde tibio-talar-

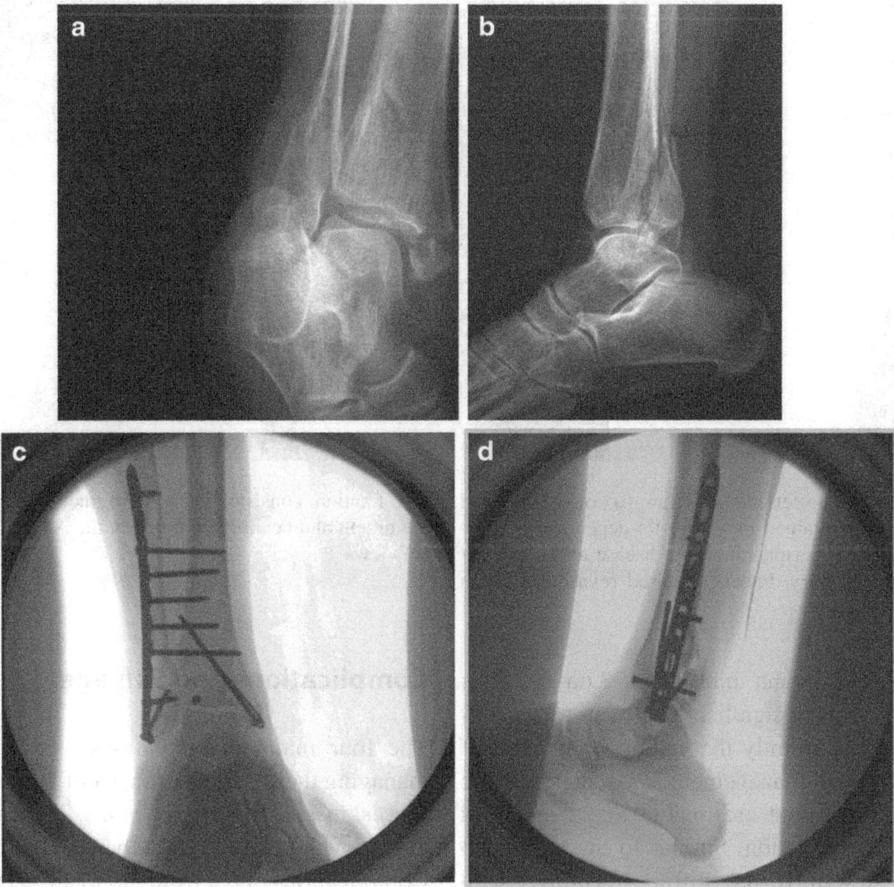

Fig. 8.3 Mortise (**a**) and lateral (**b**) views of a displaced, right trimalleolar ankle fracture in a neuropathic male. Using a *trans-syndesmotic technique*, a good reduction is noted in the postoperative mortise (**c**) and lateral (**d**) views. Note the use of bicortical screws for the medial and posterior malleolar fractures

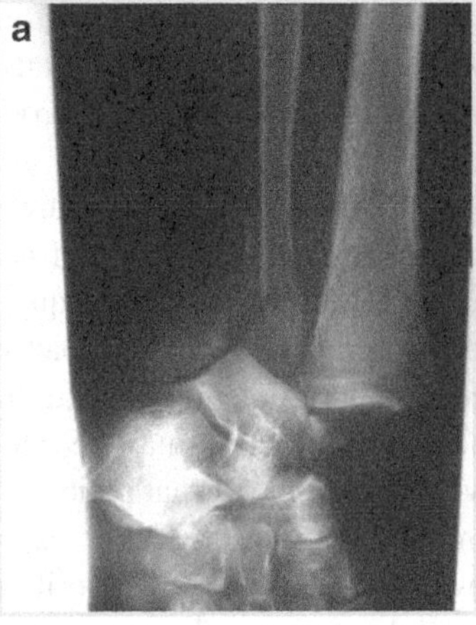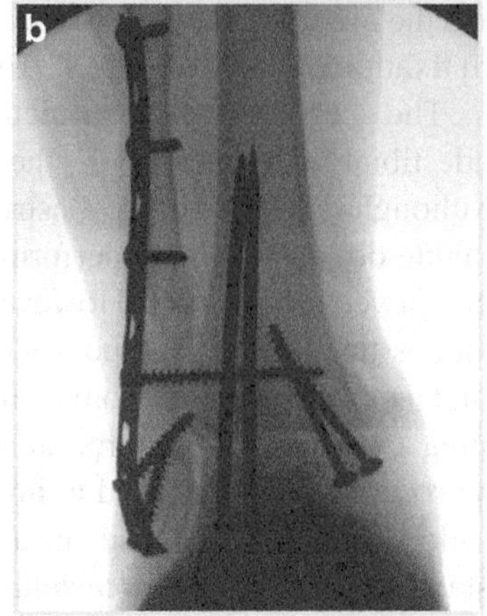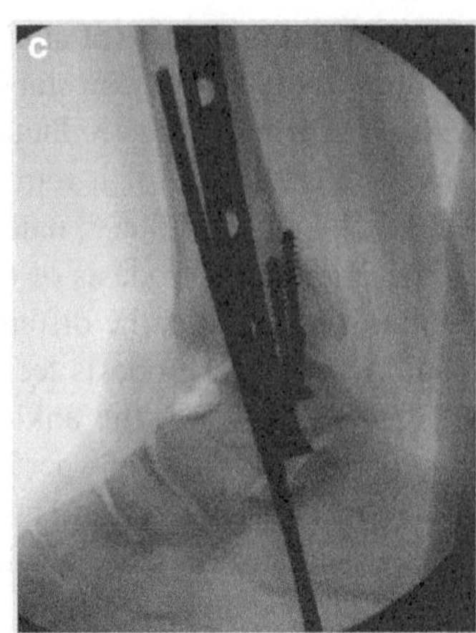

Fig. 8.4 Mortise view (**a**) of a displaced trimalleolar fracture in a patient with neuropathy and renal failure. Management consisted of a *trans-articular technique* with a good reduction noted in the mortise (**b**) and lateral (**c**) views. Pins were left in place for 12 weeks

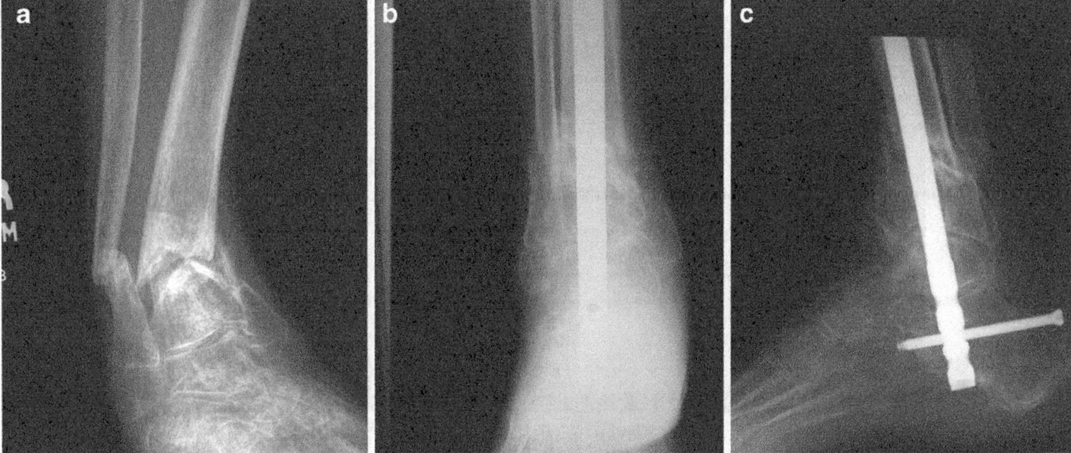

Fig. 8.5 Anteroposterior (AP) view (**a**) of a displaced pilon fracture sustained in an insulin-dependent, neuropathic male with peripheral artery disease and a 3 pack/day smoking history. Patient required revascularization and fixation consisted of a retrograde nail. Improved alignment and healing are noted in the AP (**b**) and lateral (**c**) views

calcaneal Steinmann pins (Fig. 8.6a–d). This approach provides significant stiffness to the construct and is currently the authors' treatment of choice for the management of acute diabetic ankle fractures that are unable to be managed with standard fixation. Similar to the other two methods described, the stiffness acquired with this approach does not seem to be a problem clinically because ambulation progressively restores motion between the tibia and fibula. The postoperative care is described in Table 8.1.

Complications and Salvage

The four major complications associated with managing these patients consist of failure of fixation, skin and wound problems, infections, and the development of Charcot arthropathy. Complications range from 3.6 to 43 % [8, 20, 25, 27, 29, 32, 33] and can occur individually or in any combination. It is of no surprise that the rates of complications are higher for the diabetic than in the non-diabetic population, with the highest

Table 8.2 Surgical tactic for trans-syndesmotic and combined fixation techniques of the ankle

Lateral approach to fibula

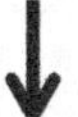

Select a 10-hole or greater locking plate, place slightly posterolateral. Plate should allow placement of multidirectional locking screws

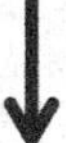

Fix to distal fibula first. Proximal to plate, place a screw and use a lamina spreader to "push" fibula out to length and to correct rotation. Reduce and hold fracture. Place 1–2 bicortical locking screws proximally to hold length

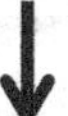

If diastasis identified, compress fibula to tibia. Proximal to articular surface, place as many tetracortical screws as possible, angled 20–30° anteriorly, through the plate and into the tibia

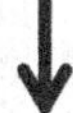

Open reduction of medial malleolus. Fixation performed using 1–2 bicortical 4.0 mm cortical screws

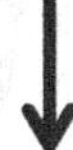

Percutaneous fixation of posterior malleolus using 1–2 bicortical 4.0 mm cortical screws. For Combined Technique, retrograde 2–3 smooth Steinman pins

risk occurring in poorly controlled diabetics [25]. Therefore, the question is, after operating on these high-risk patients can their complication(s) be treated without necessitating an amputation as the only salvageable option?

Failure of Fixation

In this context, failure of fixation is defined as a loss of the reduction early in the postoperative period, without the development of a Charcot joint (Fig. 8.7a–c). The most common reasons for this complication are often a combination of the patient's neuropathy, their inability to avoid weight-bearing on the extremity, and inadequate fixation performed at the index procedure. By far the biggest mistake is in managing these patients like a well-controlled or non-diabetic patient. Because a significant number of patients have little or no upper body strength, patients will often begin full weight bearing within hours after their surgery. In an attempt to decrease this complication, patients should be placed into wheelchairs to help them maintain a non-weight-bearing attitude, a discussion should be made with their caregivers about the importance of keeping them off their foot, and weekly visits may be necessary if non-compliance persists to make sure that displacement has not occurred.

The salvage of a failed fixation is via one of the three previously discussed alternative approaches, with the timing dependant on the health of the soft-tissue envelope. Continued conservative treatment of the malaligned extremity will result in malunions, non-unions, the development of contractures, and possible skin breakdown and/or ulcerations (Fig. 8.8a–b). It is possible that the addition of trans-articular external fixation can improve the overall alignment of the extremity but it may not produce an anatomic reduction of the mortise. If a revision fixation is unable to be performed then a salvage using an ankle or double hindfoot arthrodesis (ankle and subtalar joint), may be necessary to salvage the extremity (Fig. 8.9a–g).

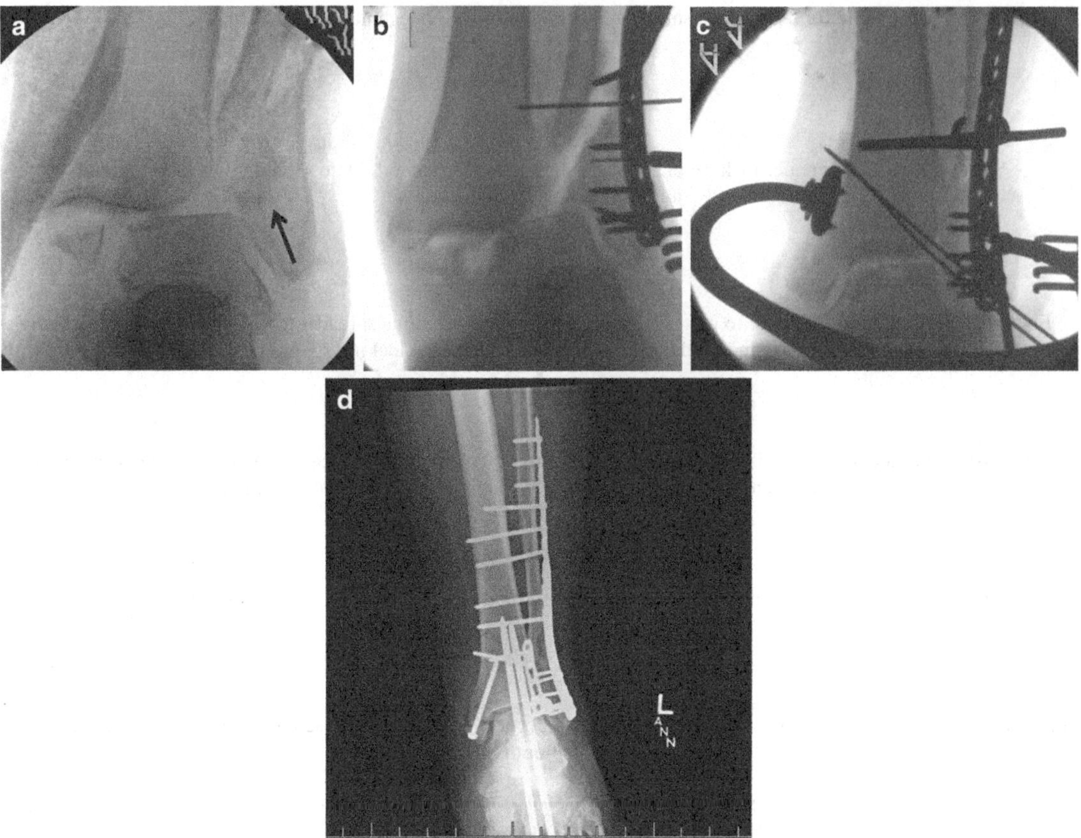

Fig. 8.6 Mortise view (**a**) of a fracture dislocation in a morbidly obese, neuropathic male. Note the displacement (*arrow*) of Chaput's tubercle. Using a *combined technique*, the fibular was lengthened using a push–pull technique (**b**) and once out to length the syndesmosis was reduced with a periarticular clamp (**c**). Postoperative reduction (**d**) shows improved alignment of the fracture. See Table 8.2 for the surgical tactic

Skin and Wound Problems

Wound edge necrosis and dehiscence, without the presence of infection, are constant concerns when managing these patients. Even without the presence of a fracture or surgery, there is a considerable challenge in trying to get things to heal in this population [27]. As has already been noted hyperglycemia decreases blood flow to both small and large vessels [22], increases blood viscosity, impairs the ability of the red blood cell to adequately flow, and decreases the amount of oxygen reaching the tissues. This resulting hypoxia inhibits fibroblasts from migrating to the wound and causes them to lose their ability to proliferate, which may last for up to 8 weeks [3]. This is in addition to smoking, hypertension, dyslipidemia, increased body-mass index, and advanced age, which have also been shown to have a negative effect on healing [3, 8–11, 14, 20].

Given the combination of fracture edema, hypoxia, and hyperglycemia one can envision a poor environment for diabetic wound healing [29] even in at-risk patients managed nonoperatively. Early salvage requires frequent (often weekly) clinic visits since these problems are usually identified during routine cast changes. During these visits, encouraging good control of their diabetes, discussing the need for elevating the extremity, and placing them into wheelchairs may all help with healing, compliance, and edema. In addition, reapplying a well-padded splint, in-lieu of the cast, may help avoid pressure to the compromised skin. When skin or wound problems are identified, a systematic approach should be used to manage these patients. For the first 3–4 weeks, after the wound has been identified, initial treatment includes local, daily wound care, through a windowed cast, and the empiric use of a broad spectrum oral antibiotic. If the wound fails to improve, irrigation and debridement and the use of negative pressure wound therapy may be necessary. If after 4–6 weeks of negative pressure therapy, worsening or no improvement is noted, a plastic surgery consultation may be necessary.

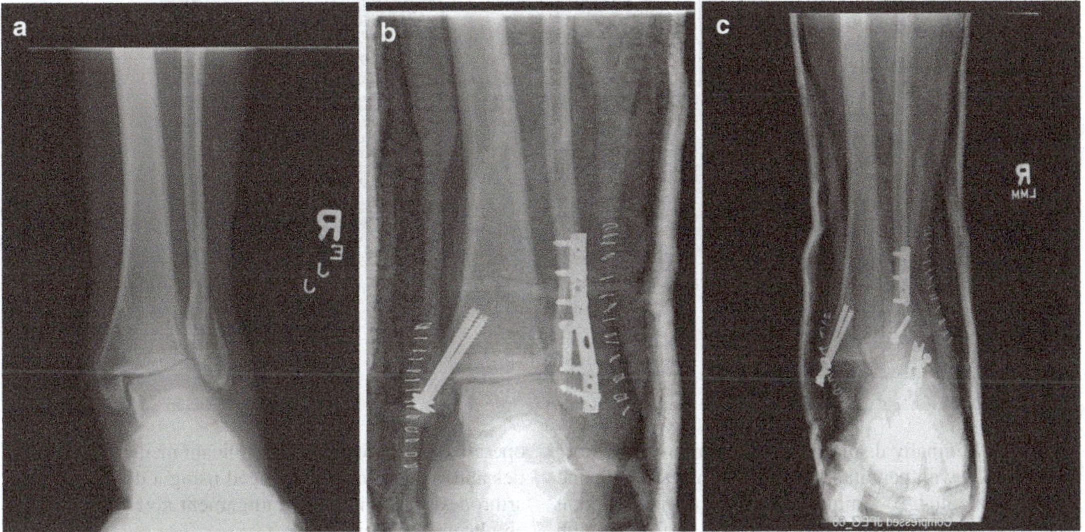

Fig. 8.7 An AP view (**a**) of an unstable bimalleolar left ankle. Immediate post-fixation in a splint (**b**) demonstrates a good reduction of the ankle. Short leg cast applied and patient returned to clinic 10 days later demonstrating a broken plate (**c**) and displacement of the fracture. Courtesy of Robert Probe, MD

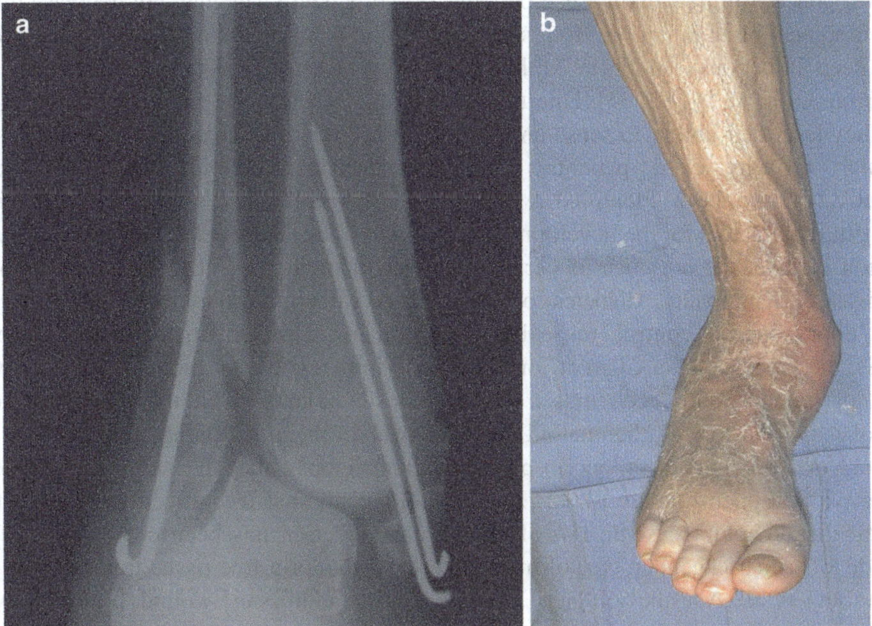

Fig. 8.8 Poorly fixed ankle fracture (**a**) that resulted in significant malalignment of the extremity (**b**)

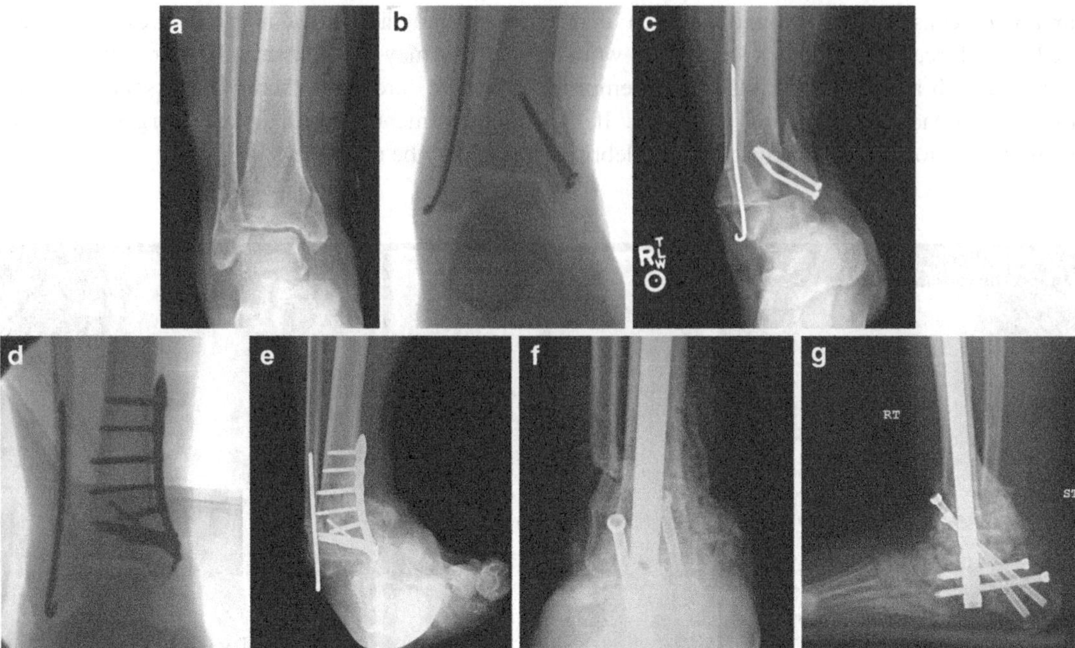

Fig. 8.9 Minimally displaced bimalleolar ankle fracture (**a**) managed with percutaneous fixation of the fibula and medial malleolus (**b**). Failure of fixation (**c**) identified at first office visit. Revision fixation (**d**) was performed with failure of second fixation (**e**) identified at that initial post-operative visit. Patient had significant medical comorbidities and was ultimately salvaged using a double hindfoot arthrodesis, with improved alignment noted in the AP (**f**) and lateral (**g**) views

Infection

The biggest concern in managing these patients is the development of an infection. Both superficial and deep infections can occur with rates ranging from 3.6 to 43 % [32, 33]. Due to neuropathy, they lose their ability to sense an infection, which is why even patients treated non-operatively have been identified with an infection [9]. Risk factors for the development of an infection include, the presence of peripheral arterial disease, neuropathy, diabetes of long duration, poor glucose control (especially a HgA_{1c} >8), the presence of a Charcot joint, the presence of edema and ecchymosis, older patients, obesity, a history of rheumatoid arthritis, a history of a previous ulcer, and in patients presenting with an open fracture [9, 11, 20, 25, 33]. Factors that do not increase the risk of infection include tobacco use, gender, type of fracture, American Society of Anesthesiologists (ASA) classification, and whether the surgery was performed as an inpatient or an outpatient [11, 20].

Frequent visits may not decrease this complication from occurring but can offer earlier treatment when they are identified. As with wound complications, the infection is often identified during a routine change of the patient's cast. For superficial infections, windowing the cast, to allow local, daily wound care, providing oral antibiotics, and weekly office visits may be sufficient to manage the problem. In contrast, all deep infections should be managed with irrigation and debridement, a minimum 6-week course of intravenous antibiotics, and removal of all loose implants. Avoid the urge to perform a local swab of the area. Rather, deep cultures or even a bone biopsy may be necessary to identify the organism(s) if osteomyelitis is suspected. Once the infection has been controlled, the use of a local flap or a free tissue transfer may be necessary to address the wound. If after bony debridement significant bone has been removed or the articular surfaces have been lost then an ankle or double hindfoot arthrodesis may be needed to salvage the extremity. If the extremity is not salvageable then an amputation may be necessary. Further discussions on reconstructions can be found in the chapter on the Management of Infections and Osteomyelitis in the Diabetic Patient.

Charcot Neuroarthropathy

Its incidence, in diabetic ankle fractures, has been reported to occur between 6 and 47 % [11, 25, 28, 33]. It is challenging to manage, especially when it presents after the surgical care of an ankle fracture, because it is often confused with infection. On initial presentation, patients often present with erythema, edema, and some warmth to palpation. The differential diagnosis can include gout, cellulitis, abscess, and osteomyelitis. However, the diagnosis of a Charcot joint should be considered in any compliant patient, who had an anatomic reduction of the mortise and presents with failure of fixation. Careful physical, laboratory, and radiographic examinations will identify whether the patient has developed a Charcot neuroarthropathy or has a postoperative infection (See Appendix, Table 1).

The salvage of these patients can be difficult because they often present late with malunions, non-unions and contractures of the extremities. Reconstructions should be considered when the extremity is in the subacute or chronic stages. Indications for surgery should include failure of conservative care, chronic deformity, instability not amenable to bracing, and evidence of abnormal plantar pressures, despite the use of an orthoses and special shoes. Reconstructions often involve bony and soft-tissue procedures in order to improve the alignment and obtain a viable extremity. Further discussions on reconstructions can be found in the chapter on the Management of the Charcot Ankle.

In conclusion, avoid managing the acute diabetic ankle fracture similar to those treated in the non-diabetic population. These patients have increased rates of complications and infections and are usually non-compliant due to their neuropathy. Careful preoperative evaluations and postoperative vigilance can improve outcomes. These patients require very rigid repair, often with some kind of adjunctive fixation, with long periods of immobilization and protective weight bearing. Significant deformities can produce abnormal plantar pressure, irritability with shoewear and malalignment of the extremity. However, good outcomes can be expected with alternative techniques and even some residual deformity does not seem to produce much disability.

References

1. Vincent AM, Russell JW, Low P, Feldman EL. Oxidative stress in the pathogenesis of diabetic neuropathy. Endocr Rev. 2004;25:612–28.
2. Paraskevas KI, Baker DM, Pompella A, Mikhailidis DP. Does diabetes mellitus play a role in restenosis and patency rates following lower extremity peripheral arterial revascularization? A critical overview. Ann Vasc Surg. 2008;22:481–91.
3. Stadelmann WK, Digenis AG, Tobin GR. Impediments to wound healing. Am J Surg. 1998;176(2A Suppl):39S–47.
4. Macey LR, Kana SM, Jingushi S, Terek RM, Borretos J, Bolander ME. Defects of early fracture-healing in experimental diabetes. J Bone Joint Surg Am. 1989;71:722–33.
5. Weinberg E, Maymon T, Moses O, Weinreb M. Streptozotocin-induced diabetes in rats diminishes the size of the osteoprogenitor pool in bone marrow. Diabetes Res Clin Pract. 2014;103:35–41.
6. Loder RT. The influence of diabetes mellitus on the healing of closed fractures. Clin Orthop Relat Res. 1988;232:210–6.
7. Boddenberg U. Healing time of foot and ankle fractures in patients with diabetes mellitus: literature review and report on own cases. Zentralbl Chir. 2004;129:453–9.
8. Ganesh SP, Pietrobon R, Cecílio WAC, Pan D, LightdaleN NJA. The impact of diabetes on patient outcomes after ankle fracture. J Bone Joint Surg Am. 2005;87:1712–8.
9. Flynn JM, Rodriguez-del Río F, Pizá PA. Closed ankle fractures in the diabetic patient. Foot Ankle Int. 2000;21:311–9.
10. Carnevale V, Romagnoli E, D'Erasmo E. Skeletal involvement in patients with diabetes mellitus. Diabetes Metab Res Rev. 2004;20:196–204.
11. Jones KB, Maiers-Yeldon KA, Marsh JL, Zimmerman MB, Estin M, Saltzman CL. Ankle fractures in

patients with diabetes mellitus. J Bone Joint Surg Br. 2005;87:489–95.

12. Centers for Disease Control and Prevention. National Diabetes Statistics Report: Estimates of Diabetes and Its Burden in the United States. Atlanta, GA: U.S. Department of Health and Human Services; 2014. http://www.cdc.gov/diabetes/pubs/statsreport14/national-diabetes-report-web.pdf.

13. Clark JL, Meiris DC. Building bridges: integrative solutions for managing complex comorbid conditions. Am J Med Qual. 2007;22:5–15.

14. Ong KL, Cheung BM, Wong LY, Wat NM, Tan KC, Lam KS. Prevalence, treatment, and control of diagnosed diabetes in the U.S. National Health and Nutrition Examination Survey 199-2004. Ann Epidemiol. 2008;18:222–9.

15. Court-Brown CM, Caesar B. Epidemiology of adult fractures: a review. Injury. 2006;37:691–7.

16. Herbst SA, Jones KB, Saltzman CL. Pattern of diabetic neuropathic arthropathy associated with peripheral bone mineral density. J Bone Joint Surg Br. 2004;86:378–83.

17. Prisk VR, Wukich DK. Ankle fractures in diabetics. Foot Ankle Clin N Am. 2006;11:849863.

18. Smieja M, Hunt DL, Edelman D, Etchells E, Cornuz J, Simel DL. Clinical examination for the detection of protective sensation in the feet of diabetic patients. International Cooperative Group for Clinical Examination Research. J Gen Intern Med. 1999;14:418–24.

19. Pham H, Armstrong DG, Harvey C, Harkless LB, Giurini JM, Veves A. Screening techniques to identify people at high risk for diabetic foot ulceration: a prospective multicenter trial. Diabetes Care. 2000;23:606–11.

20. Wukich DK, Lowery NJ, McMillen RI, Fryberg RG. Postoperative infection rates in foot and ankle surgery: a comparison of patients with and without diabetes mellitus. J Bone Joint Surg Am. 2010;92:287–95.

21. Novo S. Classification, epidemiology, risk factors, and natural history of peripheral artery disease. Diabetes Obes Metab. 2002;4 Suppl 2:S1–6.

22. American Diabetes Association. Peripheral arterial disease in people with diabetes. Diabet Care. 2003;26:3333–41.

23. Høyer C, Sandermann J, Petersen LJ. The toe-brachial index in the diagnosis of peripheral artery disease. J Vasc Surg. 2013;58:231–8.

24. Liu J, Ludwig T, Ebraheim NA. Effect of the blood HbA1c level on surgical treatment outcomes of diabetics with ankle fractures. Orthop Surg. 2013;5:203–8.

25. Wukich DK, Crim BE, Frykberg RG, Rosario BL. Neuropathy and poorly controlled diabetes increase the rate of surgical site infection after foot and ankle surgery. J Bone Joint Surg Am. 2014;96:832–9.

26. Hoogwerf BJ, Sferra J, Bonley BG. Diabetes mellitus—overview. Foot Ankle Clin N Am. 2006;11:703–15.

27. Chaudhary SB, Liporace FA, Gandhi A, Donley BG, Pinzur MS, Lin SS. Complications of ankle fractures in patients with diabetes. J Am Acad Orthop Surg. 2008;16:159–70.

28. Wukich DK, Kline AJ. Current concepts review. The management of ankle fractures in patients with diabetes. J Bone Joint Surg Am. 2008;90:1570–8.

29. McCormack RG, Leith JM. Ankle fractures in diabetics. Complications of surgical management. J Bone Joint Surg Br. 1998;80:689–92.

30. Jani MM, Ricci WM, Borrelli Jr J, Barrett SE, Johnson JE. A protocol for treatment of unstable ankle fractures using transarticular fixation in patients with diabetes mellitus and loss of protective sensation. Foot Ankle Int. 2003;24:838–44.

31. Bozic V, Thordarson DB, Hertz J. Ankle fusion for definitive management of non-reconstructable pilon fractures. Foot Ankle Int. 2008;29:914–8.

32. SooHoo NF, Krenek L, Eagen MJ, Gurbani B, Ko CY, Zingmond DS. Complication rates following open reduction and internal fixation of ankle fractures. J Bone Joint Surg Am. 2009;91:1042–9.

33. Blotter RH, Connolly E, Wasan A, Chapman MW. Acute complications in the operative treatment of isolated ankle fractures in patients with diabetes mellitus. Foot Ankle Int. 1999;20:687–94.

Plate Fixation Techniques for Midfoot and Forefoot Charcot Arthropathy

9

Eric W. Tan and Lew C. Schon

Introduction

Charcot arthropathy remains a significant deforming and destructive process affecting the bones, joints, and soft tissues of the foot and ankle. Though initially described as a complication of syphilis, diabetes mellitus has become the most common etiology of Charcot arthropathy in the United States, with a reported prevalence of 0.08–7.5 % in diabetic patients [1].

The pathophysiology of Charcot arthropathy is poorly understood. However, factors necessary for the development of neuropathic arthropathy include peripheral neuropathy, an unrecognized injury, continued repetitive microtrauma, and increased local circulation [2]. The recognition and treatment of diabetic Charcot arthropathy is important since it may result in progressive deformity and instability, skin breakdown, infection, sepsis, osteomyelitis, and potential loss of limb and life.

The presentation of Charcot changes may vary from a red, swollen foot to a subluxation, dislocation, fracture, or fracture-dislocation [3]. In general, the more proximal the Charcot changes are within the foot, the greater the possibility of long-term instability. The midfoot appears to be the most commonly affected area, presenting in almost 60 % of Charcot feet. Damage to the midfoot bones results in progressive fractures and dislocations, resulting in collapse of the foot. Charcot arthropathy in the forefoot, however, remains uncommon, but when encountered it typically affects the metatarsophalangeal joints. Despite the fact that the midfoot is site of maximal deformity, peak plantar pressures are found in the forefoot [4].

The goals of treatment for Charcot arthropathy are to preserve structural stability, to maintain a plantigrade foot, and to prevent the development of ulcers, infections, and osteomyelitis. Conservative management remains the mainstay of treatment of early changes of Charcot arthropathy and consists primarily of prolonged immobilization in an offloading total contact cast [5]. However, immobilization, with strict non-weightbearing, can often be difficult and can lead to secondary injury and deformity. In fact, nonoperative interventions have been associated with a 2.7 % annual rate of amputation, a 23 % risk of bracing worn for greater than 18 months, and a 49 % risk of recurrent ulcerations [6]. To avoid these problems, surgical fixation and reconstruction are often necessary, especially in patients with recalcitrant wound issues and gross deformities or instability. Surgery, however, is not only technically challenging, but also requires an understanding of

E.W. Tan, M.D. • L.C. Schon, M.D. (✉)
Department of Orthopaedic Surgery, MedStar Union
Memorial Hospital, 3333 N. Calvert St., JPB 400,
Baltimore, MD 21218, USA
e-mail: erictan1423@gmail.com;
lewschon1@gmail.com

© Springer International Publishing Switzerland 2016
D. Herscovici, Jr. (ed.), *The Surgical Management of the Diabetic Foot and Ankle*,
DOI 10.1007/978-3-319-27623-6_9

the appropriate fixation principles and constructs in order to avoid hardware failure, nonunion, and a recurrence of the deformity.

In this chapter, the authors' goal is to provide orthopaedic surgeons with plate fixation techniques, including surgical considerations, deformity classifications, treatment algorithms, and fixation constructs that can be useful for the management of Charcot arthropathy of the midfoot and forefoot.

Classification of Charcot Arthropathy

Diabetic Charcot arthropathy has been classified into three stages by Eichenholtz [7]. Stage I, known as fragmentation, is characterized by erythematous, hot, and swollen joints. Radiographs demonstrate osseous fragmentation with possible periarticular fracture, subluxation, or dislocation. In Stage II, the redness, swelling, and warmth begin to resolve with imaging significant for fusion of the large bony fragments and absorption of fine debris. Fusion of joints and sclerosis of the bone may also be found. Stage III, reconstruction, is the final stage and is characterized by a resolution of the inflammation, bony remodeling, and a progressive deformity of joint architecture. Though only supported by level IV and V data, surgical intervention is not usually recommended during the active inflammatory stage (Stage I) because of the increased risk of wound problems, infection, and bone fixation failure [8]. In addition, Brodsky [9] described an anatomic classification based on three areas (midfoot, hindfoot, ankle) with an additional two areas described by Trepman et al. [10] (multiple regions, forefoot) typically affected in patients with Charcot arthropathy.

Because of the involvement of the midfoot in Charcot arthropathy, Schon et al. [11, 12] developed a classification in an attempt to further delineate deformities of the midfoot and medial column (Fig. 9.1a, b). Their system combines an assess-

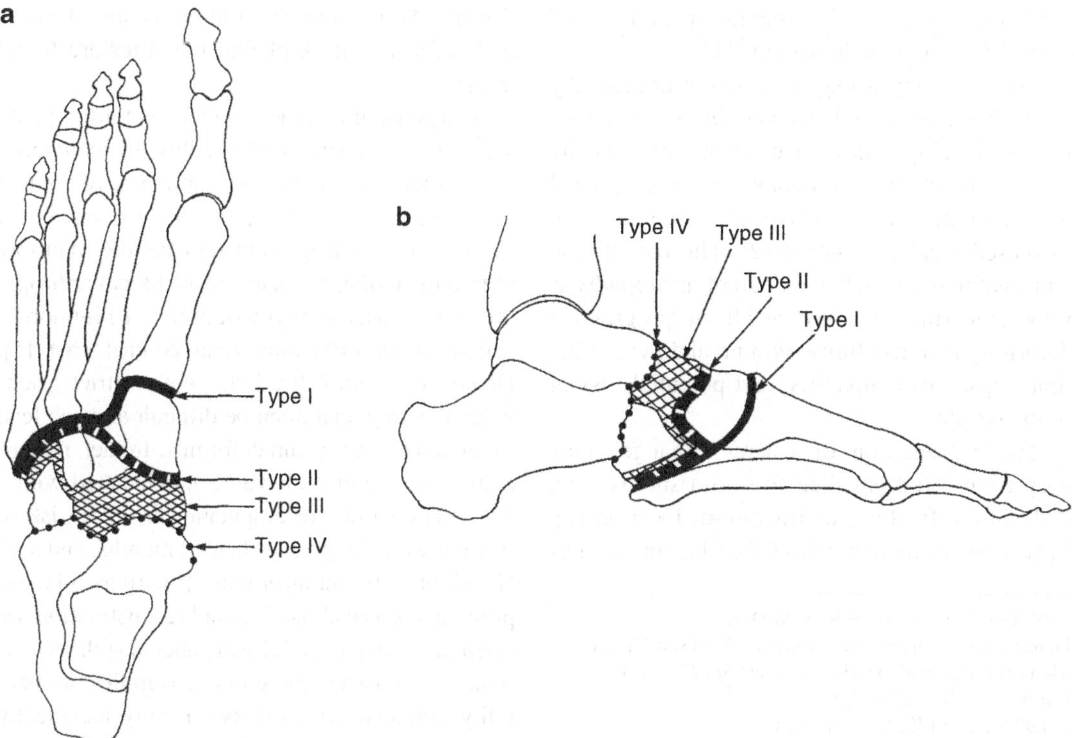

Fig. 9.1 Types of midtarsus deformities seen on the anteroposterior (**a**) and lateral (**b**) views, according to the Schon classification of Charcot arthropathy (Schon et al. [23]). → This image is from Schon et al. (1998). It is an FAI article and this is Fig. 9.3 in that paper. The publisher will need to ask for permission

ment of the clinical severity along with an anatomic-radiographic evaluation of the deformity.

Clinically, the severity of the midfoot deformity can be divided into three stages. Stage A represents a mild collapse of the midfoot arch with low risk for ulceration. In Stage B, the midfoot lies flat to the ground with the midtarsus coplanar to the metatarsocalcaneal plane. Stage C is associated with an obvious rocker-bottom deformity, as the midfoot lies below the level of the metatarsocalcaneal plane. This last stage has been shown to have the highest risk for progressive skin ulceration [12].

Radiographically, the midfoot deformities are be divided into four types. Type I deformities occur initially through the first, second, and third metatarsocuneiform (lisfranc) joints and may progress into the fourth and fifth metatarsocuboid joints. The plantar prominence progresses from medial to lateral and most of these feet are abducted. Type II deformities occur primarily in the naviculocuneiform joint with subsequent involvement of the lateral fourth and fifth metatarsocuboid joints. Here the plantar prominence progresses from lateral to medial. Type III deformities (perinavicular) begin with collapse or fragmentation of the navicular. The foot is typically adducted and supinated with the plantar prominence located laterally. Type IV deformities occur through the transverse tarsal joint. The plantar prominence may be found under the calcaneocuboid joint as well as under the talonavicular joint.

The severity of each of the above radiographic classifications can be further subdivided into two categories—alpha and beta. The beta stage represents a moderate to severe deformity defined by the presence of one or more of the following radiographic findings: (1) dislocation; (2) lateral talar-first metatarsal angle $\geq 30°$; (3) lateral calcaneal-fifth metatarsal angle $\leq 0°$; and (4) anteroposterior talar-first metatarsal angle is $\geq 35°$. If any beta features are present, there is an increased risk of ulceration, infection, and osteomyelitis. If none of the above radiographic findings are present, the alpha stage is assigned and portends a better prognosis.

Considerations for Plate Fixation of the Mid- and Forefoot

The treatment of Charcot arthropathy depends on multiple factors, including the stage of the arthropathy, location of involvement, presence of ulceration or infection, and the ability to achieve a stable, plantigrade foot [13]. Surgical treatment for Charcot arthropathy of the foot and ankle is typically reserved for chronic, recurrent ulcerations or unbraceable, unstable joints. These often present with an associated deformity or contracture of the extremity as well as with acute, displaced fractures often in patients who have adequate circulation [14, 15].

For these patients, the goal of surgery is to realign and stabilize the architecture of the foot and ankle. However, the evidence guiding the surgical management of the midfoot and forefoot is limited [2, 16–18]. Studies have shown that the surgical treatment of the midfoot, using standard methods of single joint fixation with smaller screws, has been associated with a high incidence of hardware failure, delayed unions, and, nonunions [19, 20]. Additionally, fixation constructs using large cannulated screws, one-third tubular plates, Kirschner wires, and staples have also demonstrated high rates of failure [21–23]. To avoid these problems, the surgical treatment of the midfoot will often require a combination of techniques rather than one single method of fixation.

As techniques and implants have evolved, the concept of a superconstruct has been developed to describe techniques that increase stability and reduce the risk of fixation failure [24]. The superconstruct model is based on four factors: (1) fusion extended beyond the injury to include unaffected joints; (2) bone resection to shorten extremity and allow for deformity correction while reducing tension on the soft tissues; (3) use of the strongest device tolerated by the soft tissue envelop; and (4) application of hardware in a position that optimizes mechanical function. Each of these factors represents an important detail in the treatment of Charcot arthropathy of the midfoot and forefoot.

Indications for Plate Fixation

In most cases, the management of chronic Charcot fractures and dislocations in the midfoot, in the absence of ulceration and infection, can be treated with a reduction and fixation versus arthrodesis. The major indication for plate fixation is the correction of a severe deformity, which may or may not involve a bony wedge resection. Plate fixation in this setting provides increased compression and stability. Another indication includes acute fractures of the midfoot and forefoot as plating may result in improved anatomic reduction. In addition, plate fixation is indicated for reconstructions in younger patient as it limits the damage to adjacent, uninvolved joints that can be seen with axial fixation. Because plates provide a stronger construct than axial screws or external fixation, it should be utilized in the obese patient. Good soft tissue envelopes are important for the success of plating.

Contraindications to Plate Fixation

The use of plate fixation is contraindicated in the setting of deep infection, osteomyelitis, inadequate vascularity, and severe medical comorbidities. Relative contraindications include active superficial infection, acute Charcot inflammation, presence of ulcer, a high HgA1c (greater than 7.0), malnutrition, and inadequate bone stock secondary to osteolysis, necrosis, osteopenia, or osteoporosis. Even with the advent of locking plate technology, the quality of the bone and amount of bone stock present are still important considerations; if inadequate, plate fixation may not be contraindicated.

Hierarchy and Considerations for Fixation

Stabilization of the midfoot and forefoot is affected not only by the type of the fixation chosen, but also by the way the fixation is applied to the construct. A hierarchy of fixation exists and should be followed to maximize rigidity and stability. Listed in order, from weakest to strongest, these consist of: (1) application of a dorsal plate or staple without any additional fixation, (2) use of crossed screws (2–3 screws) or compression screw combined with dorsomedial plate fixation, (3) medial-based plate fixation, and (4) plantar-based plate fixation.

The use of a dorsal plate or staple alone, without additional fixation (e.g., oblique compression screw), is not recommended and should be avoided. This construct provides little to no compression and has been demonstrated to be significantly weaker than crossed screw fixation [25]. Fixation on the dorsal aspect of the midfoot places the plate on the compression side of the construct and frequently results in a nonunion with plantar gapping.

The minimum fixation that should be used is either crossed screws or a compression screw with dorsomedial plate fixation. A crossed-screw construct requires that at least 2 screws be used in order to achieve compression at the fracture or arthrodesis site. The addition of a third screw can increase stability of the construct. Gruber et al. [26] compared crossed-screw fixation and dorsomedial plate fixation with compression screw alone for an arthrodesis of the first metatarsocuneiform and found no difference in load to failure or stiffness between the two constructs. Fixation with either a medial or, more preferentially, a plantar plate, with the addition of a compression screw, represents the ideal construct. Placing the plate on the neutral or tension (plantar) side of the midfoot will increase the stability of the construct by converting the forces to compression.

Marks et al. [20] performed a biomechanical study comparing the fixation strength of a plantarly applied midfoot plate to a construct using 3.5-mm cortical screws. Plate constructs placed medially and plantarly stabilize the tension side of the medial column and demonstrated decreased displacement, increased stiffness, and increase load to failure. Clinical studies have also demonstrated successful fusion of the midfoot bones through the use of a plate along the plantar or medial aspect of the medial column [2, 23, 27].

There are, nonetheless, disadvantages associated with plantar plating. The first is that the contour of the bone on the plantar surface is typically irregular, making plating difficult unless contouring of the plantar bony surface is performed. Secondly, the implant can be prominent if placed on the plantar lateral aspect of the fifth metatarsal, underneath the first metatarsal, or if the deformity is left under-corrected leaving the patient with a residual rocker-bottom malalignment. Lastly, placement of the plate along the plantar aspect typically requires a more extensive soft tissue dissection than is required for dorsal plating, especially if the plating is performed through a plantar incision.

Surgical Management of the Midfoot

The quality of the bone will affect he type of plates and screwed utilized. In Charcot arthropathy of the midfoot and forefoot, the quality of bone is typically tenuous. Fixation using a locking plate and screws allows the strength of the fixation to rely on the interface between the screw and the plate rather than the potentially compromised bone. Furthermore, the locking construct may help preserve (the periosteal blood supply and may assist in healing but bad dissections still compromise the anatomy. Zonno and Myerson [28] emphasized the importance of fixed-angular stability of the locking plate, which was demonstrated to be four times the strength of a conventional plate. Despite these benefits, locking plates have limited trajectories for screw placement, which can make fixation difficult in situations with limited bone stock or increased deformity.

Once the decision has been made that fixation will be necessary, a careful examination of the architecture of the midfoot and forefoot is important in determining the type of reduction necessary to correct the deformity. The management of the Charcot midfoot consists of an anatomic reduction, a wedge resection, or a combination of both techniques. In situations with instability, but minimal deformity or malalignment, an anatomic reduction of each fracture and joint is recommended. In addition, isolated bone or joint involvement is amenable for realignment and fixation or fusion. Early and Hansen [16] treated 21 ft with Charcot arthropathy with midfoot collapse. Each foot was treated with reduction and fusion to restore the shape and the mechanical

axis of the foot. Thirteen of 15 patients demonstrated improvement in their feet and in the ability to ambulate. In addition, there was no recurrence of midfoot ulcers. Simon et al. [2] reported results using anatomic reduction and primary arthrodesis on 14 patients with Eichenholtz Stage 1 midfoot Charcot arthropathy. All patients achieved successful fusion and return to walking with no complications, including postoperative ulcerations.

For more significant deformities, such as those involving multiple joints or those that are fixed and immobile, a wedge resection of bone is indicated. This will help realign the foot and correct the plantar deformities that have occurred with collapse of the midfoot. The wedge resection is performed at the apex of the deformity and may be through the medial or lateral columns or, if necessary, through the entire midfoot. In most cases, a bi-planar, plantar-based, closing wedge osteotomy is required to correct a rigid rocker-bottom deformity. The bony resection not only realigns the foot but it also decompresses the skin and joints, which assist in additional reduction of the medial column.

Surgical Approaches

Every effort should be made to preserve motion and the natural mechanics of the foot. In cases of minimal deformity and reducible joints, anatomic fixation is advocated. However, when patients present with rigid deformities and bony destruction, adequate reduction of subluxated or dislocation joints is not always possible [23, 29]. In cases of uncorrectable midfoot collapse, severe rocker bottom deformities, instability, ulceration, and pain, a wedge resection of the midfoot should be considered in order to correct the alignment of the foot. In addition, if the patient does present with a severe deformity, a combination of both medial and lateral surgical approaches may be necessary in order to obtain adequate correction of the foot.

Medial Column Fixation

When medial column fixation is necessary, the authors recommend a medial surgical incision,

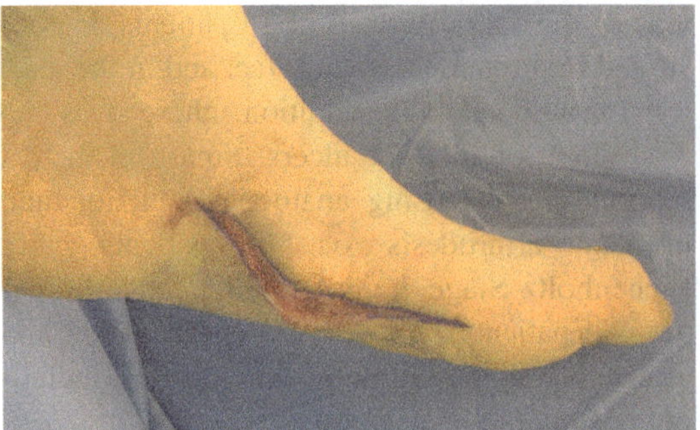

Fig. 9.2 The medial incision is located at the junction of the medial and plantar aspect of the bony contour of the medial column

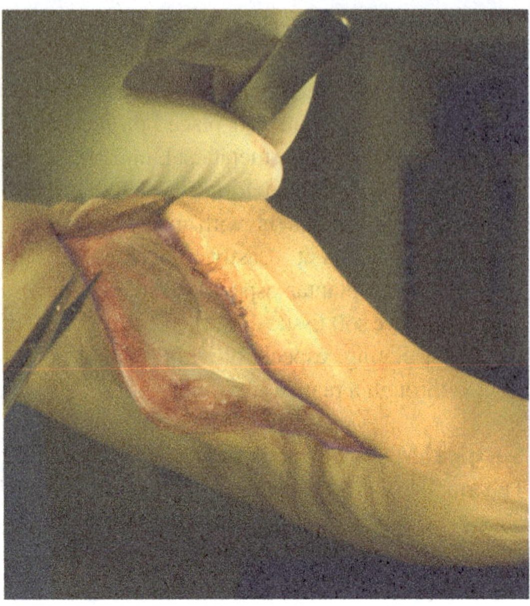

Fig. 9.3 Dissection through the fascia is performed to expose the abductor hallucis muscle

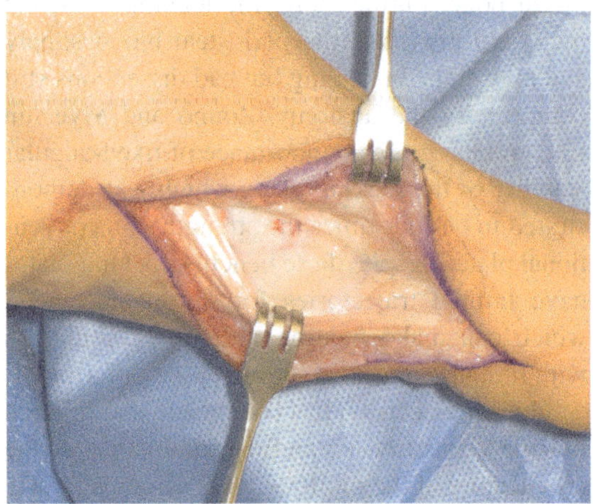

Fig. 9.4 The abductor hallucis muscle is reflected inferiorly to expose the medial periosteal capsular tissues

with subsequent dissection of the plantar tissues. This results in less of a dissection than anticipated for plate fixation of the midfoot. This approach can be used either for anatomic reductions and fixation or when a wedge resection is planned.

The surgical approach is made between the junction of the dorsal and plantar aspects of the medial column (Fig. 9.2) with a sharp dissection carried down towards the adductor hallucis muscle. The abductor fascia is then reflected dorsally with the skin revealing the abductor hallucis muscle (Fig. 9.3). The muscle is then reflected plantarly exposing the medial capsular/periosteal tissues of the first metatarsal, medial cuneiform, and navicular (Fig. 9.4). Electrocautery is then used to elevate and create a capsular periosteal flap, off the first metatarsal and medial cuneiform bones, elevating from plantar to dorsal and leaving a small area of attachment of the footprint of the tibialis anterior tendon (Fig. 9.5). Care is taken to avoid detachment of the tibialis anterior tendon and also to preserve the posterior tibialis tendon insertion on the navicular. The exposure is completed with plantar reflection of the capsular periosteal tissues. Any bony deformity or destruction as well as instability of the first MTC and medial cuneiform, navicular articulations are then clearly visualized.

An anatomic reduction and fixation can be used to manage patients if mobility is identified intraoperatively (Fig. 9.6a, b). This often requires a stress radiograph, which demonstrates some subluxation of the midfoot, irregularities at the fourth and fifth metatarsal-cuboid joints along with instability not only at the first and second MTC joints but also between the medial cuneiform and navicular joint (Fig. 9.7a, b). After the medial exposure has been performed, attention is directed towards reduction of the deformity. By placing pressure on the medial cuneiform towards the cuboid, the medial cuneiform is reduced to the navicular. Next, the cartilage and subchondral plate of the first MTC and

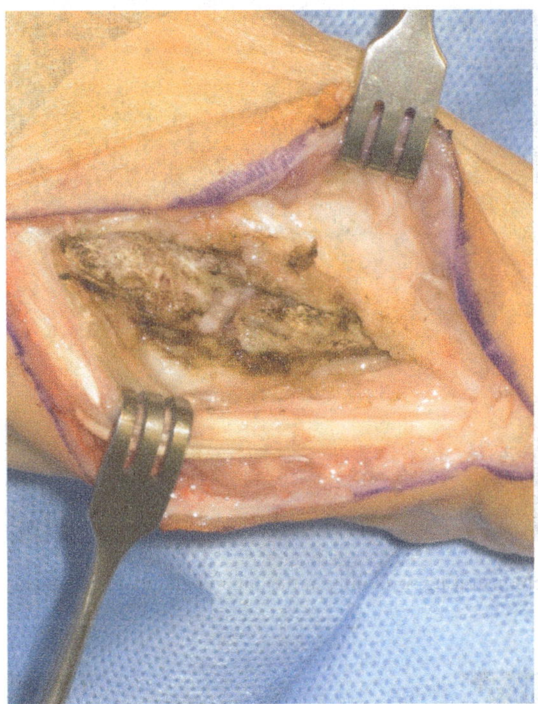

Fig. 9.5 Electrocautery is used to split and elevate the periosteal capsular tissues

medial cuneiform, and navicular articulations are removed. Once the joints are prepared, a large reduction clamp is placed from the medial cuneiform onto the base of the second metatarsal in order to reduce and compress the cuneiform into its original position. Once the reduction is confirmed, the authors' preference is to use guidewires from a 4.0 mm cannulated set to provisionally fix the medial cuneiform to the first metatarsal and the medial cuneiform to the navicular. The fixation is performed by placing the first guidewire from the medial cuneiform towards the base of the first metatarsal and a second guidewire from the medial cuneiform towards the base of the second metatarsal. Fixation across the medial cuneiform-navicular joint is then performed by placing third and fourth guidewires, respectively, from the cuneiform distally into the navicular proximally and then from the medial pole (tuberosity) of the proximal navicular into the middle cuneiform. After measuring and drilling, 4.0 mm cannulated, partially threaded screws are placed across to secure and compress the joints (Fig. 9.8a, b). The screw construct is usually supplemented with plate

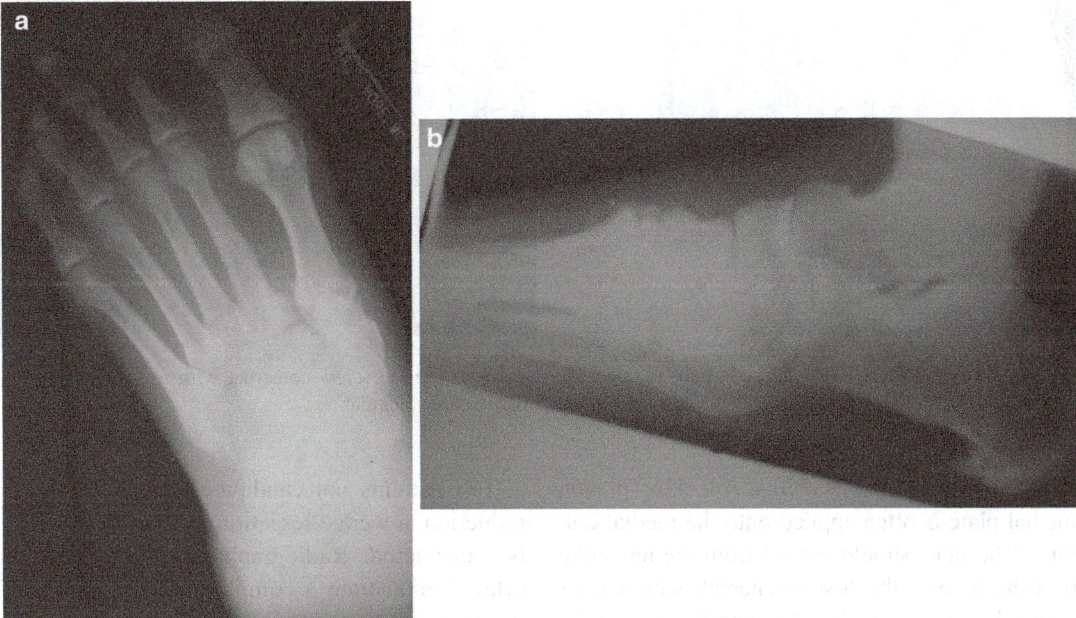

Fig. 9.6 Anteroposterior (**a**) and lateral (**b**) radiographs demonstrating subluxation of the 1st and 2nd metatarsocuneiform joints with irregularities noted at the 4/5/cuboid joint

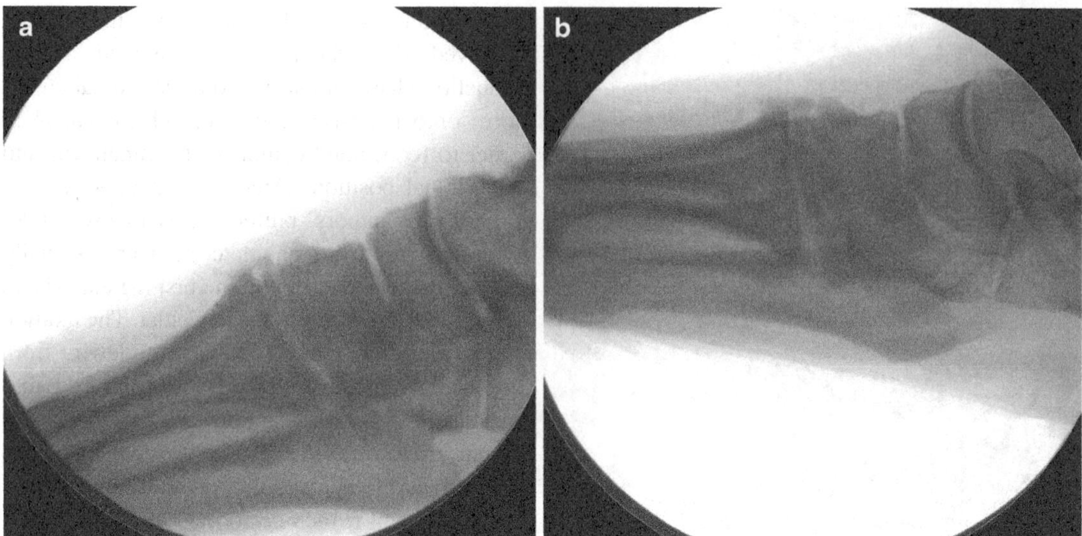

Fig. 9.7 Lateral radiograph (**a**) and stress radiograph (**b**) demonstrating instability at the 1st and 2nd metatarsocuneiform joints as well as the naviculocuneiform joints

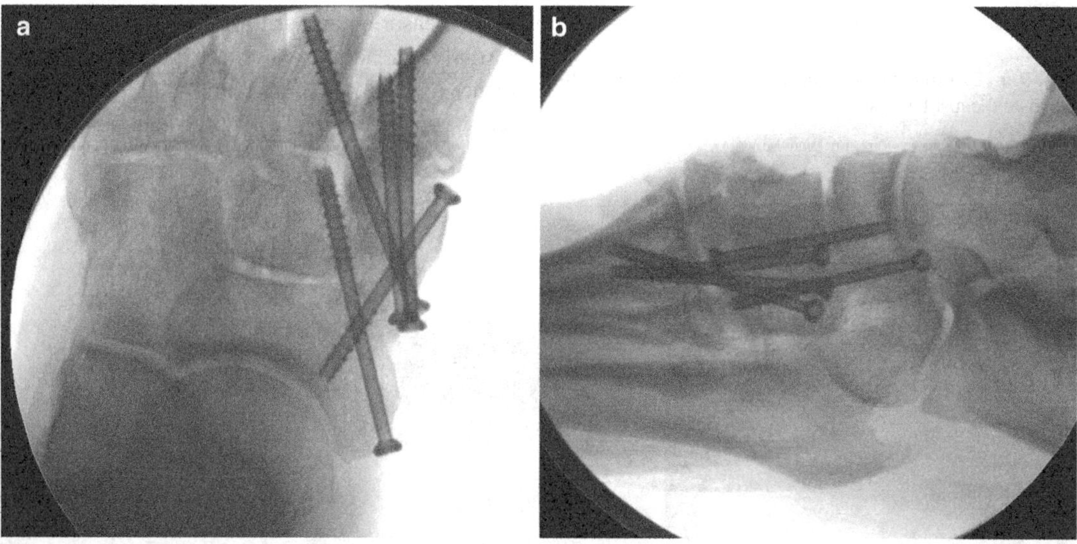

Fig. 9.8 Anteroposterior (**a**) and lateral (**b**) radiographs demonstrating the screw construct with fixation across the medial cuneiform to the 1st metatarsal and the medial cuneiform to the navicular

fixation, for additional stability. A locking plantar medial plate is often applied onto the medial column. The plate should extend from the navicular past the base of the first metatarsal, with screws placed into the navicular, the cuneiforms, and the metatarsal, creating a stable construct of the midfoot (Fig. 9.9a, b).

For patients not candidates for an anatomic reduction, a wedge resection and fixation should be considered. Radiographs for these patients often demonstrate a complete disassociation of the first and second tarsometatarsal joints, subluxation of the lateral cuneiform off the lateral aspect of the navicular, and the bases of the fourth

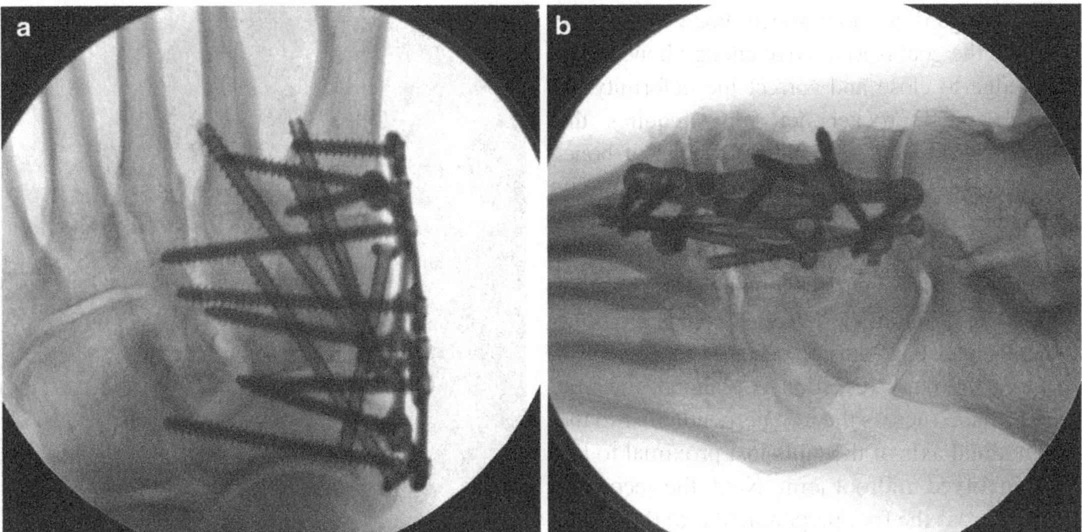

Fig. 9.9 Anteroposterior (**a**) and lateral (**b**) radiographs demonstrating the final construct after a medial plate is applied with screws from the plate into the navicular, cuneiforms, and base of the 1st metatarsal

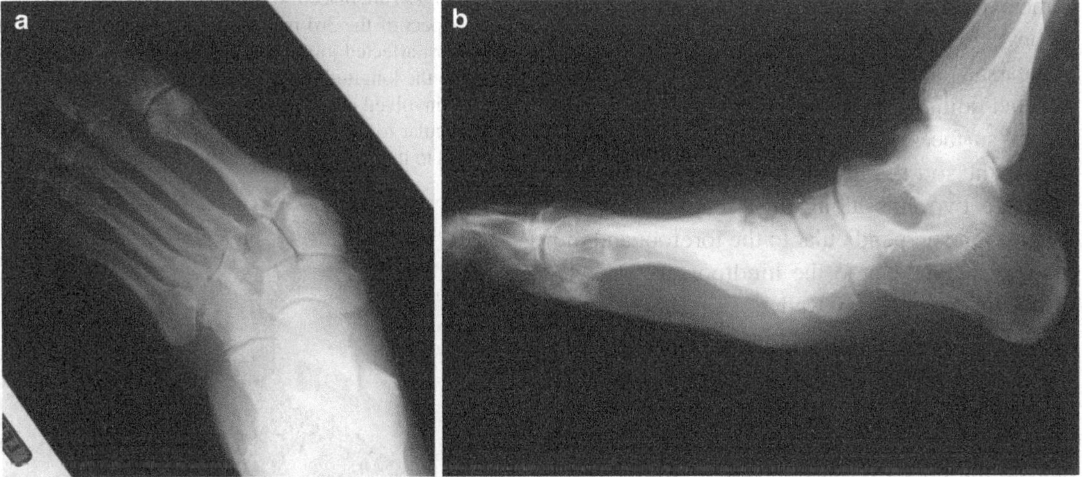

Fig. 9.10 Anteroposterior (**a**) and lateral (**b**) radiographs demonstrating 1st and 2nd tarsometatarsal dissociation and dorsal subluxation of the 4th and 5th tarsometatarsal joints

and fifth metatarsals subluxed and displaced dorsally (Fig. 9.10a, b). On the lateral view, there is often a loss of co-linearity between the talus and first metatarsal along with a negative calcaneal-5th metatarsal angle.

After the medial approach has been performed, Kirschner (k-wires) wires, usually 0.062-in. in diameter, are then placed across the foot to act as a guide for the wedge resection. The deformity is assessed on both AP and lateral views. In most cases, there is an abduction deformity on the AP view and a rocker-bottom deformity on the lateral view. Thus, a plantar-medial closing wedge osteotomy is usually planned. The resected wedge should be made at the apex of the deformity and incorporates the joints that are most affected by Charcot changes. Typically, the most affected joint is one of the following—the first metatarsocuneiform joint, the naviculocuneiform joint, or the talonavicular joint.

With regard to how much bone should be resected, the goal is to remove enough bone to get the wedge to close and correct the deformity. In general, a 30° rocker deformity requires the removal of an 8–10 mm plantar wedge of bone. However, the flexibility of the rocker deformity should be assessed; a more flexible deformity will require less bony resection for correction. In addition, in cases of a translational deformity (e.g., bayonet apposition of bones), a block of bone rather than a wedge may be need to be resected.

Once the bony resection is planned, the first wire is placed across the foot perpendicular to the longitudinal axis of the talus just proximal to the most involved midfoot joint. Next, the second is placed across the foot perpendicular to the longitudinal axis of the first metatarsal just distal to the most involved midfoot joint.

In this particular case example, the apex of the deformity occurs through the first and second tarsometatarsal joints. The wedge is planned so that it converges towards the lateral aspect of the third metatarsal, allowing for resection of the most affected joints (Fig. 9.11). On the dorsal and plantar surfaces, Homan retractors are inserted to protect the soft tissues. Next, a large saw is used to create two cuts along the previously placed k-wires, one perpendicular to the forefoot and the other perpendicular to the hindfoot, in order to resect the desired bony wedge. Dorsally, the cuts converge onto the lateral border of the third metatarsal, and care is taken not to penetrate the dorsal cortex of the midfoot and violate the neurovascular structures or tendons. The surgeon should then palpate the dorsal tissues and be mindful of the depth of the blade. Chisels and osteotomes are used to complete the cut and remove the wedge of bone that contains the first, second, and third metatarsocuneiform articulations (Fig. 9.12). The resected wedge can be morselized and used for bone graft, if necessary.

On the lateral surface of the foot, the fourth and fifth metatarsal-cuboid joints are reduced with careful attention to make certain that the metatarsal bases remain colinear with the cuboid. *See the next section discussing the surgical approach and preparation of the lateral foot.* Reduction is achieved by plantar flexing and adducting the foot through the midfoot joints. In most cases, the

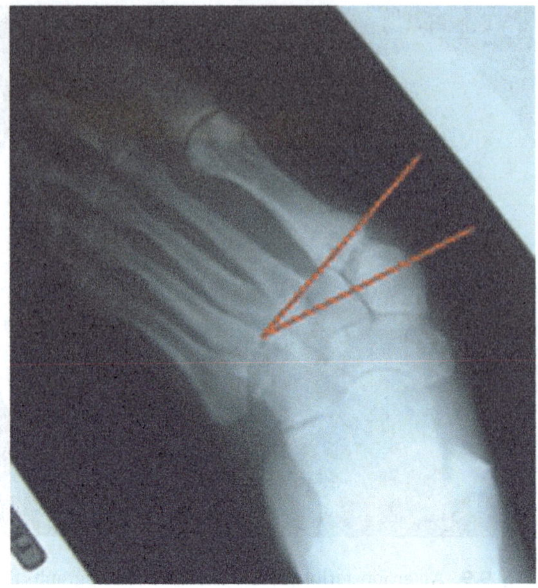

Fig. 9.11 With the apex of the deformity occurring through the 1st and 2nd tarsometatarsal joints, k-wires (shown in *red*) are placed so that they converge towards the lateral aspect of the 3rd metatarsal, allowing for resection of the most affected joints. The first wire is placed perpendicular to the longitudinal axis of the talus just proximal to the most involved midfoot joint. Next, the second is placed perpendicular to the longitudinal axis of the 1st metatarsal just distal to the most involved midfoot joint

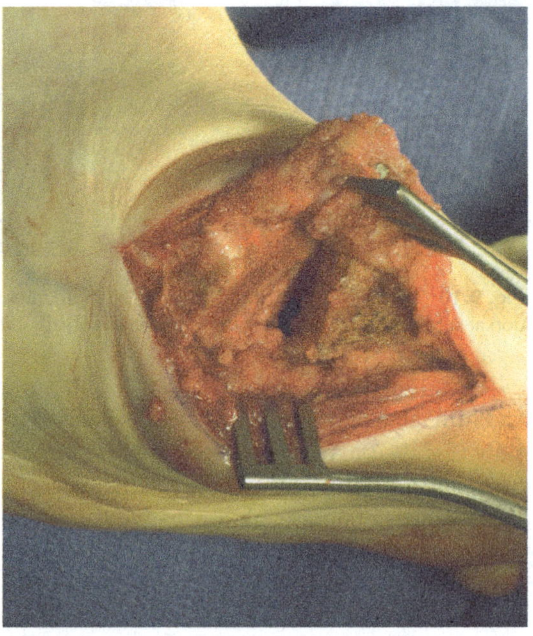

Fig. 9.12 The medial column after the resected wedge of bone containing the 1st, 2nd, and 3rd metatarsocuneiform articulations is removed

reduction is performed manually without clamps and provisionally fixed with k-wires. After the reduction has been confirmed the authors' preference is to use two parallel guidewires, from a 4.0 mm cannulated screw set and place them percutaneously at the plantar lateral aspect of the base of the 5th metatarsal at the meta-diaphyseal flare, aiming from plantar distal to proximal dorsal, and into the cuboid (Fig. 9.13). Next, the medial column is held reduced by placing two guidewires from the plantar medial aspect of the base of the 1st metatarsal into the medial cuneiform and navicular and then a second guidewire from the medial cuneiform proximally heading distally into the metatarsal. Manual compression helps during the placement of these guidewires. After the reduction is confirmed, 4.0 mm cannulated screws are placed over the guidewires. As with an anatomic reduction, a locking plantar medial plate is applied underneath the 1st metatarsal and medial cuneiform with screws going from plantar to dorsal (Fig. 9.14a, b).

Lateral Column Fixation

The lateral column of the foot is composed of the fourth and fifth metatarsals as well as the cuboid. It has been identified as having approximately 10° of motion in dorsiflexion-plantarflexion and supination-pronation [30]. The motion at the lat-

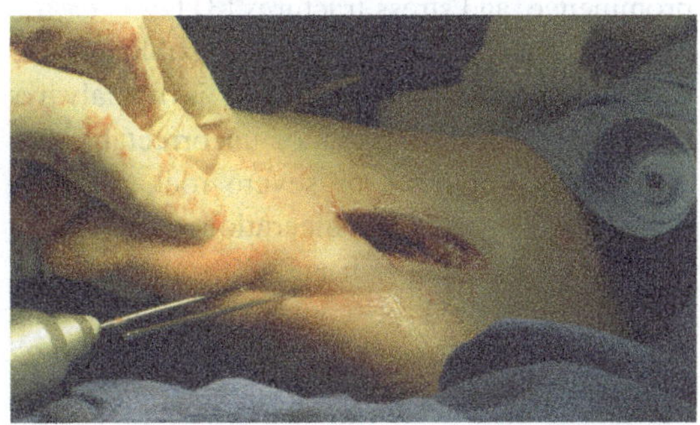

Fig. 9.13 Two parallel guidewires are placed percutaneously at the plantar lateral aspect of the foot going from the base of the 5th metatarsal at the meta-diaphyseal flare aiming from plantar distal to proximal dorsal into the cuboid

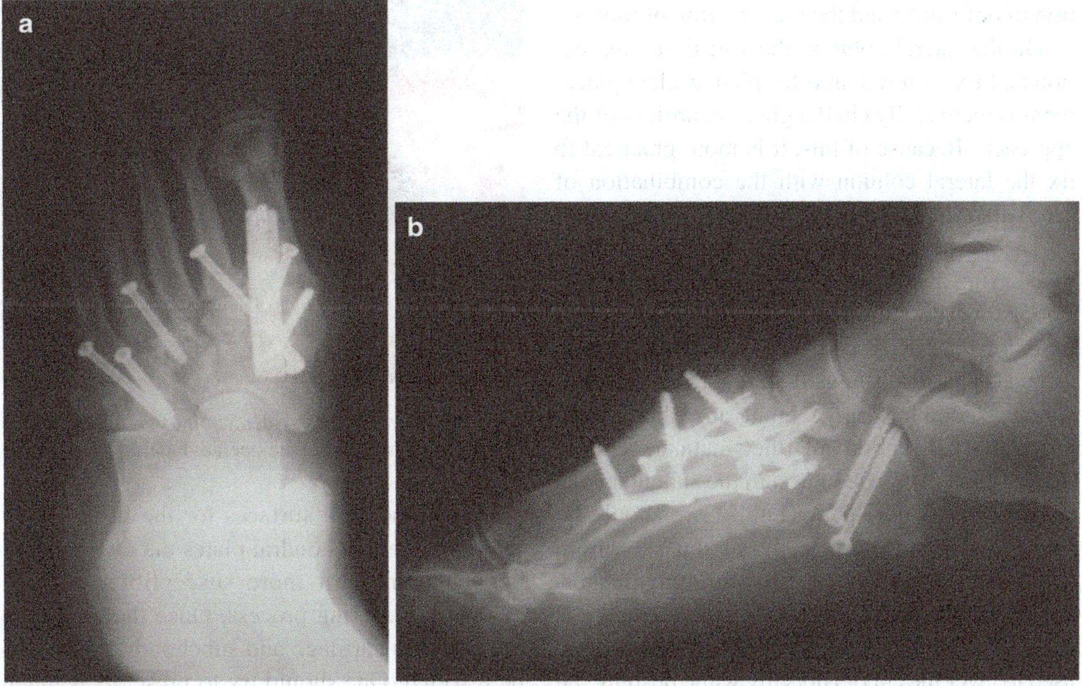

Fig. 9.14 Anteroposterior (**a**) and lateral (**b**) radiographs demonstrating the final construct after placement of a plantar medial plate underneath the 1st metatarsal and medial cuneiform

eral two midfoot joints is up to three times greater than the motion found in the medial three joints, making the lateral column responsible for almost all of the motion that occurs through the midfoot. Because of inherent motion within the lateral midfoot joints, there is concern that arthrodesis of these joints may result in complications including nonunion, chronic lateral foot pain, rigid prominence, and stress fractures [31].

However, adequate reduction of subluxated or dislocation lateral column joints is not always possible [23, 29]. In cases of uncorrectable lateral midfoot collapse or severe rocker-bottom deformity, instability, ulceration, and pain, arthrodesis of the fourth and fifth metatarsocuboid joints should be considered. Raikin and Schon [32] demonstrated good results in 26 of 28 ft treated with arthrodesis of the lateral midfoot joints (22 complete midfoot arthrodesis for Charcot rocker-bottom deformity and six in normosensate feet with painful arthritis). Significant improvements in pain, dysfunction, and AOFAS midfoot scores were achieved. Therefore, the treatment of lateral column midfoot issues involves a complex interplay between the correction of deformity and the preservation of motion.

On the lateral column, the soft tissue dissection and fixation required for plantar plate placement is technically challenging, regardless of the approach. Because of this, it is more practical to fix the lateral column with the combination of screw fixation and dorsal plating.

The surgical approach to the lateral column is made using a dorsolateral approach. The incision is begun distal to and between the subluxated bases of the fourth and fifth metatarsals and is extended proximally towards the cuboid (Fig. 9.15). Using a combination of blunt and sharp techniques, a dissection of the metatarsocuboid (MTC) joints is carried through the subcutaneous tissues down to the periosteum. Care should be used to identify and protect the sural nerve within the operative field (Fig. 9.16). Once the metatarsal bases are exposed, a periosteal elevator is inserted along the plantar aspect of the joints and used to lever the cuboid dorsally while pushing the fourth and fifth metatarsals distally and plantarly. This maneuver is performed prior to cutting or

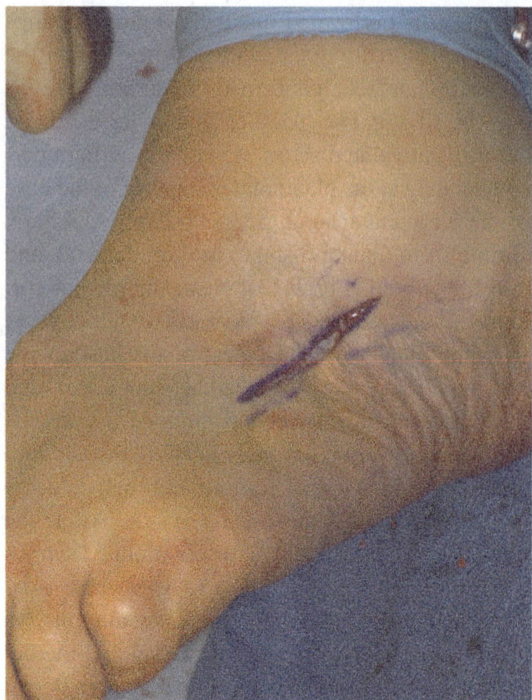

Fig. 9.15 A dorsolateral approach is made over the subluxated 4th and 5th metatarsocuneiform joints

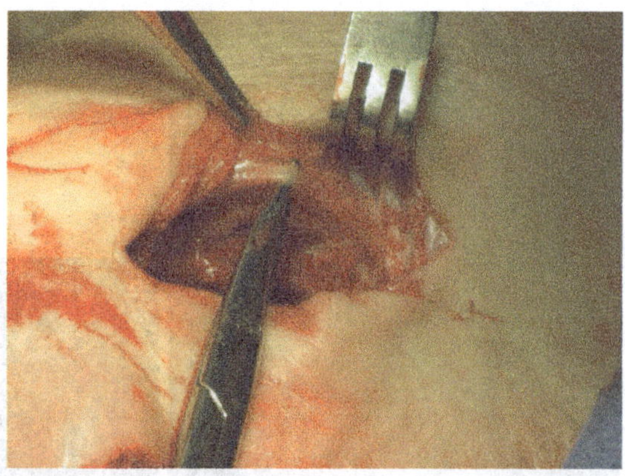

Fig. 9.16 Care is taken to identify and to retract branches of the sural nerve within the operative field

preparing the joint surfaces for the fusion since violating the subchondral plates may weaken the bone and make it more susceptible to crush during the levering process. Once the bones are reduced, the cartilage and subchondral plate can be resected. One should try to preserve as much bone stock as possible and to limit the amount of bony shortening that can occur.

Closures and Releases

During wound closure, the medial periosteal flap is reconnected, bringing back down the sleeve that contained some of the tibialis anterior tendon down to the bone. The abductor fascia is re-approximated over the abductor muscle. Finally, the subcutaneous tissues are closed with 4-0 Vicryl and skin is closed with 2-0 or 3-0 nylon stitches.

In order to decrease pressure off of the forefoot and midfoot, a Strayer gastrocnemius recession is often performed through a medial incision. This release can allow the patient up to 20° of ankle dorsiflexion. Alternatively, a tendo-Achilles lengthening may be performed. The patient is then placed into a well-padded, short-leg splint with the ankle at neutral.

Postoperative Management

At 10–14 days postoperatively, patients are seen and their wounds are assessed. They are transitioned into a cam-walker boot and instructed to remain non-weightbearing for 12 weeks. Stitches are removed between 2 and 4 weeks after surgery depending on the status of the wound.

At 12 weeks postoperatively, radiographs are taken. If the radiographs do not demonstrate any issues with healing or hardware, the patient starts partial weightbearing in the boot with advancement to full weightbearing over the next 3–6 months.

Complications and Salvage Procedures

The major complications associated with reconstructions of midfoot and forefoot include nonunions, hardware failure, the recurrence or progression of the deformity, ulcerations, and infections, any of which may ultimately lead to an amputation.

Preventing nonunions, deformity progression, and hardware failure requires adequate bony fixation, stabilization, and prolonged immobilization and limited weightbearing. These complications are, in most cases, the result of early weightbearing, as the cyclical loading will interfere with postoperative healing. When any of these three complications occur, the plate fixation should be revised. When failure occurs in the adjacent joints proximal to the surgical site, which in the authors' experience occurs approximately 10 % of the time, the new deformity should be reduced and fixed with a longer plate, with the possible placement of additional cannulated screws. In the setting of nonunion, the plate should be revised to a thicker or longer size. Furthermore, the cannulated screws should be removed and replaced with the next larger size; additional screws may be added for increased stability. Bone marrow aspirate concentrate and local autograft from resected bone may be added to the construct. The addition of a bone stimulator is not recommended and may lead to increased complications [33].

Alternatively, the construct can be supplemented or substituted with axial intramedullary screws or external fixation. In most cases, the size of the axial screws is 4.0 mm in the midfoot and 6.5 mm in hindfoot. The screws are placed either perpendicular to or obliquely across the plane of the wedge or arthrodesis site. The use of plate fixation typically obviates the need for an external fixator. However, in the setting of an infection or limited or inadequate bone stock, an external fixator may be useful. When placed, the frame is typically placed co-planar with the foot. The authors prefer the placement of a wire fixator with two wires in the hindfoot (one above and one below the frame) and two wires in the forefoot (one above and one below the frame) with compression using the bent wire technique.

Another consequence of fusion of the foot is a stress transfer to the adjacent joints, which may trigger a progression in the Charcot process. In the authors' experience, this occurs in approximately 10 % of cases. The exact mechanism of how this occurs in unclear. However, the increased stress to adjacent joints may result in increased inflammation and synovitis which may exacerbate the Charcot process. When it occurs, it is necessary to unload and rest the foot and ankle. This may be performed in different ways including bracing, casting, foot orthotics, and accommodative shoeware (rigid-soled, rocker heel, extra-depth, etc.). If conservative methods fail, further surgery may be necessary in order to extend the fusion to include the adjacent joints. Furthermore, patients need to be counseled that, in the authors' experience, 30 % of cases will develop Charcot arthropathy in the contralateral foot or ankle.

Prior to any surgical intervention, ulcerations and osteomyelitis should be treated and allowed to heal. Postoperative wound infections can often be treated with oral antibiotics and surgical debridement should be used if conservative measures fail. In the authors' experience, wound infections requiring local wound care and antibiotics occur in 5 % of cases; only 1 % of cases will require a return to the operating room. For infections without bony involvement, patients can be treated with an irrigation and debridement of the wound. In addition, the authors recommend placement of calcium sulfate dissolvable beads (Stimulan, Biocomposites, Ltd., Keele, UK) mixed with vancomycin (1000 mg) and gentamycin (240 mg) or tobramycin (240 mg). In the setting of deeper infections or osteomyelitis, surgical intervention involves removal of all hardware, irrigation and debridement, antibiotic bead placement, and possible application of a negative pressure dressing. An external fixator may be applied to maintain correction or stability of the foot. Postoperatively, an infectious disease consult is obtained and oral or intravenous antibiotics are administered as recommended. In most cases, antibiotics are required for at least 6 weeks before a return to the operating room is possible.

If ulcerations result, due to the development of a bony prominence, a limited exostectomy can be performed in order to reduce the area of increased pressure. In the authors' experience, this occurs less than 5 % of the time after initial surgical reconstruction. Initial treatment involves conservative care, such as total contact casting or accommodative shoeware. With failure of nonoperative interventions or progression of the ulceration, surgical intervention is warranted. Postoperatively, the patient is immobilized and made non-weightbearing for 4–6 weeks.

Symptomatic, painful hardware is typically not encountered after Charcot reconstructions of the midfoot and forefoot. In midfoot reconstructions, a plantar plate is typically placed on the arch of the foot making it less likely to be problematic with weightbearing. If present, the hardware may be removed once the bone is healed which is usually at 12 months postoperatively.

References

1. Reiber GE, Lipsky BA, Gibbons GW. The burden of diabetic foot ulcers. Am J Surg. 1998;176:5S–10.
2. Simon SR, Tejwani SG, Wilson DL, Santner TJ, Denniston NL. Arthrodesis as an early alternative to nonoperative management of Charcot arthropathy of the diabetic foot. J Bone Joint Surg Am. 2000; 82A:939–50.
3. Johnson JE, Klein SE, Brodsky JW. Diabetes. In: Coughlin MJ, Saltzman CL, Anderson RB, editors. Surgery of the foot and ankle. St. Louis, MO: Mosby; 2013. p. 1385–480.
4. Armstrong DG, Lavery LA. Elevated peak plantar pressures in patients who have Charcot arthropathy. J Bone Joint Surg Am. 1998;80A:365–9.
5. Myerson MS, Henderson MR, Saxby T, Short KW. Management of midfoot diabetic neuroarthropathy. Foot Ankle Int. 1994;15:233–41.
6. Saltzman CL, Hagy ML, Zimmerman B, Estin M, Cooper R. How effective is intensive nonoperative initial treatment of patients with diabetes and Charcot arthropathy of the feet? Clin Orthop Relat Res. 2005;435:185–90.
7. Eichenholtz S. Charcot joints. Springfield, Ill: Charles C Thomas; 1966.
8. Lowery NJ, Woods JB, Armstrong DG, Wukich DK. Surgical management of Charcot neuroarthropathy of the foot and ankle: a systematic review. Foot Ankle Int. 2012;33:113–21.
9. Brodsky JW. The diabetic foot. In: Mann RA, Coughlin MJ, editors. Surgery of the foot and ankle. St Louis, MO: Mosby; 1999. p. 1385–480.
10. Trepman E, Nihal A, Pinzur MS. Current topics review: Charcot neuroarthropathy of the foot and ankle. Foot Ankle Int. 2005;26(1):46–63.
11. Schon LC, Easley ME, Cohen I, Lam PW, Badekas A, Anderson CD. The acquired midtarsus deformity classification system, interobserver reliability and intraobserver reproducibility. Foot Ankle Int. 2002;23(1):30–6.
12. Schon LC, Weinfeld SB, Horton GA, Resch S. Radiographic and clinical classification of acquired midtarsus deformities. Foot Ankle Int. 1998;19: 394–404.
13. Wukick DK, Sung W. Charcot arthropathy of the foot and ankle: modern concepts and management review. J Diabetes Complications. 2009;23:409–26.

14. Burns PR, Wukich DK. Surgical reconstruction of the Charcot rearfoot and ankle. Clin Podiatr Med Surg. 2008;25:95–120.
15. Garapati R, Weinfeld SB. Complex reconstruction of the diabetic foot and ankle. Am J Surg. 2004; 187:81–6.
16. Early JS, Hansen ST. Surgical reconstruction of the diabetic foot: a salvage approach for midfoot collapse. Foot Ankle Int. 1996;17:325–30.
17. Sammarco GJ, Conti SF. Surgical treatment of neuroarthropathic foot deformity. Foot Ankle Int. 1998; 19:102–9.
18. Tisdel CL, Marcus RE, Heiple KG. Triple arthrodesis for diabetic peritalar neuroarthropathy. Foot Ankle Int. 1995;16:332–8.
19. Bono JV, Roger DJ, Jacobs RL. Surgical arthrodesis of the neuropathic foot: a salvage procedure. Clin Orthop Relat Res. 1993;296:14–20.
20. Marks RM, Parks BG, Schon LC. Midfoot fusion technique for neuropathic feet: biomechanical analysis and rationale. Foot Ankle Int. 1998;19:507–10.
21. Papa J, Myerson M, Girard P. Salvage, with arthrodesis, in intractable diabetic neuropathic arthropathy of the foot and ankle. J Bone Joint Surg. 1993; 75-A:1056–66.
22. Pinzur MS, Sage R, Stuck R, Kaminsky S, Zmuda A. A treatment algorithm for neuropathic (Charcot) midfoot deformity. Foot Ankle Int. 1993;14:189–97.
23. Schon LC, Easley ME, Weinfeld SB. Charcot neuroarthropathy of the foot and ankle. Clin Orthop. 1998;349:116–31.
24. Sammarco VJ. Superconstructs in the treatment of Charcot foot deformity: plantar plating, locked plating, and axial screw fixation. Foot Ankle Clin. 2009; 14:393–407.
25. Cohen DA, Parks BG, Schon LC. Screw fixation compared to H-locking plate fixation for first metatarsocuneiform arthrodesis: a biomechanical study. Foot Ankle Int. 2005;26:984–9.
26. Gruber F, Sinkov VS, Bae SY, Parks BG, Schon LC. Crossed screws versus dorsomedial locking plate with compression screw for first metatarsocuneiform arthrodesis: a cadaver study. Foot Ankle Int. 2008;29(9):927–30.
27. Horton GA, Olney BW. Deformity correction and arthrodesis of the midfoot with a medial plate. Foot Ankle. 1993;14:493–9.
28. Zonno AJ, Myerson MS. Surgical correction of midfoot arthritis with and without deformity. Foot Ankle Clin. 2011;16(1):35–47.
29. Schon LC, Bell W. Fusions of the transverse tarsal and midtarsal joints. Foot Ankle Clin. 1996;1: 93–108.
30. Ouzounian TJ, Shereff MJ. In vitro determination of midfoot motion. Foot Ankle. 1989;10:140–6.
31. Komenda GA, Myerson MS, Biddinger KR. Results of arthrodesis of the tarsometatarsal joints after traumatic injury. J Bone Joint Surg Am. 1996;78(11):1665–76.
32. Raikin SM, Schon LC. Arthrodesis of the fourth and fifth tarsometatarsal joints of the midfoot. Foot Ankle Int. 2003;24(8):584–90.
33. Lau JT, Stamatis ED, Myerson MS, Schon LC. Implantable direct-current bone stimulators in high-risk and revision foot and ankle surgery: a retrospective analysis with outcome assessment. Am J Orthop (Belle Mead NJ). 2007;36(7):354–7.

Treatment of Charcot Midfoot Deformity by Arthrodesis Using Long Axial Screws

10

V. James Sammarco

Introduction

Management of Charcot foot deformity in diabetics is particularly challenging because of the effects that diabetes mellitus has on multiple organ systems. There is a "perfect storm" of mechanical and biologic problems, which often leads to poor outcome in these patients. Peripheral neuropathy leads to loss of protective sensation and autonomic dysfunction, which can lead to ulceration. Even minor trauma can lead to fracture and dislocation in the foot, which may go unnoticed by the patient until a severe deformity occurs. Once the normal weight bearing architecture of the foot is lost, bony prominences increase local pressures and cause a breakdown of the soft tissue envelope. Impaired immune capability due to decreased macrophage function in glycosylated tissues makes infection more likely and also more difficult to eradicate. Atherosclerosis of both large and small vessels often accompanies diabetes and significantly complicates matters by decreasing arterial perfusion. These factors combined with poor cardiac function, venous stasis, obesity and the patients' inability to remain non-weight bearing, combine to make complications frequent. For these reasons, diabetes and related complications continue to be the leading cause of amputation in the United States with an estimated 70,000 amputations per year [1].

Conservative care of the Charcot foot consisting of offloading of ulcers with contact casting and accommodative bracing remains the mainstay of treatment. Traditionally, surgery was reserved for those cases that presented with recurrent ulceration and usually consisted of an exostectomy. Early surgical series, where surgical correction of severe deformity was done with midfoot arthrodesis, provided little evidence that a more aggressive surgical approach provided better long-term results than nonoperative care. These series used standard fixation techniques such as crossed screws, Kirschner wires, and simple neutralization plates. Complications were frequent including loss of fixation, hardware failure, and recurrence of deformity [2].

More recently, studies have questioned the validity of delaying surgical correction of progressive neuroarthropathic deformity. Saltzman and colleagues retrospectively evaluated 115 patients treated over a twenty year period [3]. One hundred and twenty seven limbs were treated with a standardized clinical protocol that emphasized nonsurgical care. Forty-seven percent of patients required extensive bracing that lasted more than 18 months and the risk of recurrent ulceration was 40 %. These authors concluded that even diligent nonsurgical treatment

V.J. Sammarco, M.D. (✉)
Reconstructive Orthopaedics and Sports Medicine,
Cincinnati, OH, USA
e-mail: vjsammarco@gmail.com

© Springer International Publishing Switzerland 2016
D. Herscovici, Jr. (ed.), *The Surgical Management of the Diabetic Foot and Ankle*,
DOI 10.1007/978-3-319-27623-6_10

133

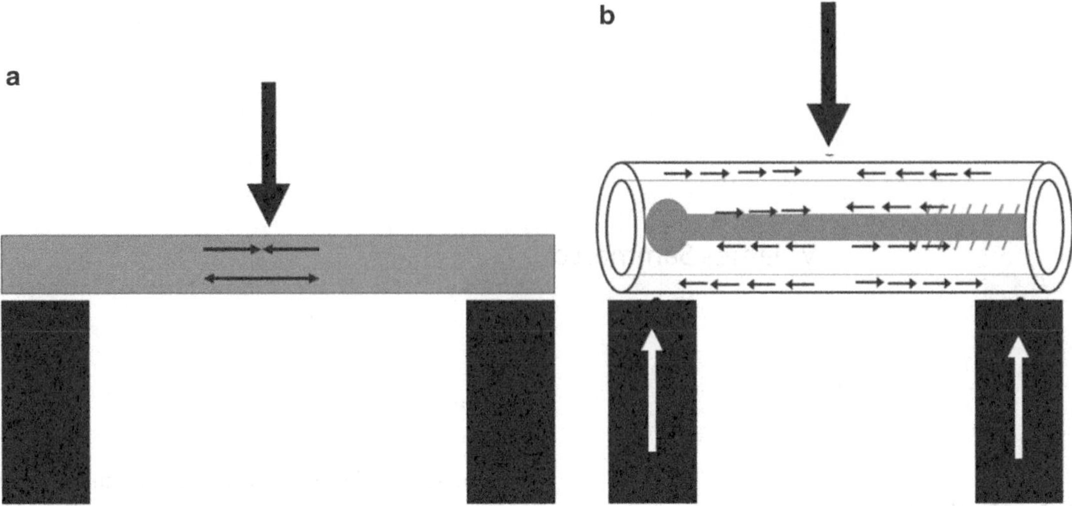

Fig. 10.1 (**a**) In a beam model of the foot, force applied centrally in the beam will generate tensile forces plantarly and compressive forces dorsally. (**b**) Screws applied axially will share compressive and tensile forces to resist deformation

can be associated with poor outcome and that better methods of treatment were necessary. Simon and colleagues reported on early surgical intervention in patients with Charcot midfoot neuroarthropathy in Eichenholtz stage I disease [4]. Fourteen patients were treated with midfoot arthrodesis. Successful results were reported for all patients. All patients returned to functional ambulation with standard diabetic and off-the-shelf shoe wear. No recurrent deformity or ulceration was reported. These and other studies suggest that corrective surgical treatment may be associated with better functional outcome than a plan which emphasizes nonsurgical care [5].

Techniques have evolved to correct Charcot midfoot deformity: plantar plating, locked plating, and axial screw fixation. The axial screw technique was developed as a method to improve fixation and stability in patients undergoing reconstruction for Charcot midfoot disease. We coined the term "superconstruct" to describe fixation techniques specifically designed for these challenging Charcot midfoot cases [6]. A superconstruct is defined by four factors: (1) fusion is extended beyond the zone of injury to include joints that are not affected to improve fixation,

(2) bone resection is performed to shorten the limb to allow for adequate reduction of deformity without undue tension on the soft tissue envelope, (3) the strongest device is used that can be tolerated by the soft tissue envelope, and (4) the devices are applied in a position that maximizes mechanical stability.

Axial screw fixation involves the placement of intraosseous screws which span the area of deformity and fix the proximal and distal fusion segments. Screws are placed such that they bridge the zone of dislocation from the intramedullary canals of the metatarsals and extending into the less compromised bone proximally. Larger diameter screws can be used without creating stress risers in the metatarsal shafts as occurs when transcortical screws are used. The intraosseous position of the screws aids in realignment of the foot. The procedure can be done through a more limited approach with less osseous stripping than is needed for plating, and the intraosseous position diminishes the risk of exposed hardware in the event of poor wound healing compared to other techniques. Biomechanically, the screws act as load sharing devices similar to steel rebar in concrete (Fig. 10.1).

Indications

The indications for surgical reconstruction of the Charcot foot are relative and must be balanced with the patient's overall health, circulatory status, their ability to control blood glucose levels, and in their ability to comply with extended periods of non-weight bearing. Diabetic medical comorbidities including cardiac disease, renal disease, and peripheral edema can contribute to poor wound healing and infection. Therefore, medical optimization by the patient's internal medicine physician is necessary prior to proceeding with surgery. In addition, peripheral arterial disease, in particular, is problematic and warrants formal evaluation with arterial Doppler examination if pulses are weak or absent. Transcutaneous oxygen perfusion can be measured as an excellent indicator of wound healing potential. If there is poor perfusion of the foot, the patient should be evaluated for revascularization by a vascular interventionist or surgeon.

Charcot midfoot deformity has been classified by Sammarco and Conti [7] and by Schon et al. [8]. Both classifications are anatomic and are based on the level of dislocation with some variation between the two. The Schon classification is subdivided with a separate designation (Beta) for cases where the deformity is severe, or where the midfoot is dislocated (Table). Schon also presented a clinical classification system with Grade C being a rocker bottom foot deformity.

We consider the indications for surgical correction of neuropathic foot deformity by midtarsal osteotomy and arthrodesis to be: (1) Patients with a non-plantigrade foot (Schon Type C) who have recurrent ulcerations despite conservative management, (2) Radiographs demonstrating a Schon type beta severity, and (3) Patients with gross instability or progression of deformity despite immobilization and casting. Ideally, patients undergoing an arthrodesis with internal fixation should be infection and ulcer free. Often Wagner Grade 1 and 2 ulcers can be effectively resolved with a period of contact casting and/or non-weight bearing. If osteomyelitis is present, or if ulcers do not show signs of healing with simple off-weighting, we prefer a staged procedure with external fixation. In the absence of ulceration, surgery can be done once medical clearance has been obtained. In the presence of significant edema, reduction of swelling by off-weighting the foot, immobilization in a cast or boot walker, and judicious use of an Unna boot wrap can improve the soft tissue envelope preoperatively.

Surgical Technique

The minimal equipment needed to perform this technique includes: (1) An image intensifier, (2) A microsagittal saw, for bone resection, and (3) Reduced head or headless cannulated screws. Multiple long length screws (up to 120 mm) should be available. A variety of diameter screws should also be available ranging from 4.0 to 8.0 mm.

The patient is positioned supine on a beanbag to allow the operative leg and the body to be supported to correct for external rotation of the leg so that foot is perpendicular to the operating table. This allows better access to the lateral aspect of the foot. A pneumatic tourniquet is placed around the proximal thigh. The leg is prepped and draped above the knee. The ankle can then be supported by stacked towels or a bump under the leg to facilitate fluoroscopy.

An equinus deformity is invariably present and must be aggressively corrected prior to performing the midfoot correction. An intraoperative Silfverskiold's test is performed and if positive, a gastrocnemius recession is done. Alternately, a three-step tendo Achilles lengthening can be performed of the deformity if equinus is present with the knee in knee flexion and extension. However, both procedures may be necessary if the equinus deformity is rigid and fixed. The goal is to achieve $10°–15°$ of ankle dorsiflexion with the knee in full extension.

Approach

The approach is tailored to the level of the dislocation. Longitudinal incisions are made medially, dorsally, and laterally as needed (Fig. 10.2).

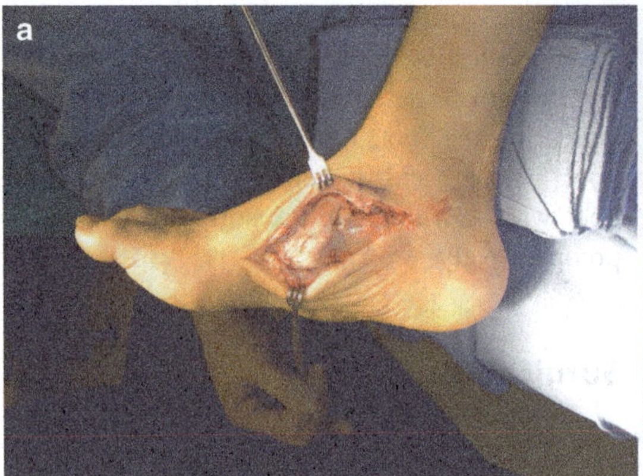
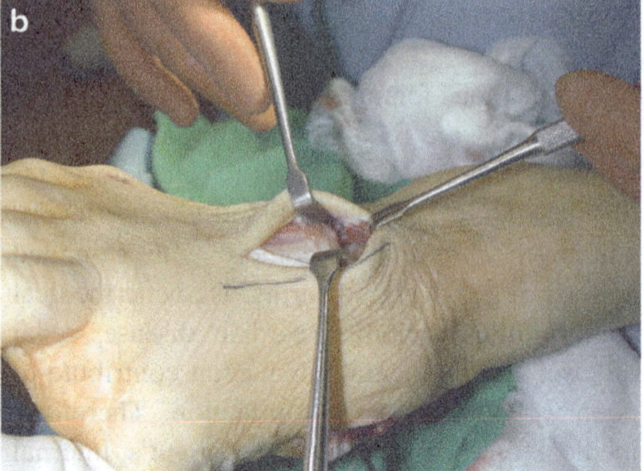

Fig. 10.2 (**a**) An extended medial approach demonstrates excellent exposure of the dislocation. Not the tibialis anterior tendon which is a deforming force causing dorsal dislocation of the midfoot. (**b**) The midline approach to the central columns demonstrating dislocation at the tarsometatarsal joint

The medial column is approached through a long medial incision centered at the apex of the deformity. The abductor hallucis is elevated as a single layer and reflected plantarly. This muscle is used as a full-thickness layer for closure at the end of the case. In most cases, the tibialis anterior tendon will need to be detached and reattached at the end of the procedure. This resolves a significant deforming force holding the forefoot dorsiflexed, which can prevent reduction if not addressed. If the navicular is fragmented, it may also be necessary to detach and tag the posterior tibial tendon for later repair.

Approaching the middle column may require a separate incision, particularly if the tarsometatarsal joints are dislocated. Typically, a longitudinal dorsal incision is made centered at the apex of the deformity. The dorsal neurovascular bundle is elevated subperiosteally and is preserved. The lateral column is often exposed through a dorsolateral incision, elevating the extensor digitorum brevis muscle as necessary. Care should be taken to create full-thickness fasciocutaneous flaps for closure, and to aid in wound healing.

Resection of Bone and Correction of Deformity

As the midfoot breaks down, one often encounters a dislocation due to the deforming forces of the tibialis anterior tendon, the posterior tibial tendon, and the Achilles tendon. These tendons cause the forefoot to sublux dorsally, which may result in the forefoot sitting in bayonet apposition on top of the hindfoot (Fig. 10.3). The apex of the dislocation will usually correspond to the most prominent area plantarly on the patient's foot. Often this is the medial cuneiform or the cuboid.

When planning a correction to the midfoot, it is helpful to think of the foot as two distinct segments, the forefoot and hindfoot. The goal of the surgery is to realign both segments and create a stable arthrodesis at the mid-tarsus.

Bone resection must be done to allow a tension-free reduction of the foot deformity. Bone resection is also done to remove articular cartilage in order to create the arthrodesis bed. It is acceptable to bridge non-involved joints without preparing them for fusion in order to preserve their vascularity and the structural properties of the bone. Bridging unprepared joints, however, increases the risk of hardware failure and screw migration. Inadequate bone resection will result in undue tension on the arterial structures and may also result in recurrence of the deformity. To correct the deformity an aggressive osseous resection is performed which incorporates a wedge resection at the apex of the deformity. This usually involves removing more bone plantarly and medially. The wedge resection of bone can be preoperatively planned by radiographs or alternately by using intraoperatively placed Kirschner wires and checking fluoroscopic

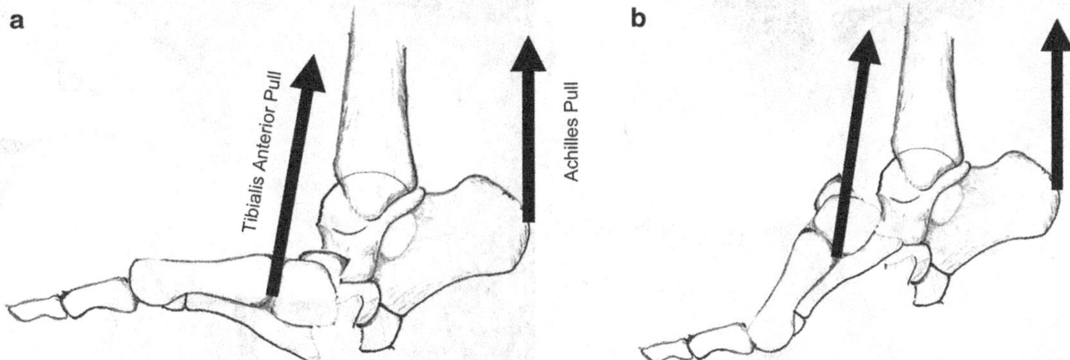

Fig. 10.3 (a) Forces of the tibialis anterior and Achilles act to induce deformity at the midfoot. (b) Dislocation may occur as the deformity progresses. Correction of these forces must be addressed at the time of surgery or reduction may not be possible

images. The medial column typically has more fragmentation than the middle and lateral columns and is therefore approached first (Fig. 10.4). Once an adequate amount of bone has been removed, a balanced resection extending laterally can be done. Care must be taken not to over-resect bone in the middle and lateral columns of the foot so to avoid gapping of the arthrodesis bed. The soft tissues must be protected during the bony resection in order to avoid transection of the arterial supply to the forefoot. This can be accomplished by placing Hohmann retractors superiorly and inferiorly to prevent excursion of the saw into the soft tissues.

Bone resection starts medially to correct the medial column first, then proceeds towards the middle and lateral columns as necessary. Resection is done in small steps, through 2 or 3 incisions, gradually removing bone until the desired foot position is achieved. A microsagittal saw and set of sharp osteotomes or chisels are ideal for this resection. The goal is to match the resection so that good opposition of the proximal and distal segments can be achieved. Once the foot can be realigned, without significant soft tissue tension, attention is directed towards fixation of the arthrodesis.

Fixation with Long Axial Screws

The goal of fixation using the axial screw technique is to span the area of Charcot dissolution and fracture, achieving fixation proximally and distally in more normal bone (Fig. 10.5). I prefer to use cannulated screws because the guidewires which are placed through the intramedullary canals of the metatarsals are used to guide overall alignment of the foot. The reduction is held temporarily with the intramedullary guidewires before placement of the final hardware.

The guidewires can be applied antegrade (from proximal to distal) or retrograde through the metatarsal heads. The antegrade technique has the disadvantage that the wires, drills, taps, and screws are passed blindly in close proximity to the neurovascular bundle. The retrograde technique is only appropriate in patients with sensory neuropathy since the technique involves passing large diameter cannulated screws through the articular surface of the metatarsal head.

My own preference is to cannulate all of the desired metatarsals retrograde to the level of the dislocation. The deformity is then reduced manually and the guidewires are advanced across the deformity into the foot proximally. The wire is checked fluoroscopically and advanced to the level of the desired correction. Once the deformity is corrected, the guidewires will hold the deformity reduced while positioning is verified radiographically. A cannulated depth gauge is used to gauge the length of the screw. The medial column is reduced first, followed by the middle and lateral columns. The fifth metatarsal can usually not be secured with axial screws because the trajectory dictated by the fifth metatarsal shaft will be lateral to the cuboid. Obliquely applied screws are used for the fifth metatarsal cuboid fusion.

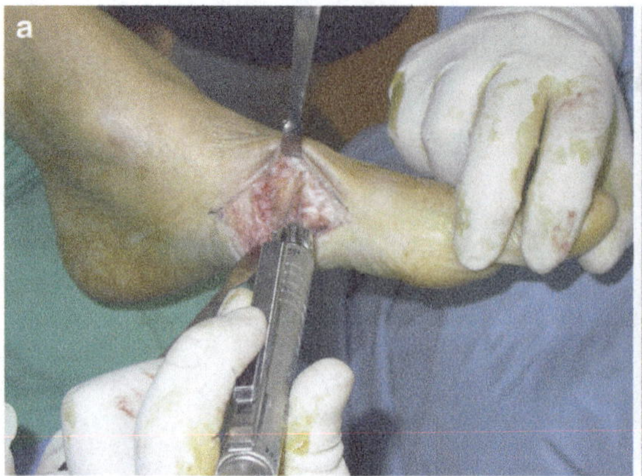 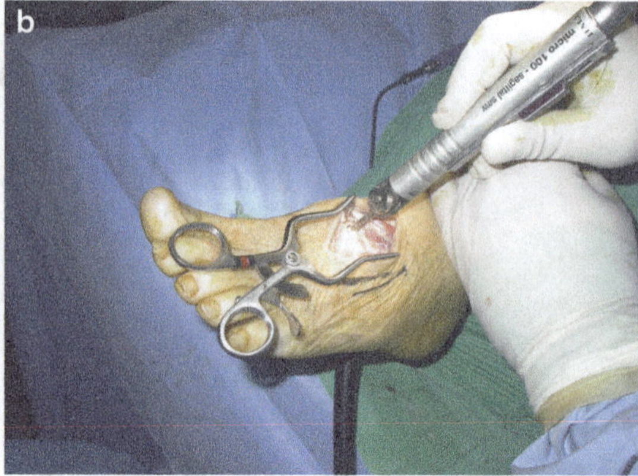

Fig. 10.4 (**a**) Resection of bone at the level of dislocation is necessary to achieve reduction. Bone resection is typically done with a plantar and medial closing wedge configuration at the apex of the deformity. (**b**) Further resection may be necessary through a dorsal or lateral incision depending on the degree of deformity

The largest diameter screw which will fit into the metatarsal shaft is used. This can be gauged by sequentially reaming the metatarsal with cannulated drills. The metatarsal shaft should be radiographically visualized during the reaming procedure to gauge the fit of the drill bit within the metatarsal. When the intramedullary canal is filled radiographically and the drill is meeting resistance, larger drills should not be applied or the metatarsal may fracture. The shaft is then tapped to prevent fracture during passage of the final hardware. The size of the tap will often dictate the size of the screw that can be used in the metatarsal shaft, and this should also be gauged radiographically. Attempting to place a screw with too large a diameter can lead to splitting or fracture of the metatarsal. Typically, the medial column will accept a screw diameter of 6.5–8.0 mm. The lesser metatarsals will accept screw diameters from 4 to 5 mm. Initial series used screws with standard heads, however at times these proved to be difficult to countersink. I have now switched to using headless screws for most procedures. It is important that the screw length should be selected so that the head is well countersunk below the level to the articular surface.

The medial column is typically fixed by passing the screw through the metatarsophalangeal joint and extending it into the tarsal navicular. If the navicular is fragmented and the transverse tarsal joint must be included in the fusion, the medial column screw can usually be advanced into the talar neck and body. The middle column is typically secured through the second and third metatarsals and is also placed into the navicular. If the transverse tarsal joint is to be fused, the second metatarsal screw can also be advanced into the talar neck. The lateral column can be secured with a screw traversing through the fourth metatarsal into the cuboid and extended into the calcaneus if necessary. This can be passed antegrade or retrograde if the calcaneocuboid joint is to be included in the fusion. The fifth metatarsal will usually not aline axially with the cuboid, and can be secured with obliquely placed screws from the fifth metatarsal metaphysis into the cuboid.

Primary apposition with compression is desirable; however, if there are gaps in the fusion site, these should be bone grafted. Often local graft obtained during the osseous resection can be used; however, I have found that demineralized allograft bone matrix is also effective for small defects. If a large amount of bone graft is required, cancellous autograft from the proximal tibia or iliac crest can be harvested.

At the time of closure, the tibialis anterior and posterior tendons, if detached for exposure, should be reattached directly to bone by suturing them through small drill holes. The fascia of the abductor hallucis is then closed over the dorsal deep fascia to cover the medial column. A layered closure of the skin is then performed.

Postoperative Management

The patient is placed into a posterior splint with a Robert-Jones type cotton wadding to allow for swelling. The splint is removed 2–5 days postoperatively and a non-weight bearing short leg cast is applied. The frequency of follow-up visits needs to be tailored to the clinical course; patients exhibiting signs of poor wound healing, excessive swelling, and those with poor compliance with weight bearing restrictions typically need more careful supervision than those that are healing without incident. The cast is changed and X-rays obtained every 2–4 weeks, until osseous consolidation is apparent radiographically.

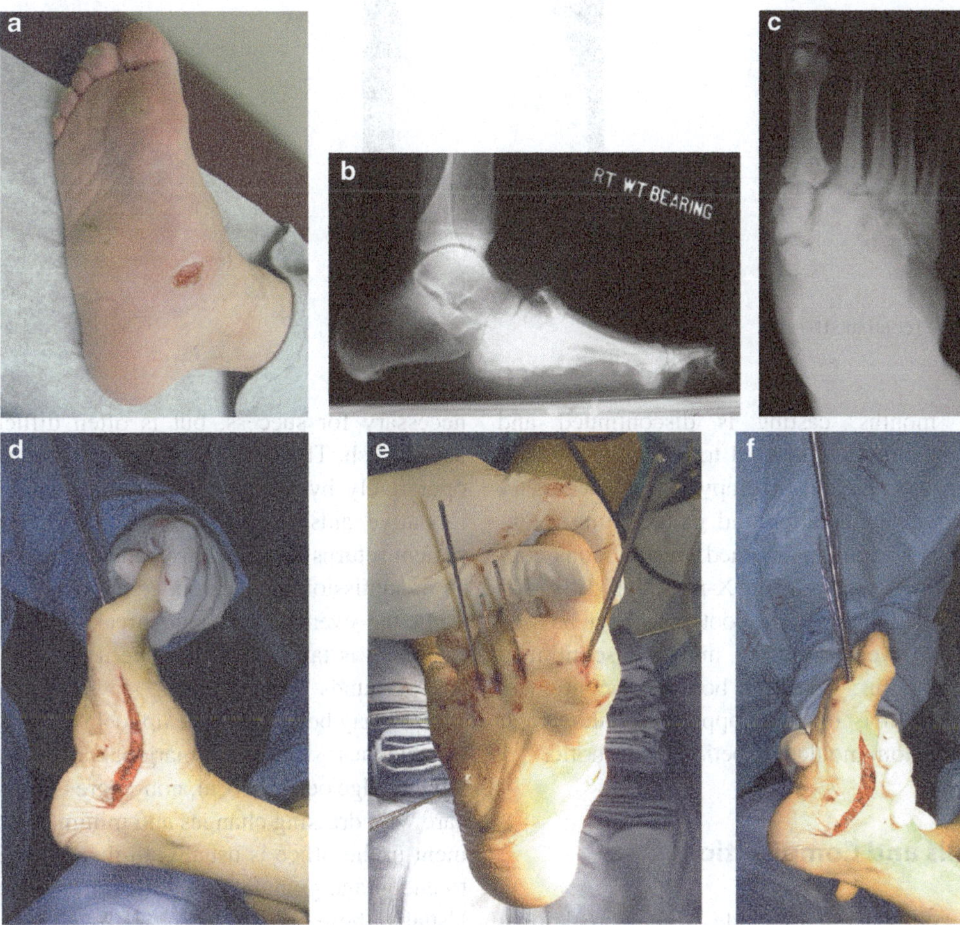

Fig. 10.5 Case study of midfoot fusion for Charcot deformity in a 56-year-old woman with diabetes mellitus: (**a**) The patient presented with a recurrent Wagner Grade 1 Ulceration medially and gross instability though the midfoot. (**b**, **c**). A/P and lateral X-rays showing chronic neuropathic dislocation of the midfoot. (**d**–**f**) Realignment is obtained and held with guidewires for cannulated screws after resection of bone at the level of dislocation. (**h**, **i**) Long axial screws are applied through the metatarsophalangeal joints over guidewires to bridge the zone of neuropathic dislocation. (**j**) Two-year postoperative clinical photograph of foot and weight bearing X-rays showing restoration of alignment and successful arthrodesis

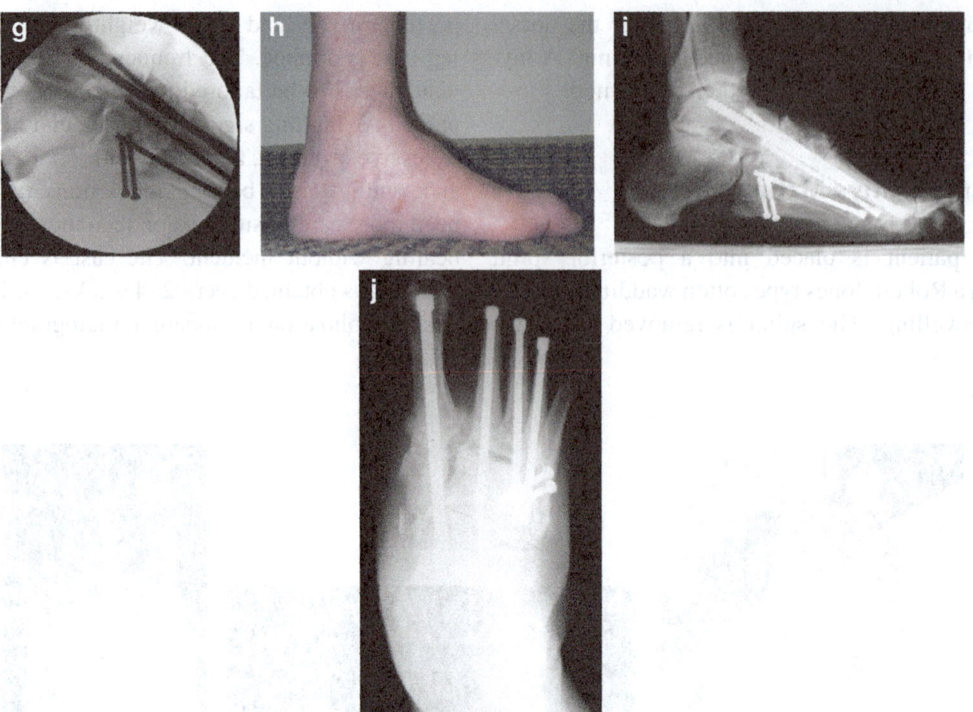

Fig. 10.5 (continued)

At 3 months, casting is discontinued and immobilization is changed to a removable cam walker boot. Physical therapy may be necessary to aid with ambulation and gait training. Non-weight bearing is maintained until osseous consolidation is apparent on X-rays, typically 4–5 months from surgery. The boot walker can be used for initial weight bearing and is discontinued after 6 months. When the boot is discontinued, the patient may return to appropriate shoe wear with a custom molded diabetic type orthotic.

Pitfalls and Complications

Early complications include wound breakdown and infections. To avoid this, it is important to have a well-vascularized foot, before proceeding with surgery, and to have the patient's blood glucose and medical issues optimized as much as possible. Ensuring that the patient complies with the strict non-weight bearing protocol is also necessary for success, but is often difficult to accomplish. The patient should be assessed preoperatively by a physical therapist and accommodative aids need to be available when the patient returns home. Many patients may benefit from admission to an extended nursing facility.

In the event that wound breakdown occurs, treatment is tailored to the severity of the problem. Wounds typically heal slowly and nylon sutures may be left in place up to 4 weeks. If partial thickness skin loss or marginal necrosis of the wound edge occurs, local, non-aggressive wound care with dressing changes and minimal debridement in the office is usually all that is necessary to encourage granulation and secondary healing. Usually, these patients are treated with more frequent cast changes with close observation of the wound. If the patient is referred to wound center, it is important to communicate with those treating the patient not to perform aggressive debridement of marginal tissue. In the event of complete dehiscence, or deep infection, return to the operating room for formal incision and debridement is necessary. We will often use negative pressure wound therapy for secondary closure in conjunction with suppressive antibiotics. Often removal of hardware and application of an external fixator are necessary.

Nonunion, hardware failure and recurrence of the deformity are more common in cases where the talonavicular joint is incorporated into the fusion. If hardware failure occurs, but the foot remains plantigrade, further surgery is not indicated. In the event that deformity recurs, the surgery can be revised by replacing the intramedullary hardware and bone grafting the nonunion site.

Long-Term Results

We reported retrospectively on 22 patients who had undergone surgical reconstruction and arthrodesis with multiple intramedullary screws, to treat Charcot midfoot deformity, using the above described techniques. Axially placed intramedullary screws, inserted either antegrade or retrograde across the arthrodesis sites, were used to restore the longitudinal arch. Radiographic measurements were recorded preoperatively, immediately postoperatively, and at the time of the last follow-up and were analyzed in order to assess the amount and maintenance of correction. Patients were evaluated clinically and radiographically at an average of 52 months. Complete osseous union was achieved in 16 of the 22 patients. There were five partial fusions and there was one nonunion with recurrence of deformity. There were eight cases with hardware failure. All patients returned to an independent functional ambulatory status without above ankle bracing using standard diabetic shoe wear and custom multidensity foam diabetic type orthotics [9].

Conclusions

Charcot midfoot deformity is a difficult disease to treat effectively. While most patients can be managed effectively with bracing, a subset of patients with significant deformity and instability exists who cannot be managed effectively without surgery. Good results have been reported with corrective arthrodesis although standard fixation techniques are often inadequate in patients with neuroarthropathy. The technique described here where fixation is achieved with long axial screws has shown successful long-term results.

References

1. National Diabetes Statistics Report. (2014). http://www.diabtes.org-basics/statistics/.
2. Munson ME, et al. Data mining for identifying novel associations and temporal relationships with Charcot foot. J Diabetes Res. 2014;2014:214353.
3. Saltzman CL, et al. How effective is intensive nonoperative initial treatment of patients with diabetes and Charcot arthropathy of the feet? Clin Orthop Relat Res. 2005;435:185–90.
4. Simon SR, et al. Arthrodesis as an early alternative to nonoperative management of Charcot arthropathy of the diabetic foot. J Bone Joint Surg Am. 2000;82A (7):939–50.
5. Hastings MK, et al. Progression of foot deformity in Charcot neuropathic osteoarthropathy. J Bone Joint Surg Am. 2013;95(13):1206–13.
6. Sammarco VJ. Superconstructs in the treatment of Charcot foot deformity: plantar plating, locked plating, and axial screw fixation. Foot Ankle Clin. 2009;14(3):393–407.
7. Sammarco GJ, Conti SF. Surgical treatment of neuroarthropathic foot deformity. Foot Ankle Int. 1998; 19(2):102–9.
8. Schon LC, et al. The acquired midtarsus deformity classification system—interobserver reliability and intraobserver reproducibility. Foot Ankle Int. 2002; 23(1):30–6.
9. Sammarco VJ, et al. Midtarsal arthrodesis in the treatment of Charcot midfoot arthropathy. J Bone Joint Surg Am. 2009;91(1):80–91.

John S. Early

Introduction

Injury to a neuropathic joint, whether it is in the foot or ankle, follows a predictable natural course where a subtle injury occurs creating a fracture of the weakened, usually osteopenic bone. When recognized early in the ankle, it is termed an ankle fracture in a neuropathic joint. This category is reserved for those ankles which still have a distinct tibial plafond or talar joint contours. Treatment of these injuries is covered in the preceding chapter. When these bones no longer exhibit recognizable articular contours, the joint is referred to as a Charcot ankle and the treatment paradigm changes. This process of joint collapse can occur whether or not the initial injury is recognized early and appropriately treated. Additionally, the patient can present as a chronic swollen ankle with or without an alignment deformity.

J.S. Early, M.D. (✉)
Clinical Professor Orthopedic Surgery, University of Texas Southwestern Medical Center, Texas Orthopaedic Associates LLP, Dallas, TX, USA
e-mail: jsearlymd@sbcglobal.net

Pathogenesis

The true incidence of spontaneous Charcot ankle is not known but reportedly occurs in 6–47 % of ankle fractures in diabetic neuropathic patients [1–3]. The actual incidence is probably higher. The difficulty in the treatment of this patient population is not the destruction of the joint but the underlying physiology of bony healing in a neuropathic patient [4–6]. The development of the bony destruction, normally seen in Charcot arthropathy, requires the loss of normal neurologic function around the affected area. Normal bone growth, repair, and remodeling are largely under the control of the local nervous system and the appropriate release of specific neuropeptides. It is these neuropeptides that modulate the interaction of the actual cells responsible for bony resorption and regeneration, which occurs during normal bone healing and remodeling. While diabetic neuropathy can involve damage to both large fibers and small fiber nerves, it appears that the selective loss of small fiber nerves around the joint, which have a significant role in controlling osteoblast and osteoclast interaction in bone healing or remodeling, is a major cause of the Charcot joint. The loss of small fiber nerves and the specific neuropeptides they produce, causes the body to lose the ability to modulate the cellular response to a bony injury. This allows the initial inflammatory response from an injury to become exaggerated, causing excessive osteolysis and instability of the surrounding bone. Activation of osteoblastic function and the formation of bone are initially delayed due to the overstimulation of osteoclasts and only slowly is the balance restored due to the loss of appropriate neuropeptide modulators. The end result is severe bony destruction of a normal joint surface with delayed and abnormal bone formation resulting in complete destruction of the joint.

Patient Presentation

Initial presentation of a Charcot ankle usually is with the complaint of a chronic swollen ankle that the patient can walk on, but after awhile, it hurts due to the swelling. Usually pain is relieved by getting off the foot and elevating the limb. Many times the patient will relate that the swelling recedes overnight. Usually there is no specifically recalled injury. Occasionally, there is a remote history of fracture treatment with initial successful recovery. Often though it has been an ongoing process for weeks to months with little urgency because of the lack of real pain [3, 7, 8].

The affected limb is indurated and has pitting edema. There can be significant crepitation noted with ankle motion or even detectible instability of the mortise. The differential diagnosis for this presentation can include gout, cellulitis, systemic issues causing dependent edema, or osteomyelitis. If there has never been a history of soft tissue ulceration in the limb, penetrating injury or previous surgery with implants in place, the presence of infection as the underlying cause is low. These patients can also present with severe deformity, soft tissue compromise at the malleoli, and even ulceration of the soft tissue due to pressure from the internal deformity.

If the patient presents weight bearing, one should obtain weight bearing films to fully assess any bony instability at the ankle joint. The degree of abnormal bone formation may also help establish a timeline to the actual onset of the Charcot process. Bony destruction with resorption and little new bone formation is seen early on in the Charcot process, as described by Eichenholz in his general classification. The visualization of significant bony contour changes and heterotopic bone formation is evidence of a much longer time frame.

In a patient who is a known diabetic, with a history of neuropathy or suspected neuropathy, the problem should be presumed a Charcot ankle until proven otherwise. Initial management should begin at the time of presentation, even as a medical workup is initiated to rule out other causes.

Management Overview

Treatment of the Charcot ankle is a very time-consuming and difficult process for both the patient and treating clinician. The goal is *a stable well-aligned limb that can be safely and permanently braced to allow weight bearing with a plantigrade foot*. At best, a fusion of the involved joints can be performed but will result in a permanent alteration of gait mechanics to the patient. On the patient's end, independent of the treatment choice, a prolonged period of non-weight bearing and confinement is often needed if there is to be any chance of success. Successful fusion and stabilization of the Charcot ankle is only the first step in the long-term care of these patients. Because of the natural stress seen at the ankle joint with normal walking, long-term care should also include permanent bracing, to help shield the fused joint from pressures that can create a new stress injury and start the process all over again [3, 6–9].

Medical Management

The issues on the importance of maximizing the patient's medical health, in order to achieve success in treatment, have been stressed throughout this book. Baseline labs to document the patient's diabetic health and nutrition status are a must. Obtaining a baseline hemoglobin A1c (HgA1c) value is important to assess the patient's long-term control of their diabetes [10]. Albumin, total protein, and leukocyte levels serve as markers of the patient's nutrition status and should be monitored throughout the course of treatment [6, 7, 11, 12]. Medical management, using a team approach, should be ongoing to improve and maintain values, as discussed in earlier chapters, for optimum healing.

Obtaining a baseline vascular profile is also important. A Charcot joint is an evolving process and any potential vasculopathy may also be evolving. Prior to any surgery and even with palpable pulses, obtaining a Doppler toe pressure assessment is recommended as a better first line to measure small vessel perfusion in the affected limb [3, 7, 13]. This can successfully be done even with a cast in place. Other testing regimens are discussed in earlier chapters and can be used to supplement initial findings. Any correctable vasculopathy detected should be treated before surgery in order to give the limb its best chance of recovery. Uncorrectable vasculopathy may be a reason to consider amputation as a treatment option, especially if nonoperative treatment is not possible due to the presence of a deformity or creates significant soft tissue compromise during treatment.

Nonoperative Management

All patients presenting with a Charcot ankle should, at least initially, be treated with nonoperative management [3, 6–9]. The author's preference is the application of a well-molded, total contact cast with an extension that includes the femoral condyles, much like a patella bearing cast (PTB). The reason for this is to help control the rotational instability that is usually present because of the loss of mortise stability. A regular cast without inclusion of the femoral condyles may allow the foot to rotate on the tibia, even when just positioning the foot on the bed or in non-weight bearing transfers. Inclusion of the condyles will afford some improvement in resistance to the rotation and may also afford some sensory feedback to the patient about any ongoing irritation to the ankle. Even if the initial determination is to proceed with surgery, initial protection from further damage is important.

Secondly, and again it can never be stressed enough, it is the author's preference that, in the case of ankle Charcot, the patient needs to be immediately and permanently made non-weight bearing on that limb until the Charcot process has coalesced. This is probably the most critical step in their care because without total protection from weight bearing pressure any treatment option sees an exponential increase for the chance to fail, leading to amputation. This is the most difficult part for a patient to both comprehend and follow. The patient and caregivers will need to understand that this period of non-weight bearing for a Charcot ankle is continuous for a minimum of three months and usually longer. Failure to impress this upon a patient can take a salvageable ankle and make it an amputation. A frank discussion with the patient and family about the real possibility of a below knee amputation, and the ramifications of that to their independence and health, needs to happen early and be repeated often. To facilitate this, a wheelchair with a leg extension is often necessary. Allowing the patient to have the foot down in a normal sitting position leads to inadvertent weight bearing, even if it is nothing more than the weight of the leg when shifting or repositioning in the chair, and can be a source of treatment failure. Securing home health or even a stay in a skilled nursing facility may also be necessary to assist these patients in simple transfers and daily care while under acute treatment and strict non-weight bearing.

Nonoperative management of the Charcot ankle, in its simplest form, is stabilization of the limb until bony maturation of the Charcot process is complete and the soft tissue envelope has improved. Candidates for this should present with axially aligned limbs (Fig. 11.1). One way to assess this is to have the limb hang off the examining table to assess the limb alignment without weight. A fixed deformity, whether varus, valgus or equinus, even if healed successfully will be a challenge for the patient and pedorthist when it comes time to bear weight. Anterior or posterior displacement of the talus under the tibia is usually well tolerated if stable plantigrade healing occurs. If more than mild pressure is needed to realign the limb, surgical stabilization should be considered.

The course of treatment is labor intensive for both the patient and treating clinician.

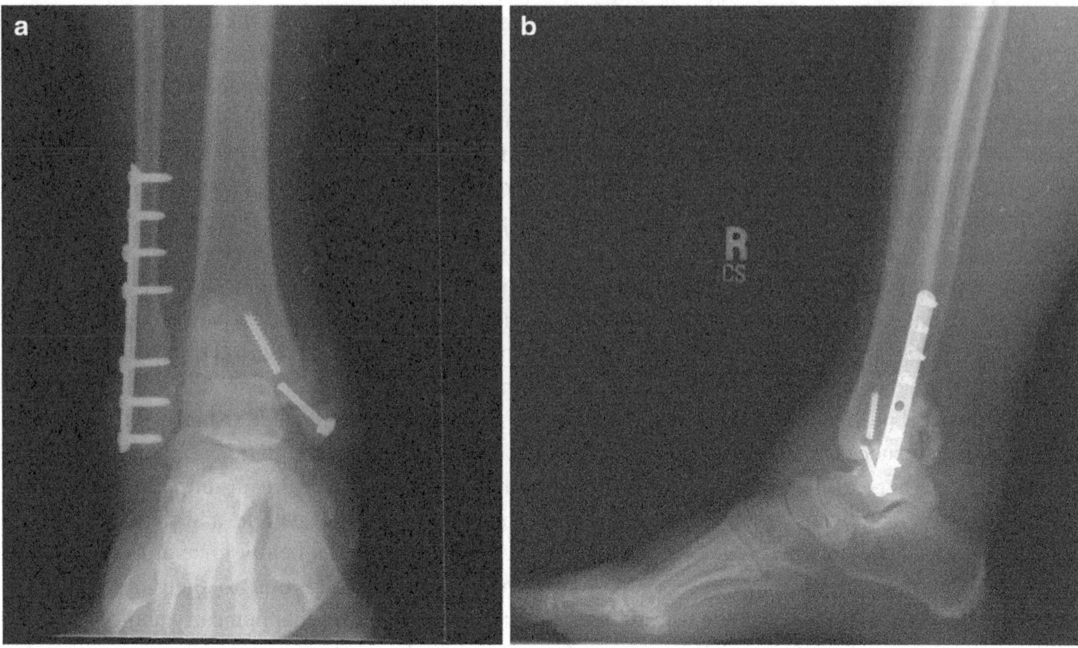

Fig. 11.1 (**a**) Anteroposterior (AP) view. (**b**) Lateral view. Example of aligned Charcot ankle from a failed ORIF. Though the talus is posterior to the tibial axis, the foot rests in a plantigrade position suitable for casting and bracing

Initially, weekly cast changes are needed to both control limb position effectively and check for early signs of soft tissue compromise. Once immobilized and protected from weight bearing forces, the soft tissue edema disappears creating space in the cast. This can be very harmful to both maintaining limb position and soft tissue integrity and will need to be changed regularly until no further shrinkage is seen. The appearance of soft tissue ulceration during this phase of treatment, when not vascular in origin, is due to abnormal pressure. This is either caused by a shifting cast, due to looseness, or inadvertent weight bearing. The appearance of any soft tissue breakdown during casting is a sign of nonoperative failure and should lead to consideration that the patient may require surgical stabilization.

Weekly radiographs are also important to assess bony alignment and stability. Once the Charcot ankle enters the consolidation phase, casting can be extended to every other week. Because of the difficulty with the patient being unable to sense pressure on the limb, they should be prevented from weight bearing until there is radiographic evidence of consolidation of the bony mass. This represents a fusion of the joint and not just clinical evidence of limb stability. As with all bony healing, there are two phases: injury repair or stabilization followed by bony remodeling to accept and resist patient-applied stress. Stabilization of the limb is the first half of the battle in protecting the limb from another injury. Returning the patient to independent weight bearing is a second, slow process. Once the patient achieves both radiographic consolidation and limb stability with manual testing, they should transition to a period of weight bearing in a total contact cast for 4–6 weeks to allow stress maturation of the bone. Inability to successfully weight bear in the cast with either recurrent swelling or radiographic evidence is late signs of instability and may need surgical intervention.

Once the patient has successfully advanced to weight bearing in a cast, they should be transitioned into a custom solid ankle brace for permanent use. This aids in shielding the neuropathic ankle from stress overload. This can be a solid ankle ankle-foot orthosis (AFO), a clamshell AFO, or a Charcot restraint orthotic walker (CROW) boot (Fig. 11.2). Consideration for an

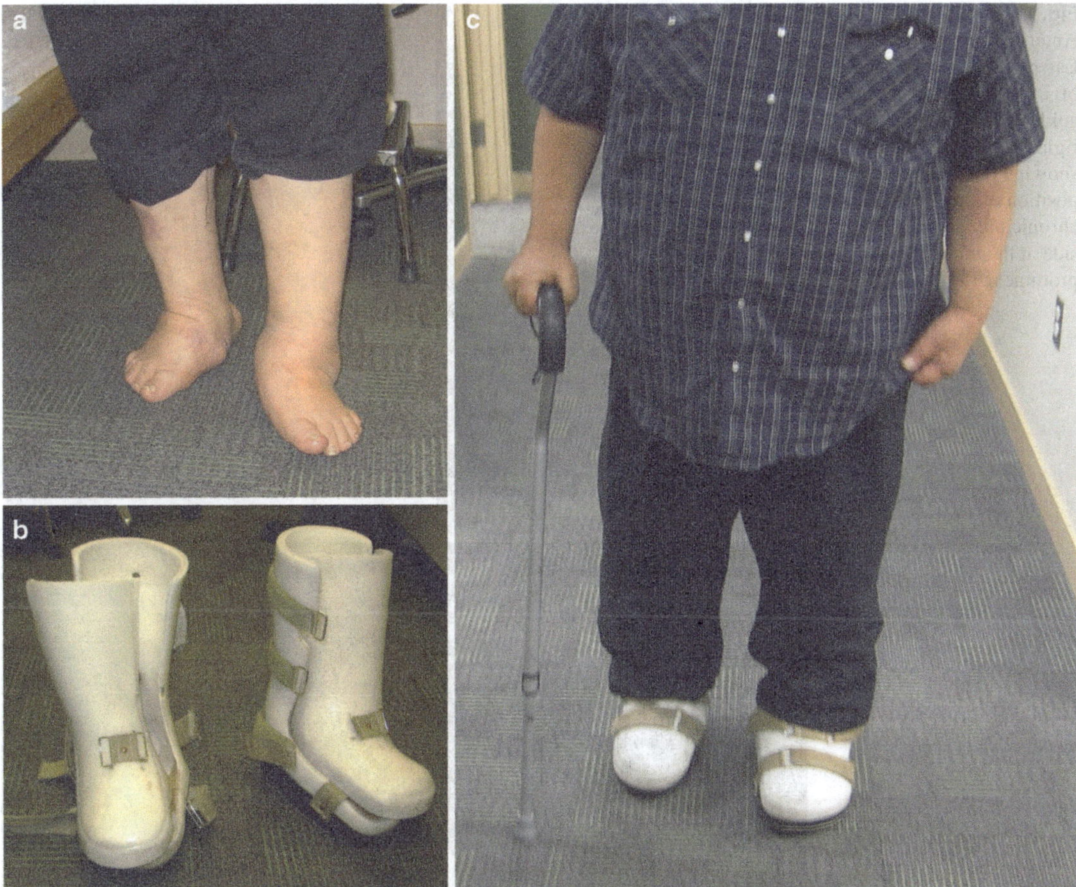

Fig. 11.2 (**a**) Clinical view of patient with stable bilateral Charcot ankles. (**b**) Custom molded Crow walker boots to protect ankle position. (**c**) Patient ambulating in bilateral Crow walker boots

enclosed brace may be necessary based on any perceived instability in the fusion mass. It may also be necessary if it is also due to issues with the foot, if accommodative shoe wear is not possible, or finally just for convenience of the patient. Failure of this treatment regimen can occur and should be addressed in a timely manner with surgical intervention.

Operative Treatment

Surgical stabilization of a Charcot ankle is truly a salvage surgery [7, 9, 14–20]. The purpose of the surgery is to provide alignment and stability to the limb while the Charcot process is consolidating.

The goal, as with nonoperative care, is to achieve a plantigrade foot axially aligned under the tibia so the patient can bear weight. Often there is no ankle architecture to reconstruct. The ability to preserve ankle motion is lost with the start of the Charcot process and no amount of surgery will restore normal function. Indications for surgery are presentation of an ankle with a severe varus, valgus or equines deformity, or even a mild deformity in these planes, that is not easily correctable without significant pressure applied to the soft tissues (Fig. 11.3). A leg with soft tissue ulceration, not related to vasculopathy, should also be considered for surgical stabilization. This is because ulcers are usually a result of significant bony instability, which is difficult to control

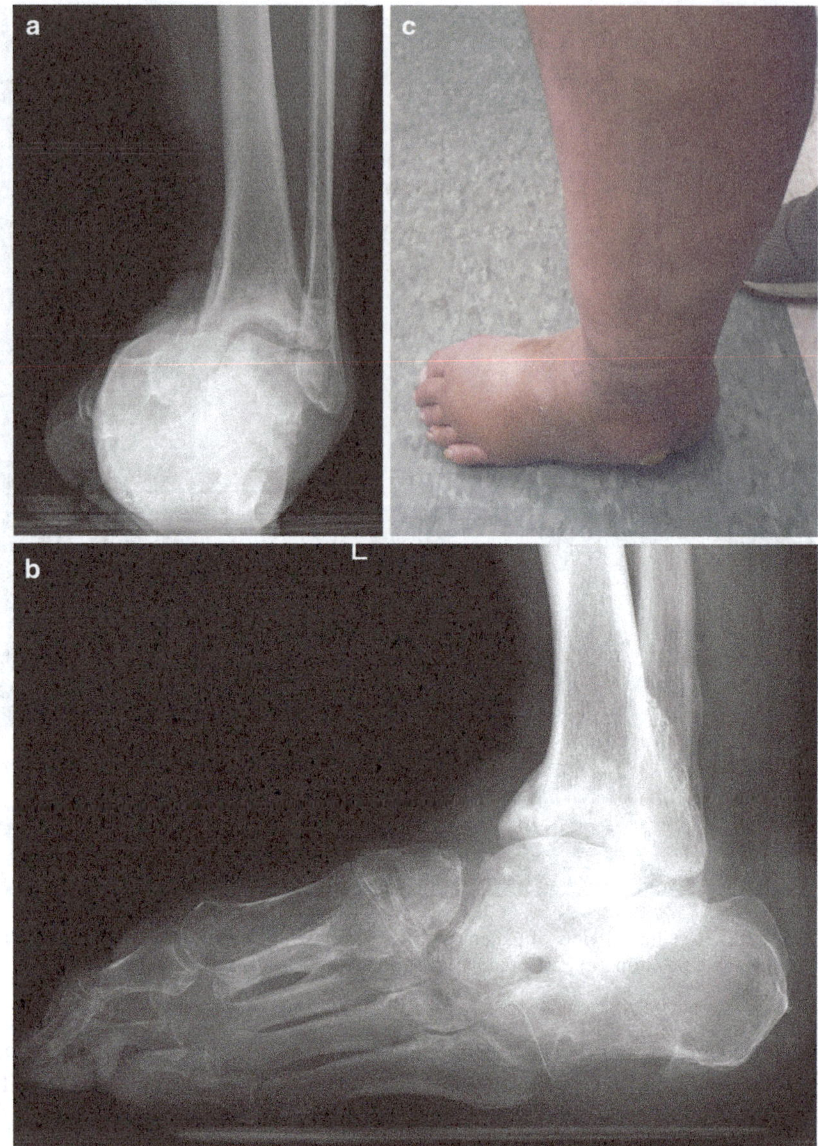

Fig. 11.3 (a) Anteroposterior view. (b) Lateral view. Radiographs of a non-braceable Charcot ankle. The foot position is rigid. (c) Clinical picture showing the weight bearing position of the foot. Note chronic ulcer on lateral side at the malleolar prominence

in a cast without placing additional pressure on the soft tissues. Again, as discussed in previous chapters, medical management of the underlying disease process is as important in determining not only the health of the patient for the surgery but also the outcome of the treatment regimen.

Surgical intervention can be broken into two categories. Internal fixation can be used to align and stabilize the foot under the tibia. External circular ring fixation can also be employed to achieve the same result. Often there may be a melding of both methods to achieve the desired result [21]. The choice of stabilization is based mainly on surgeon preference but can also be based on soft tissue considerations. Discussion of the use of circular thin wire external fixation will be addressed in the next chapter. One should remember that surgery does not change the long-term nature of the problem or the need for protracted immobilization and non-weight bearing. It merely offers a way to stabilize the bony anatomy of the leg during the Charcot process.

Preoperative Planning

There is literature to support the use of plates and screws to stabilize and fuse the ankle joint, undergoing Charcot destruction, and there are presently new plate designs which may offer a more stable, complete hindfoot fusion. In the author's opinion however, the most successful method of fixation involves the use of an intramedullary nail placed retrograde through the calcaneus, talus, and tibia to realign and stabilize the foot, allowing consolidation and a solid fusion of the hindfoot under the tibia [14–20].

When surgical intervention is chosen to control the position of a Charcot ankle, the treatment usually begins early in the Charcot process because of the instability, deformity, and soft tissue issues that occur. This is because there is often a tendency to have ongoing bony resorption before significant bony stabilization is achieved. The stability provided by a static plate placement can be lost if the bony edges reabsorb and this usually leads to implant failure and loss of stability. However, this can also be the fate of rigidly locked nails. Currently, there are intramedullary devices that allow for proximal dynamization so that the nail and foot can maintain bony contact. In the implants that do not provide for proximal dynamization, the treatment plan should include a possible dynamization of the rod by planning to remove the proximal fixation once the patient is permitted to bear weight. Initially, proximal screw fixation of the nail is vital to protect the fusion mass from rotational forces between the foot and tibia, but once stable, the ability for the nail to axially migrate is important for the maturation of the fusion mass.

The goal of the surgical treatment is to provide limb stability and to obtain a solid fusion mass of the hindfoot. This includes obtaining a fusion of both the ankle and subtalar joints. Therefore, it is critical that the subtalar joint is also addressed. In preparing both joints, removal of tissue, such as cartilage and subchondral bone, is an important step when trying to obtain a fusion mass as large as possible. Consequently, part of the surgical technique should include an aggressive exposure of those surfaces of both joint surfaces to remove tissue and bone fragments that may be blocking solid bone contact. Removal of one or both of the malleoli may also be necessary to regain alignment of the limb and remove bony contours that may be causing or potentially cause local pressure ulcers.

Surgical technique

The patient can be placed either supine or prone on the operating table. In the prone position the patient should be positioned so that the foot hangs off the end of the table to help facilitate a plantigrade foot position. The prone position also allows a posterior approach to debride and prepare both joint surfaces. However, the standard position is with the patient supine with the foot at the end of the bed. Bolsters or blankets are placed under the lower leg to elevate the limb above the other side to allow easier fluoroscopic viewing. A bolster under the thigh is also placed to maintain flexion of the knee, effectively removing any gastrocnemius contracture from interfering with the reduction. The need for gastrosoleus lengthening is usually reserved for after joint debridement and soft tissue release. The utility approach is through the lateral side as access to both the ankle and subtalar joint is possible. The incision begins about 15 cm above the distal tip of the fibula and moves distally along the long axis of the fibula. Just before the fibula tip the incision is curved into the sinus tarsi space. The incision is taken down to the periosteum and elevated off the anterior aspect of the fibula to expose the ankle and subtalar joint as well as the anterior syndesmosis. The fibula is transected above the syndesmosis or at whatever level appears necessary so that it will not interfere with final tibial talar contact. Based on the condition of the hindfoot, there are many times that preservation of the distal fibula is possible. If this is the case, the distal fibula is left attached to the surrounding soft tissue posteriorly and longitudinally sectioned removing the medial half.

Preparation of the fusion surfaces includes removal of all bone preventing tibial talar contact, as well as all cartilage and subchondral bone from the tibiotalar and subtalar joints.

Shortening or removal of the medial malleolus may also necessary to achieve solid bony contact. If it cannot be effectively reached through the lateral incision, a second medial approach can be made.

If a medial incision is necessary, it is made longitudinally along the anterior margin of the medial malleolus. This allows access into the medial gutter, to remove the cartilage and fibrous tissue, and permits the use of a sagittal saw to remove the appropriate amount of proximal malleolus needed to gain alignment and contact. If the medial malleolus requires shortening, as it usually does, the medial approach should consist of a subperiosteal dissection around the medial malleolus and placing a retractor to protect the skin. A sagittal saw then is used to make two cuts directed from anterior to posterior. The first is performed at the level of the plafond and the second at a more distal level that correlates with the desired amount of bone to remove to achieve good bony contact without interference of a malleolus that is now too long due to Charcot bone loss (Fig. 11.4). The posterior tibialis tendon can be damaged by this method but is of little functional value at this stage of neuropathic disease. Sectioning of the medial malleolus will also allow medialization of the talus and foot if it becomes necessary for axial alignment.

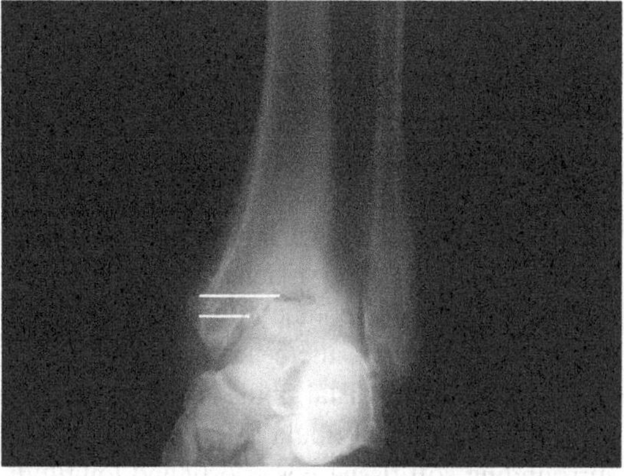

Fig. 11.4 AP radiograph of displaced Charcot ankle with medial bone block and shortening of Plafond. Illustrated are the two cuts that can be made in the medial malleolus to allow both good axial apposition and alignment of the tibiotalar joint. Cuts in this manner help avoid the difficulty of dissecting out the malleolar tip from surrounding soft tissue

When the fusion surfaces have been prepared and adequate bone has been removed to regain axial alignment and bony contact, the retrograde intramedullary device is placed according to the technique for the particular nail chosen. It is important to ream proximally at least 1–2 cm beyond the planned proximal end of the implanted nail. In addition, reaming of the bone should be at least 1–2 mm larger than the diameter of the implant. Cortical interference for any migration of the nail, either during initial compression or with late settling of the construct, can lead to failure of the nail to migrate proximally. This can result in stress fractures at the level of the nail tip or failure of the implant.

Critical to the long-term success of this surgery is the placement of the foot. A plantigrade to slight dorsiflexion is necessary to help prevent stress overload when weight bearing on the forefoot. Determining the correct position of the foot is obtained by evaluating the lateral fluoroscopic view of the foot and ankle. On this view, the position of the plantar plane of the weight bearing portion of the foot should be perpendicular to the long axis of the tibia so that posteriorly any remaining talus is in line with the posterior cortex of the tibia. If there is no recognizable talus left, in order to provide viable bony contact, the anterior surface of the tibia is decorticated and placed in contact with the navicular. The posterior half of the tibial plafond is reshaped to make maximal bony contact with the posterior facet of the calcaneus.

While all the intramedullary nails have screw fixation holes, often they do not line up as intended because the anatomy at this point is no longer normal. It is important to obtain fixation between the bone and the nail at the calcaneal level distally and then again proximally in the tibia. Ideally, the tibia hole will be dynamic, rather than static in nature, and will prevent nail rotation but will allow proximal migration in the event that bony resorption occurs. In the event it is not have a dynamic hole, eventually removing the proximal tibial screw may be necessary if further bony contact is needed.

Supplemental fixation, outside of that normally designed with the intramedullary nail, should also be considered especially if there is no real fixation in the talus. Secondary screw fixation away from the nail and crossing the subtalar joint, either from the tuberosity or talar neck, can add significant stability to the construct. This is accomplished using 4.0, 4.5, or 6.5 mm screws. The purpose of these screws is to prevent rotation of the talus around the nail and to offer independent stabilization of the subtalar fusion.

The healthy bone removed earlier can be morselized and is an easy way to provide bone graft around the joint to fill any remaining gaps. If the lateral malleolus was salvaged, it can be effective as a lateral strut across the fusion mass. When using this technique, be sure to remove adequate bone so that there is a centimeter gap between the fibular strut and the distal end of the proximal fibula so that inadvertent contact is not made in the event axial shortening occurs. The use of 3.5 mm cortical screws can be used to fix the fibular strut to the calcaneus and tibia in such a position they do not contact the nail (Fig. 11.5).

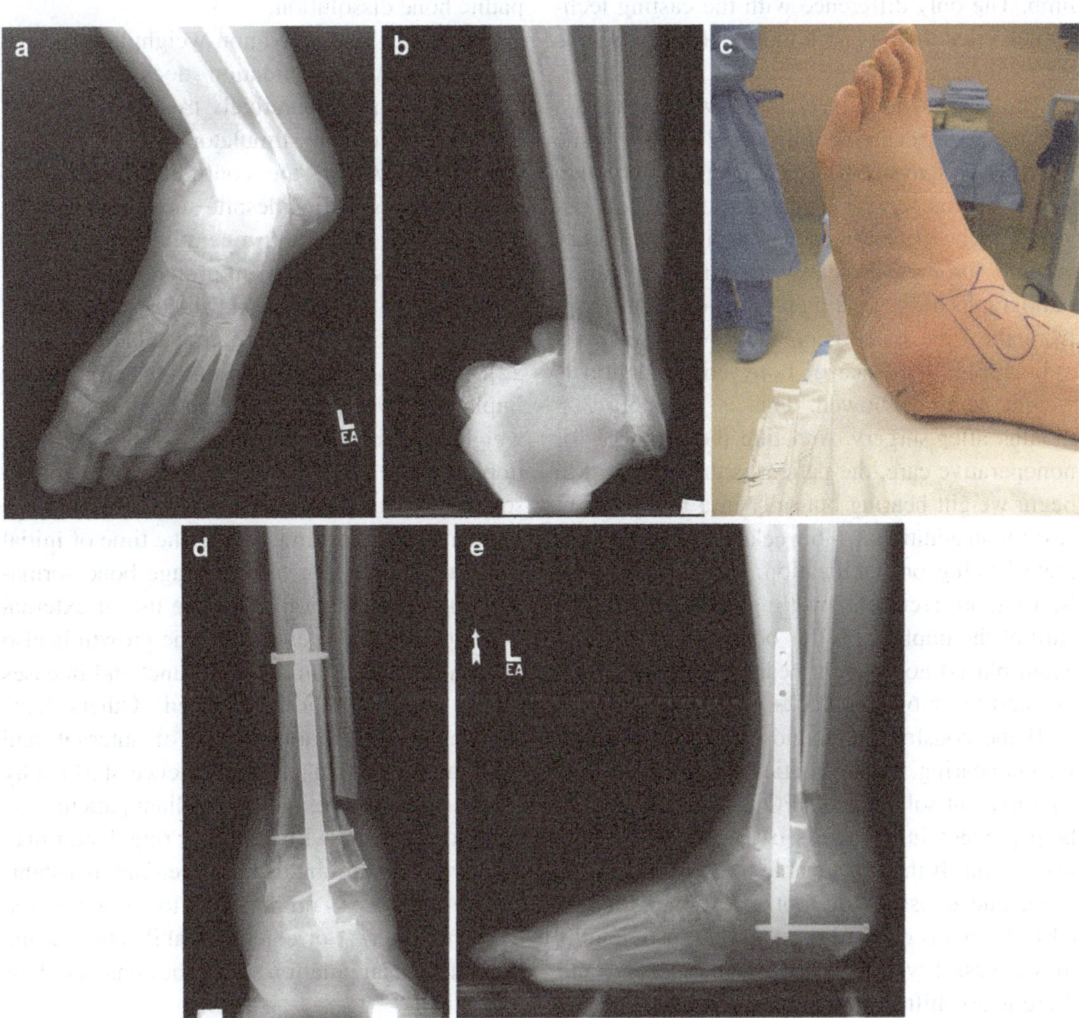

Fig. 11.5 (**a**, **b**) AP radiographs of the foot and ankle of non-braceable Charcot ankle. (**c**) Clinical picture of foot position with chronic recurring lateral skin breakdown. (**d**, **e**) Postoperative AP and lateral X-rays of foot repositioned and stabilized with retrograde tibial-calcaneal fusion nail. Lateral approach through the fibula was used to realign joint. 3.5 mm screws were used to fix the distal fibula to the tibia and talus

Postoperative Care

These patients can be placed directly into a well-padded splint or well-molded plaster cast while still on the operating table, after the tourniquet has been down for 5 min or more. In the recovery room the cast, when dry, is split anteriorly. It is then widened 3–4 mm and overwrapped with fiberglass. These patients require three months strict non-weight bearing for the best chance of success [14–20]. Routine use of a well-molded total contact cast is recommended to help control external factors and to protect the position of the limb. The only difference with the casting technique is that there is no longer a need to include the femoral condyles.

The cast is initially changed weekly with a new total contact cast, applied until the soft tissue edema has stabilized, then changed every two weeks so that regular inspection of the soft tissues can be performed. Monitoring the radiographic progress usually requires obtaining radiographs of the healing process every 4 weeks from the time of surgery. Only when there is radiographic evidence of bony consolidation is weight bearing allowed. This is routinely 2–3 months after surgery. And like the protocol for nonoperative care, the patient is then allowed to begin weight bearing but only in a total contact cast for an additional 4–6 weeks. Signs of incomplete healing or stabilization, seen with weight bearing, are recurrent swelling and radiographic shift of the implants. If this occurs, the patient is again placed non-weight bearing in a total contact cast for 4–6 more weeks.

If the construct is found to be stable while weight bearing, then the patient is transitioned to a permanent solid ankle AFO and rocker shoe to help prevent future stress overload at the now fused joint. If they are unable to accommodate a shoe, due to issues of foot size or position, a CROW boot is ordered for use. If after 6 months of successful weight bearing with a brace, and there is no shift in fixation or significant unilateral swelling, the patient is cleared to come out of the brace as long as there is no increase in swelling or pain. They are also cautioned that going without the brace, even at this point in their care, can lead to pressure overload and loss of limb stability without much warning, due to their underlying neuropathy and loss of protective sensation.

Complications and Salvage

There are four major complications associated with managing these patients: failure to obtain weight bearing stability, breakdown of the soft tissue envelope, the development of deep infection, and the recurrence or progression of neuropathic bone dissolution.

Even with prolonged non-weight bearing and casting, bony consolidation does not always occur. In the non-operatively treated patient, the use of external bone stimulators may be of benefit [21]. However, the continued presence of underlying instability, despite successful casting, usually leads patients to operative stabilization, which restarts the treatment protocol.

Failure of stabilization can also occur with surgical treatment of the Charcot ankle [7, 12, 17, 22]. Continued bony dissolution around the implants as well as poor patient compliance with weight bearing can cause both failure of the implants and loss of alignment. For this reason some have advocated the routine use of an implantable bone stimulator at the time of initial surgical intervention to encourage bone formation and consolidation [23]. The use of external bone stimulators to enhance bone growth is also advocated both as an initial adjunct and in cases where healing appears delayed. Others have advocated the combined use of internal and external fixation [21]. In the presence of a healthy soft tissue envelope and a compliant patient, surgical stabilization with a circular ring fixator may help preserve a limb that has failed internal stabilization. If there is no bone left to allow fixation for either internal or external stabilization of the foot, then an amputation should be considered for the patient.

The presence of soft tissue breakdown often occurs in the non-operatively treated patient when the pressure on the tissues, necessary to maintain limb stability, is great enough to cause ulceration. Inadvertent weight bearing by the patient will amplify the problem, even in a well-molded total contact cast. Changing the cast weekly will help catch the problem before a full thickness breakdown occurs. If skin breakdown occurs and the patient is a surgical candidate, the stabilization of the Charcot ankle should be undertaken by either internal or external fixation. The use of negative pressure wound therapy will also help in healing the pressure-damaged soft tissue.

Wound dehiscence and necrosis are an ever present concern when surgical intervention is undertaken. It has been well documented that the diabetic patient's hyperglycemia decreases blood flow to both small and large vessels, increases blood viscosity and decreases the ability of oxygen to reach the tissues [11]. The presence of local hypoxia adversely affects the ability of fibroblasts to migrate to the wound and proliferate slowing normal wound healing. With routine weekly cast changes and wound inspections incisional problems can be caught early. Also the use of negative pressure wound therapy has been found to be of aid in the healing of these wounds.

As discussed earlier in chapter on ankle fracture care, the presence of a Charcot joint, poor diabetic control, or peripheral arterial disease are all risk factors for the development of infection. The difficulty is in recognizing the presence of an infection at an early stage. Radiographic views are of little help because the Charcot healing process itself can look exactly like a bony response to infection. The use of a combined bone scan/white cell labeled 111-indium scan may be helpful in identifying a deep infection if the hot zone of the indium scan matches up anatomically with the late phase of the bone scan. Usually the appearance of the soft tissue is the clinician's best clue to underlying deep infection. If a deep infection is suspected, the best treatment is early irrigation and debridement of the area with deep bony cultures obtained to help identify the organism so appropriate antibiotics can be given [11, 24, 25]. In the presence of internal fixation the hardware should be removed. In most cases salvage of this situation will require at least the temporary use of a circular frame fixator to salvage

the limb. In the face of significant bone loss or soft tissue compromise an amputation should be considered.

Even after successful stabilization of the limb and a return to weight bearing, the threat of a recurrent Charcot process is still present. Any seemingly small overload to the limb can create a stress fracture leading to the dissolution of surrounding bone. In both the nonoperative and operative patient populations this is seen by progressive loss of limb alignment. More often in the surgically stabilized patient, there is significant bony dissolution of the hindfoot leaving little to fix with either internal or external devices. In an effort to minimize this late complication the routine full time use of a well-molded solid ankle AFO, to help shield the stable limb from abnormal stress forces generated by weight bearing on a neuropathic limb, should be considered. Early recognition of Charcot recurrence before significant deformity occurs requires that the patient restart the treatment cycle of casted non-weight bearing. Significant bone loss will most likely lead to amputation of the limb.

In conclusion, managing a Charcot ankle requires both patience and significant effort on the part of both the physician and patient. Prolonged non-weight bearing is necessary to preserve limb alignment until the bony mass has consolidated. Treatment success is measured by the patient having a stable limb with a plantigrade foot that will safely allow protected weight bearing without damage to the surrounding soft tissues. Failure to provide a stable, braceable limb may lead to amputation.

References

1. Jones KB, Maiers-Yeldon KA, Marsh JL, et al. Ankle fractures in patients with diabetes mellitus. J Bone Joint Surg Br. 2005;87:489–95.
2. Wukich DK, Kline AJ. Current concepts review. The management of ankle fractures in patients with diabetes. J Bone Joint Surg Am. 2008;90:1570–8.
3. Van der Van A, Chapman CB, Bowker JH. Charcot neuropathy of the foot and ankle. J Am Acad Orthop Surg. 2009;17:562–71.
4. Mabilleau G, Edmonds ME. Role of neuropathy on fracture healing in Charcot neuro-osteoarthropathy.

J Musculoskelet Neuronal Interact. 2010;10(1): 84–91.
5. Macey LR, Kana SM, Jingushi S, et al. Defects of early fracture-healing in experimental diabetes. J Bone Joint Surg Am. 1989;71:722–33.
6. Trepman E, Nihal A, Pinzur MS. Charcot Neuroarthropathy of the Foot and Ankle. Foot Ankle Int. 2005;26(1):46–63.
7. Meyerson MS, Edwards WHB. Management of Neuropathic Fractures in the Foot and Ankle. J Am Acad Orthop Surg. 1999;7(1):7–18.
8. Pinzur MS. Benchmark analysis of diabetic patients with neuropathic (Charcot) foot deformity. Foot Ankle Int. 1999;20(9):564–7.
9. Pinzur MS. The development of a neuropathic ankle following successful correction of non plantigrade Charcot foot deformity. Foot Ankle Int. 2012;33(8):644–6.
10. Liu J, Ludwig T, Ebraheim NA. Effect of the blood HbA1c level on surgical treatment outcomes of diabetics with ankle fractures. Orthop Surg. 2013;5: 203–8.
11. Wukich DK, Crim BE, Frykberg RG, Rosario BL. Neuropathy and poorly controlled diabetes increase the rate of surgical site infection after foot and ankle surgery. J Bone Joint Surg Am. 2014;96:832–9.
12. Lowery NJ, Woods JB, Armstrong DG, Wukich DK. Surgical Management of Charcot Neuropathy of the Foot and Ankle: A Systematic Review. Foot Ankle Int. 2012;33(2):113–21.
13. American Diabetes Association. Peripheral arterial disease in people with diabetes. Diabet Care. 2003;26:3333–41.
14. Cinar M, Derincek A, Akpinar S. Tibiocalcaneal arthrodesis with posterior blade plate in diabetic neuropathy. Foot Ankle Int. 2010;31(6):511–5.
15. Alvarez RG, Barbour TM, Perkins TD. Tibiocalcaneal Arthrodesis for Nonbraceable Neuropathic Ankle Deformity. Foot Ankle Int. 1994;15(7):354–9.
16. Caravaggi C, Cimmino M, Caruso S, Noce SD. Intramedullary compressive nail fixation for the treatment of severe Charcot deformity of the ankle and rear foot. J Foot Ankle Surg. 2006;46(1):20–4.
17. Caravaggi C, Sganzaroli AB, Galenda P, et al. Long term follow-up of tibiocalcaneal arthrodesis in diabetic patients with early chronic Charcot osteoarthropathy. J Foot Ankle Surg. 2012;51:408–11.
18. Paola LD, Volpe A, Varatto D, et al. Use of a retrograde nail for ankle arthrodesis in Charcot neuropathy: a limb salvage procedure. Foot Ankle Int. 2007;28(9):967–70.
19. Pinzur MS, Noonan T. Ankle Arthrodesis with a Retrograde Femoral Nail for Charcot Ankle Arthropathy. Foot Ankle Int. 2005;26(7):545–9.
20. Siebachmeyer M, Boddu K, Bilal A, et al. Outcome of one- stage correction of deformities of the ankle and hindfoot and fusion in Charcot neuropathy using a retrograde intramedullary hindfoot arthrodesis nail. Bone Joint J. 2015;97B:76–82.
21. DeVries JG, Berlet GC, Hyer CF. A retrospective comparative analysis of Charcot ankle stabilization using an intramedullary Rod with or without application of circular external fixator- utilization of the retrograde arthrodesis intramedullary nail database. J Foot Ankle Surg. 2012;51:420–5.
22. DiDomenico LA, Brown D. Limb Salvage: Revision of Failed Intramedullary Nail in Hindfoot and Ankle Surgery in the Diabetic Neuropathic Patient. J Foot Ankle Surg. 2012;51:523–7.
23. Hockenbury RT, Gruttadauria M, McKinney I. Use of implantable bone growth stimulation in Charcot ankle arthrodesis. Foot Ankle Int. 2007;28(9):971976.
24. Blotter RH, Connolly E, Wasan A, Chapman MW. Acute complications in the operative treatment of isolated ankle fractures in patients with diabetes mellitus. Foot Ankle Int. 1999;20:687–94.
25. Wukich DK, Lowery NJ, McMillen RI, Fryberg RG. Postoperative infection rates in foot and ankle surgery: a comparison of patients with and without diabetes mellitus. J Bone Joint Surg Am. 2010;92: 287–95.

Exostectomy for Charcot Arthropathy

12

Steven Anthony and Gregory Pomeroy

Introduction

Charcot arthropathy (CN) is a destructive process of the bones and joints. In developed countries, this is most commonly seen in the diabetic population. The primary goal in the treatment of CN is to preserve or achieve, and then maintain, a stable and plantigrade foot that is shoeable and ulcer-free. Exostectomy of bony prominences is a viable treatment option for the stable Charcot foot, presenting with an ulcer or impending ulceration [1–4]. When indicated, an exostectomy has the potential to cure dangerous ulcerations while avoiding the morbidity and complications that can be seen after performing reconstructions and fusions in the foot and ankle [1–4]. The primary concerns with this procedure are an inadequate resolution of ulceration and iatrogenic destabilization of a previously stable foot, through overly aggressive bony resection. (Fig. 12.1a, b)

The midfoot)is the area most commonly affected by CN and is likewise the area of the foot most commonly treated with surgical measures [1–6]. The hindfoot is the second most commonly affected and the ankle third [5]. The ankle, though, is operated on more frequently than the hindfoot [6]. Given that the midfoot is the area most commonly affected, when discussing exostectomy exclusively, it is overwhelmingly the most common area treated [1–4, 6]. We present a discussion on indications and how to use an exostectomy in the treatment of Charcot neuroarthropathy.

Etiology

The etiology of)bony prominences arises from complete bone displacement after joint subluxations/dislocations, displacement of a bone fragment, or excessive bony formation during the healing and consolidation phases. These bony prominences are most commonly unfractured bones, which are malpositioned, due to collapse of the foot, rather than displaced fractures or new bone formation [1]. In our experience, there is often a combination of these etiologies, where bone fragmentation and subsequent healing creates a bone bridge between fractured and

S. Anthony, D.O. (✉)
Advanced Orthopedic Center,
1641 Tamiami Trail, Port Charlotte, FL, USA
e-mail: steveanthonydo@gmail.com

G. Pomeroy, M.D.
Orthopaedic Foot & Ankle, Mercy Hospital,
195 Fore River Parkway, Suite 210,
Portland, ME 04102, USA
e-mail: gpome40@hotmail.com

© Springer International Publishing Switzerland 2016
D. Herscovici, Jr. (ed.), *The Surgical Management of the Diabetic Foot and Ankle*,
DOI 10.1007/978-3-319-27623-6_12

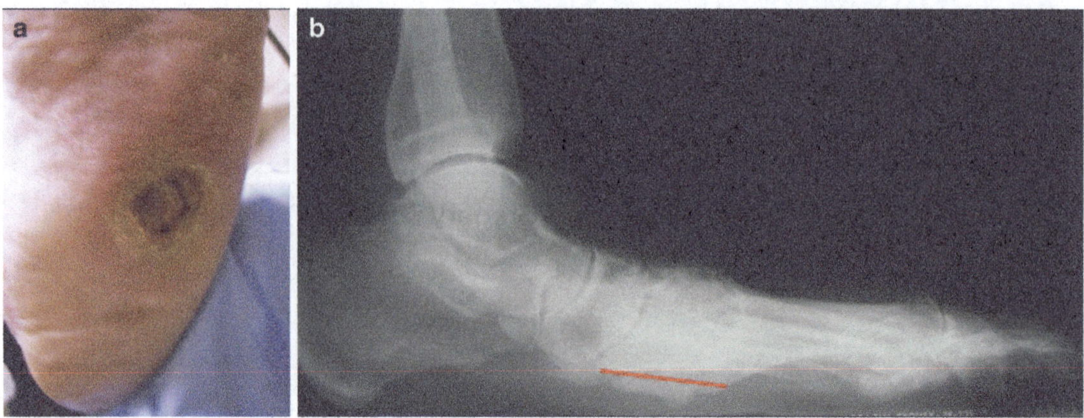

Fig. 12.1 (**a**) Plantar foot ulcer overlying a plantarly subluxed medial cuneiform. (**b**) Lateral X-ray demonstrating the exostosis, a subluxed medial cuneiform and the suggested level (line) of where the exostectomy should be performed

unfractured bones. This creates a large, inflexible bony mass, which is often malpositioned plantarly. Soft-tissue calcifications may also be noted. While they are not true exostoses, they do contribute to ulcer formation by limiting skin flexibility and blood supply.

Staging

The two most commonly used classification systems for Charcot arthropathy are the Eichenholz system and the Brodsky classification. The Eichenholz classification is a temporal classification system that discusses Charcot arthropathy as it progresses through three stages: Stage 1 (dissolution/fragmentation), Stage 2 (coalescent/healing), and Stage 3 (resolution/consolidation) [7]. Stage 0 has been added and is used to describe an early charcot reaction where the foot is red, hot, and swollen, but without any fragmentation [8].

The Brodsky classification organizes the arthropathy by anatomic location. Type 1 is located in the midfoot (tarsometatarsal or naviculocuneiform). Type 2 affects the hind foot (subtalar and/or Chopart joint). Type 3A involves the ankle joint and type 3B affects the posterior tuberosity of the calcaneus [5]. This classification has been modified by Trepman et al. to include type 4 (combination of areas) and type 5(the forefoot), respectively [9].

Indications/Contraindications

A conservative approach should be the initial treatment for any patient presenting with Charcot arthropathy. This should consist of temporary immobilization and off-loading techniques such as total contact casting or Charcot Restraint Orthotic Walking (CROW) boot, until the arthropathy has stabilized (Eichenholtz stage 2 or 3). The patient should then be fitted for protective shoe wear with accommodative orthotics or braces. In addition, an Achilles tendon stretching program should be instituted, either with a physical therapist or at home with appropriate education and guidance. If an ulcer develops, conservative treatments such as total contact casting and custom off-loading braces (Charcot Restraint Orthotic Walker(CROW)) should be utilized. Antibiotics should be instituted if an infection is identified or subsequently develops. Broad spectrum oral antibiotics are acceptable for superficial infections. If osteomyelitis is suspected, broad spectrum or bone culture-specific IV antibiotics should be instituted with assistance from an Infectious Disease specialist. If these measures fail to prevent or resolve the ulceration, surgical options should be considered.

When the problematic deformities are stable and shoeable and/or braceable, reconstruction and/or arthrodesis may not be necessary. An exostectomy of the offending bony prominences should be considered for these patients. This procedure can eliminate a prominence causing the ulcer with limited morbidity and minimal risks [1–4].

Another indication for an exostectomy is an unstable Charcot arthropathy in a patient with ulceration over a bony prominence and underling osteomyelitis, which has not resolved with appropriate antibiotic and off-loading treatments. In this circumstance, a reconstruction is not advised due to the high risk of developing a postoperative infection or a subsequent infected nonunion. The purpose of the exostectomy is to relieve pressure by reducing the size of the prominence, but also to remove any necrotic or infected bone which may be recalcitrant to antibiotic treatment. The goal is to heal the ulcer and clear the infection, allowing for later reconstruction of the foot to a stable, plantigrade position. Advanced imaging, including magnetic resonance imaging (MRI) and/or white blood cell (WBC) bone scan, should be performed prior to any surgery to document the extent of the infection and to guide the bony resection. Exostectomies should also be considered in an unstable Charcot foot which would be best treated with reconstruction or fusion, in cases where the patient is medically unstable or is at too high a risk for postoperative complications. In these circumstances, chronic ulceration can lead to osteomyelitis and ultimately amputation. While an exostectomy will not correct the instability of the foot, it may help resolve any chronic or impending ulceration and thus lower the risk of amputation.

The only absolute contraindication to exostectomy is in a foot that presents during Eichenholz stage 1, with bony edema and fragmentation. Clinically, edema, warmth, and erythema should first be resolved and radiographically, bone healing and stability should be evident. Relative contraindications include instability (subluxation or dislocation which would worsen if the offending bone were excised), severe peripheral vascular disease and an unbraceable/unshoeable deformity that cannot be resolved with exostectomy, who are medically stable.

Preoperative Evaluation

The preoperative decision making should always begin with a basic history and clinical examination. The history should identify the patient's symptoms (onset, history of trauma, sensation changes, discoloration, deformity, pain, swelling, discharge, previous episodes), how long the symptoms have been present and what previous treatments have been employed. Additionally, the surgeon should gain an understanding for the patient's satisfaction with the foot (Does it fit in regular shoes or braces? Are they able to ambulate effectively? Are they able to examine the foot daily and manage minor problems such as calluses and skin abrasions?). Any patient comorbidities should also be discussed, evaluated, and managed by their medical doctor preoperatively and postoperatively.

The clinical examination should evaluate the structure and stability of the foot, as well as searching for signs of active Charcot arthropathy or infection. As stated above, instability, active charcot, and nonplantigrade foot are contraindications to exostectomy. Instability is defined as a deformity which is dynamic and progressive over serial X-rays, or as a deformity which will recur or worsen after the exostosis is removed. An example of the latter is a lateral plantar ulcer, often the cuboid being forced plantarly. If there are no bone bridges fusing the cuboid to surrounding bones, resection of the plantar bone will only lead to the remaining cuboid subluxing further plantar and creating the same pressure to the plantar lateral skin. Resection of the entire cuboid will destabilize the lateral column of the foot. If the patient presents with findings suggestive of a superficial or deep infection, advanced imaging modalities and appropriate lab values are necessary to evaluate the exact extent of infection. If osteomyelitis is present, a surgical debridement should be performed and samples of affected bone should be sent for gram stain and culture with sensitivity to guide antibiotic treatment. Without concern for infection, surgery should be delayed in order to allow for the patient's medical doctors to stabilize the patient's comorbidities and optimize the chances for a good outcome.

Vascularity of the extremity should also be carefully evaluated. If there are any signs of vascular compromise, such as diminished pulses, temperature changes, or cyanosis of the toes, a vascular surgery consult should be obtained in order to determine the viability of the affected area. If blood flow is compromised, restorative procedures should be performed prior to performing any bony surgical interventions.

Imaging of the foot and ankle should begin with basic weight-bearing radiographs. Bony coalescence and sclerosis should be identified and any bony prominences seen on the radiographs should correlate clinically with areas of ulceration. Computed Tomography (CT) should also be considered to more accurately correlate bony protuberances with skin ulcerations.

Superficial and deep infections should be fully investigated prior to performing an exostectomy. If bone can be easily identified at the base of the ulcer, a working diagnosis of osteomyelitis is assumed to be present and MRI should be performed to determine the extent of infection [10, 11]. Without exposed bone, a WBC-labeled bone scan or combined bone scans may be more specific and sensitive than MRI for ruling out osteomyelitis [11, 12]. Swabbing the ulcer for cultured yields unreliable information is not recommended, but deep tissue samples may provide more accurate culture and sensitivity results. Superficial infections and ulcerations can be expected to resolve with oral or IV antibiotics once the pressure causing prominence is removed. The use of oral versus IV antibiotics has many factors, such as the virulence of the suspected organism (history of MRSA?) and the vascularity of the foot. An infectious disease expert should be involved to guide this aspect of the treatment. A deep infection may require multiple debridements with possible bulk resection of deep tissues, including bone in patients with osteomyelitis.

Surgical Approaches

General Considerations

Incisions should be planned so that they avoid the plantar surface and the ulcerated skin, while providing good access to the bony prominence.

Dissection should be full-thickness, avoiding any undermining of the skin and subcutaneous tissues. Excising a plantar ulcer should only be considered for small lesions with no evidence of infection. (Figs. 12.2 and 12.3) Once removed, the bony prominence should be sent to pathology to evaluate for osteomyelitis. If a superficial or deep infection is present, deep tissue and/or bone cultures should also be obtained. Swabbing the ulcer is likely to lead to misleading culture results, and thus is not recommended. Great care must be taken to avoid excessive bony resection, which can subsequently result in iatrogenic destabilization of a stable foot. Lengthening the achilles tendon should always be considered for plantar or heel ulcerations. This has been shown to lower peak pressures on the plantar foot during ambulation, and likewise may lower the risk of recurrent ulceration [13].

Forefoot

The metatarsophalangeal (MTP) joints are the area most commonly affected in the forefoot. The destruction seen at these joints may not be secondary to the same unique Charcot disease process that is noted in the midfoot, hindfoot, and ankle. Rather, the problem is often believed to be from chronic overloading of the forefoot and subsequent bone and joint destruction. In addition, there is often an associated deep infection. Most patients present neuropathy producing an insensate forefoot along with an equinus contracture, both of which causes an overload of the forefoot. Either due to excessive pressure, infection, or a combination of both, one can often see bone destruction and subsequent bone growth during repair. This combination of bony overgrowth and excessive loading of the forefoot can lead to ulceration of the plantar skin over the MTP joints.

For the second- third- and fourth metatarsals, there are two available approaches: dorsal and plantar. A dorsal approach is preferable, as ulcerations are typically plantar, it is best to place incisions away from the ulceration, and an exostectomy of a plantar bony prominence is

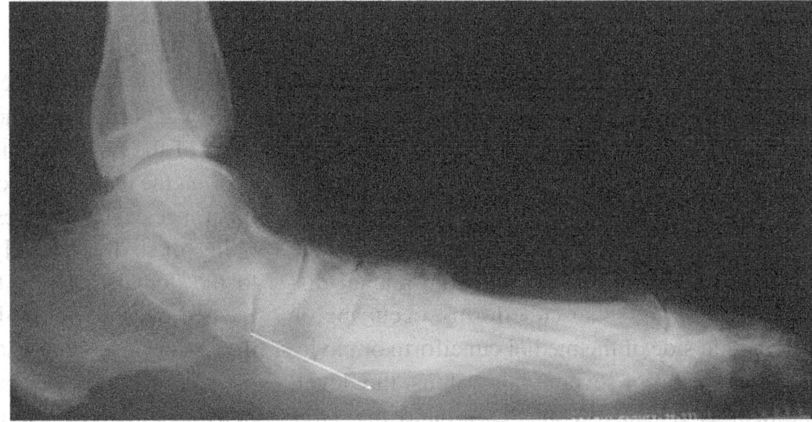

Fig. 12.2 Lateral X-ray demonstrating another level of exostectomy (line) how much bone should be excised for bony problems at the level of Chopart Joint

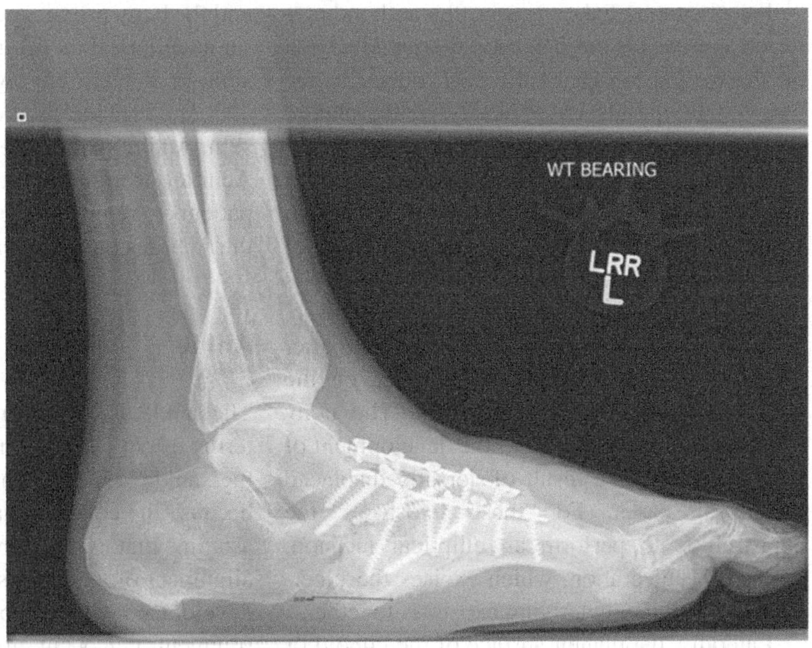

Fig. 12.3 Lateral X-ray demonstrating an exostosis that has developed after fixation of the midfoot and the proposed (line) exostectomy

technically difficult. There is no clinical research to guide decision making but the authors prefer a complete metatarsal head resection for ulcers greater than 1 cm which are recurrent or have failed to resolve with conservative care for 3 months. For impending ulcerations or smaller ulcers with no signs of infection, a plantar approach, excising the affected area, can be performed provided there is adequate healthy skin to close without tension. When approaching the first or fifth metatarsals, a medial incision for the first or lateral incision for the fifth may also be utilized, respectively.

In addition to the exostectomy, irrigation and debridement of necrotic tissues should be performed and a percutaneus achilles tendon lengthening should also be considered. Lengthening the achilles tendon has been shown to lower peak pressures on the plantar forefoot during ambulation, and likewise may lower the risk of ulceration [13].

Midfoot

The midfoot is the area of the foot most commonly affected by CN [1]. The most common problematic bony prominences in this area are the plantarly displaced medial cuneiform and first metatarsal base [1], often presenting in conjunction with a plantar ulcer. Other problematic protuberances are seen arising from plantar displacement of the other cuneiforms, occurring on the medial side of the medial cuneiform or navicular as a result of severe planovalgus, the development of dorsal osteophytes around the TMT joints, and exostoses that occur at the base of the fifth metatarsal or cuboid laterally [1–4].

For plantarmedial exostoses, the authors' preferred approach is through a longitudinal incision on the medial border of the foot, dorsal to the ulcer. Since the ulcer is typically on the plantar surface, the incision will allow for a direct access to the midportion of the subluxed cuneiform. A small oscillating saw is then used to cut through the bone, from medial to lateral, removing all of the offending plantar prominence. A bone rasp is then used to smooth down any rough edges.

Dorsal exostoses typically result in smaller ulcerations, since they are not located on the weight-bearing surface of the foot. The bony prominences are often due to the development of osteophytes or as a result of dorsally displaced metatarsal bases. For these exostoses the approach is to perform an elliptical incision, beyond the ulceration, which excises the ulcerated skin and the underlying exostosis together.

Laterally, the plantar surface of the cuboid or the lateral surface of the fifth metatarsal base can be problematic to treat. The approach for these lateral ulcers is preferred on the lateral border of the foot, performing a full-thickness approach to the exostosis (Fig. 12.4a–e). The longitudinal incision used is dorsal to the ulceration will allow complete exposure of the bone through healthy skin and allow removal of the exostoses. One should be cognizant that there may be a higher risk of ulcer recurrence with lateral exostectomy, as compared to treatment of medial exostoses [2]. An achilles tendon lengthening procedure should be considered when treating plantar ulcers of the midfoot if an equinus contracture is present.

Hindfoot

The hind foot rarely requires surgical intervention for CN. In the authors' experience, displacement of the posterior tuberosity of the calcaneus is often the cause for most problematic bony protuberances. This can result in ulcerations developing medially, laterally, or posteriorly. Similar to the dorsal midfoot, these ulcerations are not located on any weight-bearing surfaces. Rather, they occur secondary to friction produced from the patient's shoes or braces rubbing against the bony protuberance. An exostectomy can often be performed directly over the exostosis, with an elliptical incision, again excising both the ulcer and the bony prominence. If the ulcer is too large for an elliptical incision to be closed without tension, or if there are signs of deep infection, an alternate incision should be used through healthy skin. Additionally, a percutaneous release of the Achilles tendon should be considered in these patients to remove the excessive proximal pull of the Achilles on the calcaneal tuberosity.

Ankle

The ankle is least commonly affected area in terms of patients presenting with CN. However, the ankle is frequently managed surgically because the collapse that occurs is often so devastating that it frequently affects the anatomic alignment of the other structures in the foot. The development of osteophytes or displaced bony fragments can occur anywhere. These most commonly occur medially or laterally, can cause anterior or posterior impingement, or result in ulcerations anywhere about the ankle.

The ulcerations that occur are not overweight-bearing surfaces. Most often they occur secondary to pressure necrosis or abrasion from shoes and braces. For these patients, an exostectomy should be as minimal as possible in order to avoid iatrogenic instability. In particular, surgeons should be careful not to detach the origins of the deltoid or lateral ligaments with overly aggressive bony resection. Incisions should be longitudinal and away from the ulceration in an area which is anatomically safe and allows for access to the exosto-

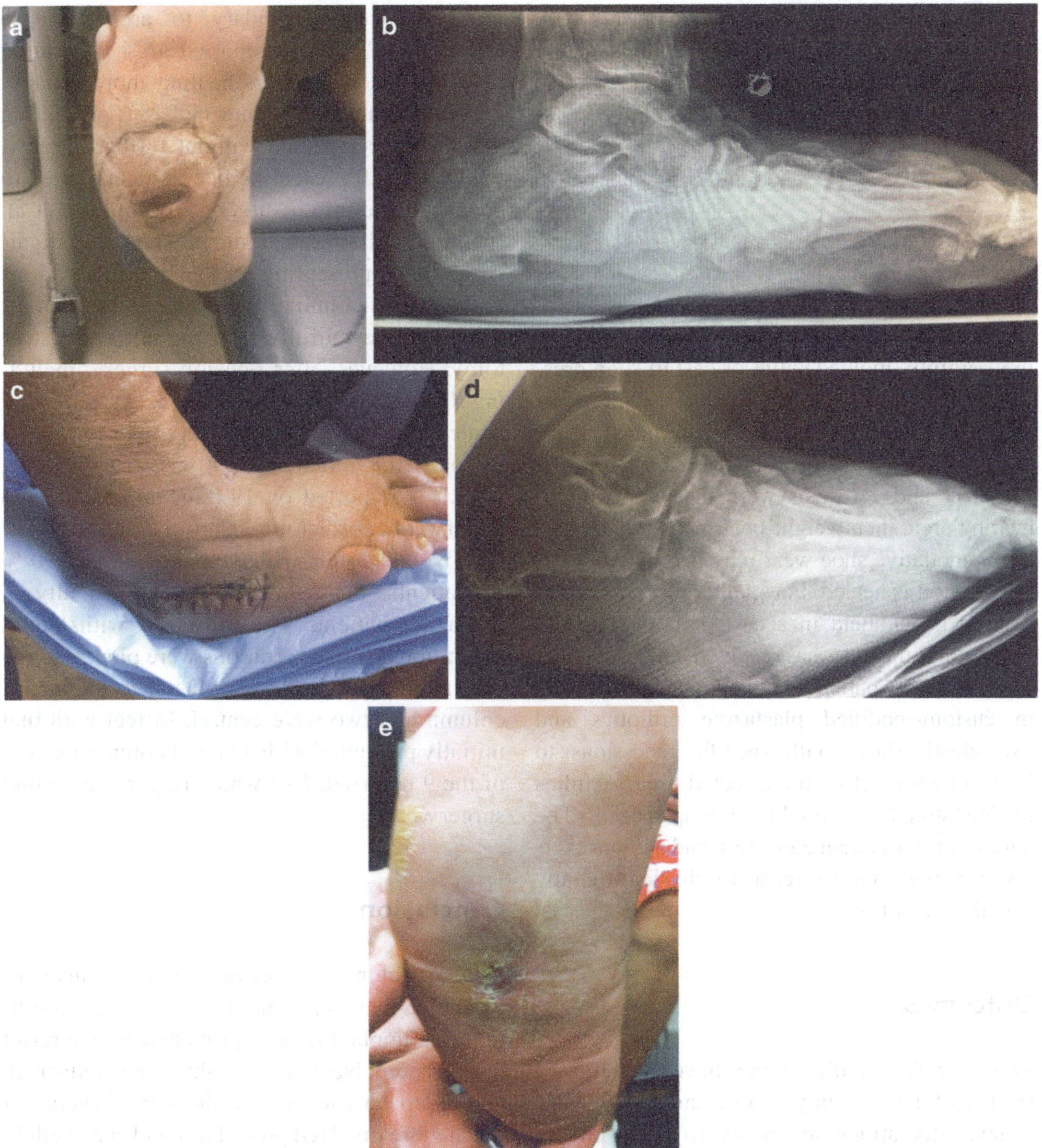

Fig. 12.4 (**a**) Plantar foot ulcer that has developed overlying a subluxed cuboid and lateral cuneiform. (**b**) Preoperative lateral X-ray demonstrating the subluxed cuboid and lateral cuneiform. (**c**) Surgical incision used to approach and perform the exostectomy. (**d**) Postoperative lateral X-ray demonstrating resection of the exostoses. (**e**) Resolved plantar ulcer status post exostectomy

sis. Patients presenting with displaced bony fragments also frequently present with impingement of the soft tissues and limited motion around the ankle. If a large posterior exostoses is identified, it should be removed, if it causes any decrease in motion, produces impending skin problems, or has already resulted in the development of an ulcer. When patients are identified with either anterior tibial and talar osteophytes, they often demonstrate difficulty in dorsiflexing the ankle along increased pressures to the plantar forefoot and midfoot, and often develop secondary arthritic changes to the ankle joint. When an exostectomy about the ankle is performed, an Achilles tendon release should also be considered, in order to increase dorsiflexion at the ankle and lower plantar peak pressures.

Postoperative

All patients should be immobilized postoperatively and made non-weight-bearing for 2 weeks in a carefully molded splint or cast to keep pressure off the foot. If there was concomitant osteomyelitis, antibiotics should be continued under the guidance of an infectious disease expert. If the ulcer and exostosis were in a non-weight-bearing area, then weight-bearing as tolerated in accommodative shoe wear may begin as soon as the incision is healed. For plantar ulcers, weight-bearing is withheld in a cast or boot (CROW, CAM) until the ulcer has resolved. Once the ulcer has healed, the patient may begin weight-bearing in custom-modified plastazote orthotics and extra-depth shoes with specific recessions to keep pressure off of the affected area. Achilles tendon stretching should be emphasized. The authors prefer patient education and a home exercise regimen, but a referral to physical therapy can also be utilized.

Outcomes

There are few studies which have investigated the use of exostectomy as a means to surgically relieve ulcerations secondary to bony prominences in Charcot Arthropathy of the foot and ankle. Brodsky and Rouse [1] reported on 12 patients with problematic plantar bony prominences. One patient had a problem affecting the hindfoot and the remaining eleven had arthropathy affecting the midfoot. Eight involved the medial foot and four were lateral. Eleven of the twelve patients remained free of ulceration throughout the follow-up period. Catanzariti, et al. [2], reported on 20 patients (27 ft) who underwent exostectomy for the treatment of midfoot ulcers secondary to arch collapse caused by CN. They reported a 74 % healing rate, with medial ulcers healing more reliably than lateral ulcers. Seventeen of 18 ft presenting a medial ulcer healed without further surgery, while 6 of 9 ft presenting lateral ulcers failed to heal after the initial surgery. Rosenblum, et al. [4], reported similar findings when investigating patients presenting with plantar ulcerations to the lateral column of the foot. Only 21 of 32 ft healed uneventfully after the initial exostectomy. However, after revision surgery, including flap coverage, 29 of the 32 ft remained healed and functional throughout the follow-up period (20.8 months). Lastly, Laurinaviciene, et al. [3], reported on 19 patients (20 ft) who underwent exostectomy. They also found excellent overall results with wound healing in 90 % of patients, but again noted the difficulty in managing patients who presented with lateral ulcerations. Nine ulcerations were plantar to the medial column, nine were plantar to the lateral column and two were central. In feet with that initially presented with a lateral column ulcer, 6 of the 9 recurred, 5 of which required a second surgery.

Conclusion

An exostectomy is a proven minimally invasive technique that can be used to treat ulcers resulting from impinging bony prominences that result from Charcot Neuroarthropathy. When indicated, this approach can provide the same benefits of much more involved procedures and can result in excellent outcomes, while producing fewer complications. Incisions should be made away from the ulcer but in small ulcers an excision of both the ulcer and exostosis can be combined. It appears however, that that lateral ulcers are more difficult to heal than medial ulcers. At the time of surgery, consideration should also be given to performing an Achilles lengthening in these patients in order to improve ankle dorsiflexion while limiting the plantar peak pressures that occur in the mid- and forefoot region.

References

1. Brodsky JW, Rouse AM. Exostectomy for symptomatic bony prominences in diabetic Charcot feet. Clin Orthop Relat Res. 1993;296:21–6.
2. Catanzariti AR, Mendicino R, Haverstock B. Ostectomy for diabetic neuroarthropathy involving the midfoot. J Foot Ankle Surg. 2000;39:291–300.
3. Laurinaviciene R, Kirketerp-Moeller K, Holstein PE. Exostectomy for chronic midfoot plantar ulcer in Charcot deformity. J Wound Care. 2008;17:53–8.
4. Rosenblum BI, Giurini JM, Miller LB, Chrzan JS, Habershaw GM. Neuropathic ulcerations plantar to the lateral column in patients with Charcot foot deformity: a flexible approach to limb salvage. J Foot Ankle Surg. 1997;36:360–3.
5. Brodsky JW, Klein SE, Johnson JE. Diabetes. In: Coughlin MJ, Mann RA, Saltzman CL, editors. Surgery of the foot and ankle. 9th ed. MO, Mosby: St. Louis; 2014.
6. Lowery NJ, Woods JB, Armstrong DG, Wukich DK. Surgical management of Charcot neuroarthropathy of the foot and ankle: a systematic review. Foot Ankle Int. 2012;33:113–21.
7. Eichenholtz S. Charcot joints. Springfield, IL: C. C. Thomas; 1966.
8. Shibata T, Tada K, Hashizume C. The results of arthrodesis in the ankle for leprotic neuroarthropathy. J Bone Joint Surg Am. 1990;72:749–56.
9. Trepman E, Nihal A, Pinzur MS. Current concepts review: Charcot neuroarthropathy of the foot and ankle. Foot Ankle Int. 2005;26:46–63.
10. Ma LD, Frassica FJ, Bluemke DA, Fishman EK. CT and MRI evaluation of musculoskeletal infection. Crit Rev Diagn Imaging. 1997;38:535–68.
11. Tehranzadeh J, Wong E, Wang F, Sadighpour M. Imaging of osteomyelitis in the mature skeleton. Radiol Clin North Am. 2001;39:223–50.
12. Sella EJ, Grosser DM. Imaging modalities of the diabetic foot. Clin Podiatr Med Surg. 2003;20:729–40.
13. Armstrong DG, Stacpoole-Shea S, Nguyen H, Harkless LB. Lengthening of the Achilles tendon in diabetic patients who are at high risk for ulceration of the foot. J Bone Joint Surg Am. 1999;81A:535–8.

Use of External Fixation for the Management of the Diabetic Foot and Ankle

Bradley M. Lamm and Dror Paley

Introduction

Charcot arthropathy is an overwhelming complication of peripheral neuropathy. It occurs in approximately 30 % of those individuals afflicted with peripheral neuropathy, with diabetes mellitus being the most common cause in the United States [1]. The consequence of this progressive and debilitating condition is pedal joint subluxations, dislocations, fractures, and extensive osseous architecture destruction resulting in deformity of the foot and ankle and ulcerations. When evaluating patients, the authors assess the foot and ankle for the stage and location of arthropathy, the presence of any ulcers, and whether the patient has any soft tissue and the bone infections.

As explained in Chap. 4, the temporal classification system of Eichenholtz [2] discusses Charcot arthropathy as it progresses through three stages. These are described as developmental, coalescence and reconstruction, with Shibata et al., adding an additional phase (stage 0) to describe the foot at risk, which precedes the developmental phase and which radiographic findings are negative [3]. Treatment often consists of nonoperative treatment including a total contact cast immobilization until bony consolidation occurs. Non-weightbearing produces an increased load on the contralateral foot, which can then lead to ulceration, precipitation of Charcot arthropathy, and osteopenia. Maintaining non-weightbearing status is difficult for this patient population for various reasons including obesity, diminished proprioception, and muscle atrophy. Despite early recognition and treatment, the disease process can result in osseous and soft tissue deformities, which can lead to a deformed foot position and the presence of equinus, all of which can be difficult to properly shoe, brace, and/or offload. This places the individual at risk for ulcerations, infections, and subsequent limb loss [1, 4]. Once the stage of Charcot has been determined, it is important to note the anatomic location of the Charcot deformity. Various authors have classified the Charcot foot and ankle based on its anatomic location [5–7]. Although useful, none have been validated as predictive of outcomes. However, the authors feel that the Charcot location has a significant determination on the type and success of treatment rendered for the deformity.

B.M. Lamm, D.P.M., F.A.C.F.A.S. (✉)
International Center for Limb Lengthening,
Rubin Institute for Advanced Orthopedics,
2401 West Belvedere Ave., Sinai Hospital,
Baltimore, MD 21215, USA
e-mail: bradankle@yahoo.com

D. Paley, M.D., F.R.C.S.C.
Paley Advanced Limb Lengthening Institute,
St. Mary's Hospital, 901 45th Street, Kimmel
Building, West Palm Beach, FL 33407, USA

© Springer International Publishing Switzerland 2016
D. Herscovici, Jr. (ed.), *The Surgical Management of the Diabetic Foot and Ankle*,
DOI 10.1007/978-3-319-27623-6_13

Next, it is important to identify the presence of an ulcer. Ulcers become more common when patients present with midfoot Charcot deformities, especially if the deformity progresses proximally. The key to managing these deformities is to allow for bony consolidation of the dislocation. However, when this consolidation results in a significant deformity, or recurrent ulceration occurs, surgical intervention is typically performed. A collapse of the medial column of the midfoot tends to produce ulcers along the plantar medial aspect of the foot. This often occurs when there is peritalar dislocation of the navicular-cuneiform joint causing the talus to dislocate medially and plantarly. Lateral ulcers are due to a disruption of the lateral column. This collapse is exacerbated by the effect of the ground reaction vector that is initiated at heel strike. In addition, the presence of an equinus contracture and the pull of the tibialis anterior tendon further exacerbate the lateral column disruption. This produces a "bayoneting" affect of the forefoot on the hindfoot, which produces a classic "rocker bottom" deformity of the foot. Prolonged weightbearing on these unstable midfoot deformities acts to produce further dislocation of the lateral column, leading to an ulceration of the lateral plantar foot. Additionally, ankle and hindfoot Charcot deformities can also occur, either as an isolated event or in combination, and can also lead to the development of an ulcer. Regardless of its location, ulcers often respond well to offloading of bony prominences and conservative management. When conservative management is unsuccessful, and if the deformities are unstable or non-braceable, the authors feel that they must then be addressed surgically in order to create a stable foot and ankle complex. The goal of the surgery is to create a stable or fused foot and ankle. Regardless of the location of any Charcot deformities, it is important to rule out any infective process that may have resulted from the previous ulceration. This chapter will hopefully provide useful information for the management of the Charcot foot and ankle using external fixation.

Indications and Preoperative Surgical Approach

As stated, the primary goal of surgery is to obtain a plantigrade foot that can be placed into an appropriate shoe and/or brace to minimize the risk for further breakdown or infection [7, 8]. Reconstruction of Charcot midfoot deformity is traditionally recommended during the coalescence or healing stage of the patient's arthropathy. Clear indications for surgery include an unstable deformity, a non-healing or infected ulcer, with or without the presence of osteomyelitis, a patient presenting with an equinus deformity, and a stable foot with a deformity that is at risk for ulceration in a shoe or brace.

One of the most challenging aspects in treating patients with Charcot arthropathy is in determining which patients are suitable candidates for reconstruction. One problem is in treating the neuropathic patient because the risks for complications are higher than for the non-neuropathic patient. A second problem is that these are often unhealthy patients presenting with significant comorbidities, such as cardiopulmonary disease, peripheral vascular disease, and immune dysfunction, all of which need to be addressed and optimized by the patient's medical specialists, including cardiology and endocrinology, before attempting any reconstruction. Lastly, the surgeon must be cognizant of the patient's psychosocial state and family support. Both the patient and their family should be educated about the risks and benefits of surgery, in addition to the importance and scope of the procedures needed for limb salvage [1, 4].

During the preoperative assessment, the clinician should obtain a thorough history that includes the duration and progression of the deformity, any history of ulceration or infections, and history of previous interventions, surgical or otherwise. The physical examination should include observing the patient's gait and stance, evaluating for any equinus, and evaluating the plantar surface of the foot to look for any areas of compromise that may lead to the development of skin breakdown or ulceration. Radiographic examination should consist of multi-planar foot and ankle weightbearing radiographs (anterior–posterior, lateral, and axial) to assess the foot and ankle alignment. These radiographic views aid in the planning that is needed to correct the deformity. Radiographs of the foot and ankle also allow the surgeon to determine the severity of the collapse and the amount of soft tissue edema that is present. If a proximal deformity is clinically observed, the radiographic evaluation should also include a standing radiograph of the patient's entire lower limb, which should include the pelvis, femur, and tibia, in order to assist in measuring lower extremity alignment, joint orientation angles, and limb length discrepancies [9]. The use of a computerized axial tomography (CT) scan is helpful for determining the quality and position of the bone. Also, a 3D reconstruction CT image provides beneficial information about morphology of the bone deformity. These radiographs are essential to accurately locate the center of rotation of angulation (CORA), or apex of the deformity for preoperative surgical planning [9]. Supplemental imaging studies such as bone scan or magnetic resonance imaging can also aid in the preoperative assessment and are helpful in identifying the extent of bone loss or infected bone segments [10]. Lastly, laboratory data, such as C-reactive protein or erythrocyte sedimentation rate, can be helpful in identifying osteomyelitis.

Surgical Management of the Patient

Various surgical methods have been described for the management of Charcot collapse. Large open incisions and wedge bone resections are typically performed to correct Charcot foot deformities [11, 12]. The disadvantages of this approach are the large amount of bone resection required, which shortens the foot, and the large incisions required to accomplish reduction. These approaches can also increase the rate of infection and create potential wound healing problems. We have developed minimally invasive techniques utilizing gradual distraction with realignment, in order to obtain and achieve an anatomic position of the foot and ankle during

fusion of the Charcot joints. This technique also allows one to employ the use of an acute wedge resection, if necessary, in order to improve the alignment and attain a reduction and fusion of the Charcot foot and ankle. Deformity planning and principles are presented based on the authors' extensive experience in Charcot foot and ankle deformity correction. These general principles can hopefully help guide the surgeon when addressing the patient who presents with a Charcot deformity.

Management of the Soft Tissues

Before, during, and after treatment, one needs to respect the soft tissue envelope of the entire leg. During stage I of the arthropathy, the soft tissue swelling in the foot and ankle is extensive and should be managed before any surgical intervention is performed. During stages II or III, enough of the soft tissue edema and erythema has resolved that the clinician can really assess the foot and ankle to determine a treatment plan. During this preoperative planning, one should again carefully evaluate the foot and ankle and take notice of any ulceration that has developed, assess the stability of joints, identify the presence of any equinus deformity, and look for any bony prominences that may aid the surgeon in determining whether a conservative or surgical plan should be used. If conservative treatment is chosen, the goal is to maintain a closed, durable skin envelope that prevents ulcerations and infections. This approach consists of using protective shoes, braces, inserts, orthotics, and boots in any combination to assist in the offloading during weightbearing. For further information, please refer to Chap. 5. If surgery is contemplated, the dissections should consist of full thickness skin flaps that are raised in an atraumatic technique. Minimal incision techniques should be utilized when possible to minimize the soft tissue compromise in this unique patient population. Retraction of skin is limited, and should be used only when needed. Also, all postoperative edema must be controlled with elevation and appropriate fluid balance. At times admission into the hospital may be required to ensure strict elevation and medical fluid rebalancing.

Equinus Correction

Any equinus correction should be performed prior to the construction and application of the external fixation device. Charcot patients without an equinus deformity tend to fare better than those with a contracture. This is because an equinus deformity tends to produce ulceration over bony prominences on the plantar surface of the foot and can prevent one from obtaining an improved alignment of the foot and ankle. For these patients, a tendo-Achilles lengthening is recommended. The lengthening is performed at a level based on the Silversköld test. A gastrosoleal recession, using either a Vulpius or Strayer procedure, is preferred over the use of a Hoke triple hemisection tenotomy, because it allows the patient to maintain push-off strength and decreases the risk of a calcaneus gait. A gastrocnemius recession, using either a Baumann or Silversköld, is performed as an alternative if an isolated gastrocnemius equinus is present or if the patients possess a poor distal soft tissue envelope [13]. Alternatively, a gradual correction of the equinus can also be obtained using external fixation via gradual soft tissue distraction. This is performed by placing a hinged external fixator along Inman's axis of the ankle joint or by using a Taylor Spatial Frame to gradually correct the equinus, which typically is done in combination with the Charcot reconstruction procedure.

External Fixation Advantages

External fixation has many advantages when managing a Charcot foot or ankle deformity. First, its application is minimally invasive but the correction of deformity can be extensive. Second, because the correction can be obtained by gradual distraction, it can be used with or without the use of an adjunctive, limited open technique. Third, in cases of acute deformity correction, the external fixation allows for fine-tuning of residual defor-

mity outside the operating room. In contrast, patients treated with internal fixation require that a precise correction of the deformity be obtained at the time of surgery, which cannot be altered during the postoperative period. Fourth, external fixation constructs allow for immediate weightbearing with an assistive device during the postoperative course. The use of early weightbearing can lessen disuse osteoporosis and minimize contralateral limb overload, which is typical in the Charcot patient. Fifth, the use of external fixation may allow for access to the soft tissues for wound care that is often utilized during treatment of osteomyelitis. Lastly, fine wire fixation avoids placing large implants through the bone, which can lead to stress risers or iatrogenic fractures.

External Fixation Disadvantages

The disadvantages of external fixation include the need for special surgical expertise required for construction. Second, pin site infection is a common complication, but this can often be handled with oral antibiotics. Third, failure of fixation can occur through the wire, ring, or half pin resulting in breakage or deflection. This can result in destabilization of the external fixation. Lastly, external fixation treatment may have to be left on for long periods of time to ensure complete osseous healing has occurred. This can result in loosening of wires and half pins. Although complications are seen with the use of any surgical approach, most complications using external fixation are minor, when recognized in a timely manner, and can be addressed non-operatively. Typically, when operative intervention is required, the external fixation can be left in position while the complication is addressed [14].

Construction of Stable External Fixation

Charcot neuropathic patients often present with one or more of the following problems: decreased healing potential, poor bone quality, obesity, altered osseous alignment, inability to maintain a non-weightbearing gait, vascular problems, lower extremity edema, and may present with ulcers, infections, or osteomyelitis, either as isolated problems or in any combination. Thus, constructing a stable and sustainable external fixation is a challenge. In order to obtain a rigid construct, one often needs to construct ring fixation blocks, and then place them on each side of the Charcot joint. A ring fixation block consists of two circular rings that are connected together using 4 or 5 threaded rods, telescoping rods, or sockets. The size or span of a ring fixation block can be the entire length of the tibia (150–250 mm threaded rods connecting the tibial rings) or can be only as high as the foot (40–60 mm sockets connecting the foot rings). The ring fixation block is then connected to the bone with at least four smooth wires and/or half pins. Half pins are reserved only for the tibia and in the Charcot patient the authors recommend using a 6 mm diameter half pin. In addition, the number of connections to the bone should be greater than what is generally used to manage the non-neuropathic patient, thus in general we add an additional point of fixation (half pin or smooth wire) per ring. When selecting rings to construct the fixation block, it is important that the ring size selected is able to accommodate any increased postoperative edema. Typically, full rings are preferred over 2nd/3rd rings because of the increased strength. Also rings that are one size larger than the ones used on a non-neuropathic patient are recommended so as to accommodate for postoperative leg swelling. Thus, normally the author's two fingers distance circumferentially between the ring and the patient's skin in normal patients. We use three fingers for the neuropathic population. The authors prefer the full Taylor Spatial rings (made of aluminum) for the leg (155–230 mm) and long foot closed rings completed with half rings for the foot (155–180 mm). The authors do not use composite rings (carbon fiber) as we feel these have less strength. A large span of tibial fixation is required to increase the stability. Any postsurgical tibial fractures have been noted by the authors to occur just proximal or at the proximal fixation point of the frame, thus we typically span

most of the tibia. (see Fig. 13.3). The wires and half pins should be placed as close as possible to the ring fixation block to decrease cantilever (loading) of the bone. A foot block or "bumper" is two completed foot rings connected with sockets or threaded rods. The foot block (two completed foot rings) holds all foot, digital, and talar wires as well as it provides a walking surface by the addition of a bolted on cast shoe with the upper portion of the cast shoe cut off (Fig. 13.3c). This provides increased stability and protects the digits from accidental injury during the external fixation treatment period. The authors do not recommend half pins in the foot for neuropathic patients as the cortical bone in the foot is thin. In addition, we typically avoid the use of olive wires unless necessary for a dynamic correction. Olive wires create a periosteal reaction which can lead to pin site infection. The authors' recommend at least two points of fixation per bone segment with maximum obliquity of the two 1.8 mm Ilizarov wires, to ensure stability without the use of olive wires.

The ring foot block should be mounted parallel to the sole of the foot by using two crossed calcaneal wires: one perpendicular wire below the ring, from medial to lateral, and one obliquely placed wire above the ring, also placed medial to lateral. The calcaneal wires should be started medial and posterior to the lateral plantar nerve and medial to the Achilles tendon insertion. Tensioning on the two calcaneal wires should be approximately 110 mmHg using the tensioning device. In the midfoot, one wire is inserted across the cuneiform cuboid level and is tensioned (110 mmHg) and fixed. Next, two smooth wires are inserted into the talus. One is placed medial to lateral, through the talar neck, and the other from anteromedial in the neck of the talus to posterolateral to the Achilles tendon. The position of the wires should be monitored with fluoroscopy to make sure they do not enter the subtalar or ankle joints. The two wires are connected to the foot ring and tensioned (90 mmHg). Additional midfoot, metatarsals, and digital smooth wires (1.8 mm) are inserted as needed.

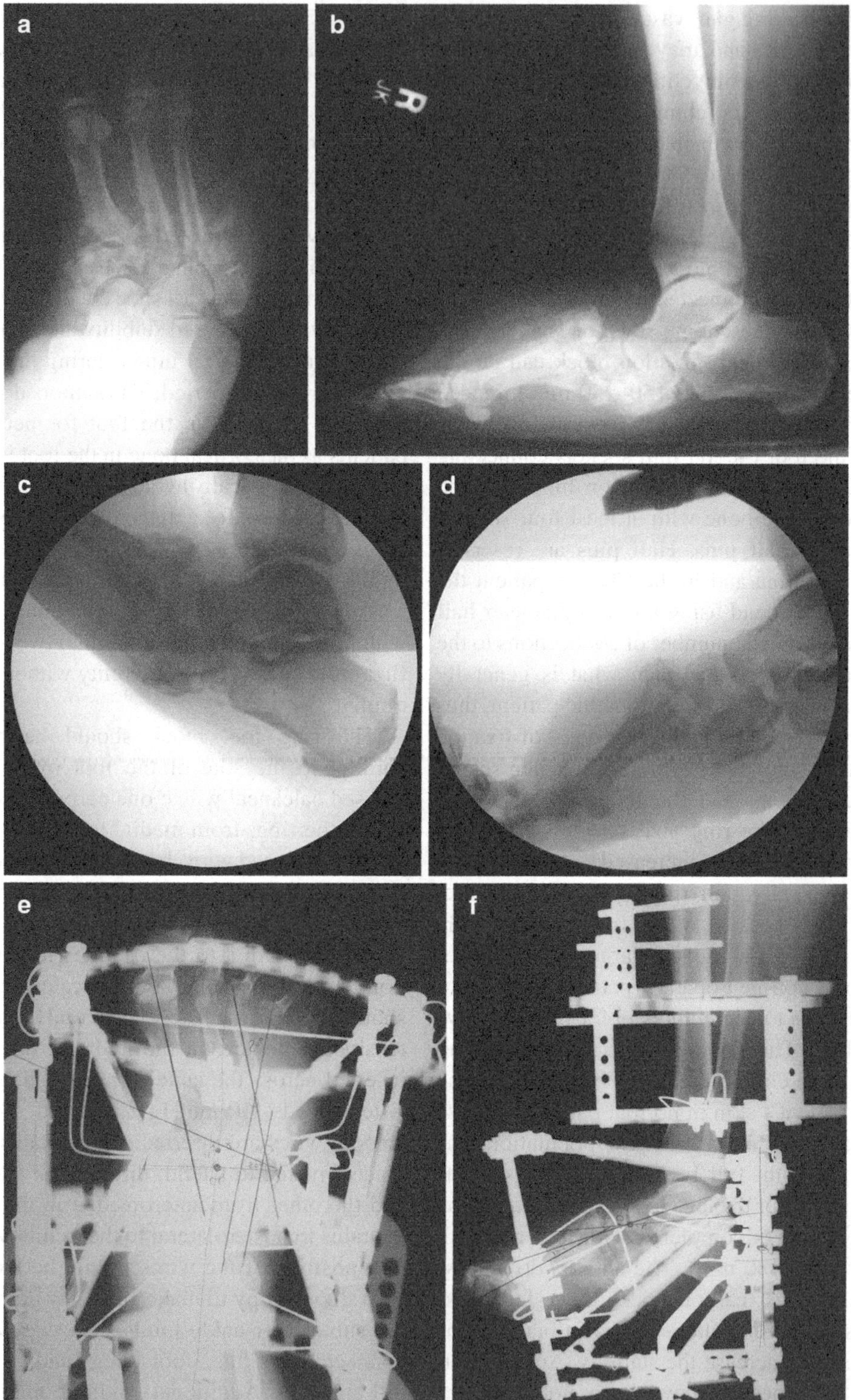

Fig. 13.1 (**a**) Anteroposterior radiograph view of a patient with midfoot Charcot neuroarthropathy deformity (Eichenholtz stage II, unstable) who also presented with a superficial plantar medial ulceration and previous resection of the 4th and 5th metatarsals. X-ray shows midfoot adduction deformity. (**b**) Lateral radiographic view shows rocker bottom and equinus deformities. Note the dorsal displacement of the forefoot and the break in Meary's

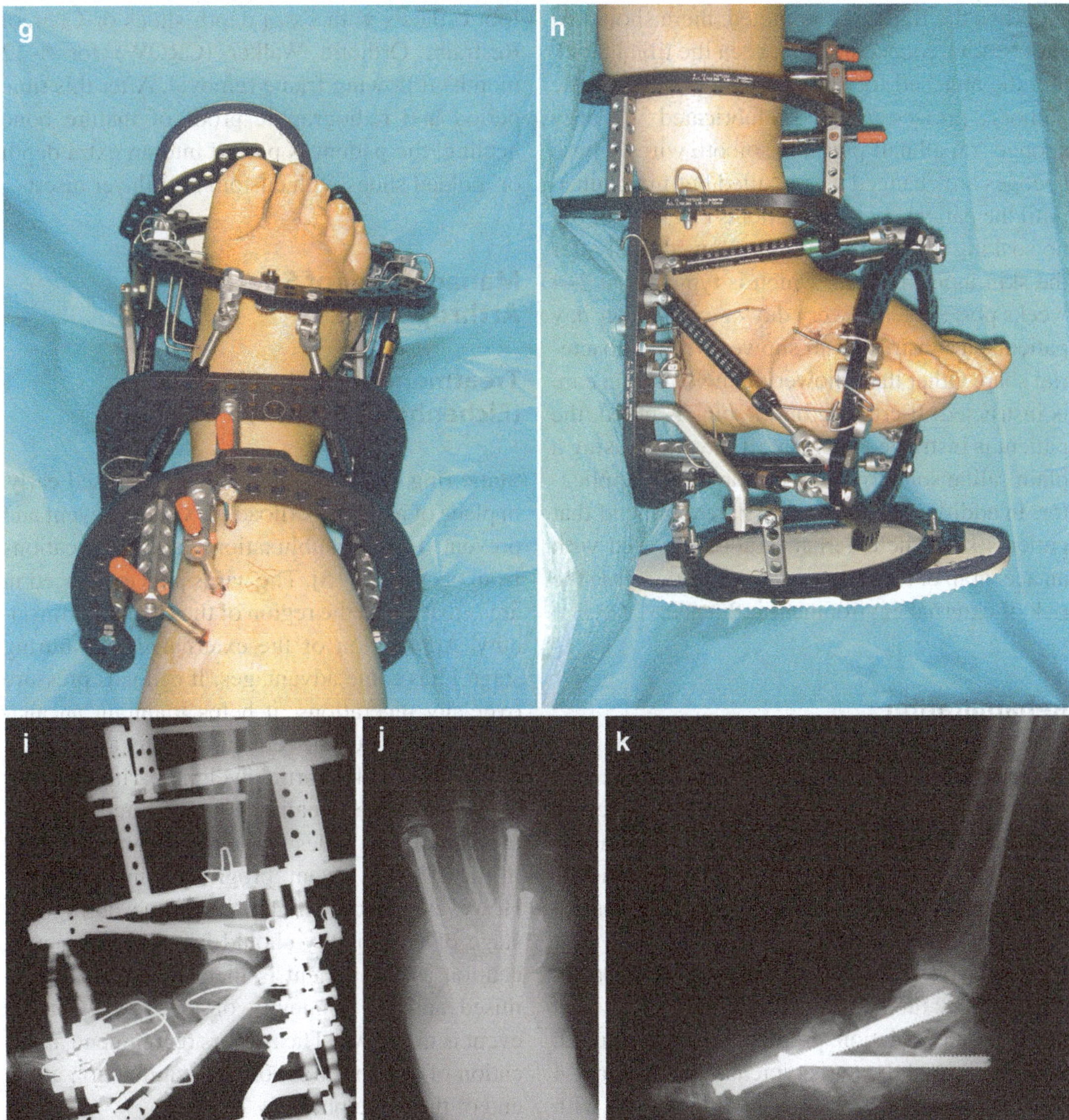

Fig. 13.1 (continued) angle. (**c**) The lateral fluoroscopic view image confirming instability of the midfoot Charcot demonstrating forefoot dorsiflexion. (**d**) The lateral fluoroscopic view demonstrating instability of the midfoot with significant forefoot plantarflexion. (**e**) Immediate postoperative anteroposterior radiographic view demonstrating midfoot adduction (*black lines*). Stirrup wires (90° bent wires that are not tensioned) are placed adjacent to the region of distraction and realignment (midfoot). (**f**) Immediate postoperative lateral radiographic view demonstrating some plantarflexion of the forefoot. The stirrup wires (90° bent wires that are not tensioned) are placed adjacent to the region of distraction and realignment (midfoot). (**g**) Clinical photograph demonstrating an applied Taylor spatial frame (forefoot 6×6 butt) applied. Note the delta configuration of the tibial half pins and the build out area of the distal foot ring in order to allow for soft tissue clearance. (**h**) A clinical lateral photograph shows the Taylor spatial frame (forefoot 6×6 butt) applied. Note the stirrup wires adjacent to the distraction region (midfoot). (**i**) Lateral radiographic view in which gradual Taylor spatial frame correction showing a near normal or zero Meary's angle. At this time the foot ulcer healed and the foot is correctly positioned. (**j**) After removal of the external fixator, a minimally invasive fusion of the midtarsal joint was performed. A weightbearing anteroposterior view radiograph shows three percutaneous intramedullary metatarsal screws that were inserted for stabilization of the fusion of the midtarsal joint. Note the improved anatomic reduction compared to the initial radiograph. (**k**) Lateral postoperative radiograph during weightbearing which shows a plantigrade foot with intact intramedullary metatarsal screws

When the frame is completed, there should be at least four connections between the tibial block and the attached foot block. Postoperatively, the authors prefer using prefabricated Ilizarov sponges on all half pins and smooth wires. These sponges are changed when soiled but maintained until the patient showers. Patients can shower but no soaking of the extremity is allowed until after the skin incisions heal, which is typically at 3–4 weeks post surgery. Every day or every other day patients are instructed to shower with antibacterial soap. Other than showering, no daily pin care is instructed. If crusting on the pins is noted, the patient is instructed to clean off the pin(s) using a plain saline solution and a cotton tipped applicator. In addition, the authors also recommend that patients keep the external fixation covered with an ace wrap or some kind of cover to decrease the risk of external environment influence.

Rehabilitation

Before, during, and after any treatment, the patient, family, and friends should be educated and recruited to assist in the success of healing. Frequent follow-up visits and close home or rehab monitoring are essential for a successful outcome. In addition, the surgeon's support staff must be well versed on the protocols and easily reachable by the patient. When an issue arises in this patient population, prompt action is required.

The external fixator is typically left on for 3–4 months. Patients are instructed to begin with immediate 50 % weightbearing with an assistive device (crutches or walker). Patients are seen in the clinic weekly or biweekly and radiographs are taken at this time to determine the time for removal of external fixation. Advanced imaging, using a CT scan, is considered to evaluate the fusion mass when visualization of the osteotomy/fusion is difficult via radiograph or to assess bone healing prior to removal of the external fixation. After removal of the external fixation in the operating room, the patient is then placed into a cam walking boot for 1 month. The patient is then transitioned into a custom molded ankle foot orthosis with extra depth shoes or Charcot Restraint Orthotic Walker (CROW) for 8–12 months following frame removal. After this time period and radiographic proof of mature bone healing, the patient is placed into an extra depth or molded shoes with custom multilayer inserts.

Management of Specific Arthropathies

Treatment of Acute Charcot (Eichenholtz Stage 1)

Static ring external fixation has been used early, in place of a cast, to offload the Charcot event and prevent further subluxations and dislocations from occurring [15]. The wires/pins are placed in areas that avoid the region of the Charcot arthropathy. Application of the external fixator during stage I has some advantages. It offloads pressure over any ulcerations, it helps maintain an anatomic position of the remaining bony anatomy, it allows for early partial weightbearing, it may provide quicker healing of the acute Charcot event, and it provides for an easier reconstruction if the Charcot event progresses into stage 2. However, the use of this technique during this stage of arthropathy should be undertaken with caution as the patient is metabolically compromised and the longevity of the acute Charcot event is unknown. The authors recommend application of external fixation for stabilization at the end of the acute phase.

Acute Midfoot Correction with External Fixation

A nonmobile malunited Charcot joint will often need the addition of an osteotomy to obtain correction of the deformity. In contrast, the mobile Charcot joint will need anatomic reduction and formal fusion. Factors such as poor vascularity, reduced bone mineral density, due to long periods of strict non-weightbearing, and impaired nutrition all decrease the patient's ability to heal [16–18]. Although internal fixation can be used, it is often used to add stability and to augment the external fixation.

An acute correction can be obtained by performing a wedge resection at the apex of the deformity. The correction shortens the skeleton, allows the bony segments to be realigned and decreases tension on the soft tissue structures to allow for easier wound approximation. The approach is made through medial and/or lateral incisions utilizing full thickness flaps. The type of incision varies depending on the type of deformity and the presence of an ulceration. Medial/lateral vertical incision are used when foot shortening osteotomies are employed and a plantar transverse incision is utilized when a large plantar ulcer is present with a rocker bottom foot deformity. Using fluoroscopy, Kirschner (K-wires) wires are inserted from medial to lateral to act as cutting guides for the biplanar wedge resection. See Glossary for description. The resection is performed with a combination of a large saw and sharp osteotomes, with care taken to protect dorsal and plantar neurovascular structures. The resected bone can be used for grafting if viable or allograft stem cells can be added for improved osseous consolidation. Provisional fixation is obtained using axially placed 2.0 mm K-wires or larger Steinman pins. Layered skin closure is performed and a drain is utilized as needed.

A static circular external fixator is then applied using a tibial ring fixation block, with at least 3 points of fixation per ring (combination of 1.8 mm wires and 6 mm half pins). The foot ring block is then constructed and mounted parallel to the sole of the foot, by placing two 1.8 mm wires into the calcaneus and two 1.8 mm wires in the talus (these wires are inserted medial to lateral). Next, a 1.8 mm wire is inserted distal to the wedge resection and is tensioned as a bent wire, by walking the wire onto the foot ring posteriorly by one or two holes from where it was inserted and exited the skin. This bent wire tension technique allows for compression of the midfoot with the wires that were placed in the talus and calcaneus. Two additional tensioned metatarsal wires are inserted for additional stability, one placed from medial to lateral and capturing the first and second metatarsals and one placed from lateral to medial from the fifth through second metatarsals. In cases of mobile severe Charcot deformity, where osseous and soft tissue problems prevent acute correction, the authors will also utilize gradual distraction with the external fixation to correct any residual deformities.

Gradual Midfoot Correction with External Fixation

This minimally invasive 2-stage approach, to correct a midfoot Charcot deformity, was initially described by Lamm and Paley [19]. It can be used for both rigid or mobile deformities and utilizes gradual correction of the deformity through soft tissue distraction utilizing external fixation. It is then followed with either static compression, applied through the external fixator, or by removing the external fixation and achieving an arthrodesis using percutaneously placed intramedullary foot fixation (IMFF) [20]. These two approaches obtain and maintain anatomic realignment, avoid large incisions, limit neurovascular compromise, preserve foot length, and reduce the risk of infection.

The first stage consists of gradual deformity correction achieved by ligamentotaxis. The majority of Charcot midfoot deformities can undergo distraction without the need for an osteotomy to realign the pedal architecture. However, a stable or coalesced Charcot deformity may require an osteotomy before gradual correction can take place. The authors perform this osteotomy by using a Gigli saw that is placed percutaneously through the midfoot. Of note is that no bone is removed, just the osteotomy is performed. When the midfoot is mobile, no osteotomy or open surgery is required other than a posterior muscle group Achilles lengthening prior to application of the external fixation. The authors prefer using a Taylor Spatial Frame (TSF) in which a 6×6 butt frame is constructed and applied to the foot. The butt portion of the frame is where the tibial and calcaneal rings meet at a 90° attachment. A second forefoot ring is mounted to the forefoot and the 6 struts are placed between the butt ring (calcaneal and tibia) and the forefoot ring. A reference ring must be chosen by the surgeon from the computer based software analysis, which can either be the proximal or distal ring. A second more proximal tibial ring can be applied for additional stability. It is essential to first fix the hindfoot and the ankle in neutral within the TSF. The forefoot is then fixed to a distal foot ring. Finally, the TSF struts are applied and final radiographs are obtained orthogonal to the reference ring. The reference ring radiographs are significant because they allow one to obtain accurate measurements postoperatively that will then allow the surgeon to enter it into the computer web-based program for deformity correction. Gradual distraction of the forefoot on the fixed hindfoot is performed using the TSF to realign the pedal anatomy. This first stage should be accomplished within 2–3 weeks or less [19]. During this phase of treatment the patient is instructed to be non-weightbearing or heel touch down only, as the forefoot ring is moving to correct the deformity.

The second phase of the correction consists of performing a minimally invasive arthrodesis of the affected joints. Minimally invasive arthrodesis is easily preformed because the Charcot joint(s) are already distracted. The arthrodesis is achieved by making small transverse incisions (2–3 cm in length) over the affected joint(s). An important step during this part of the procedure is to first remove any remaining articular cartilage and then prepare the joints for an arthrodesis. At this time, the Charcot midfoot can be stabilized using some kind of internal fixation or the external fixation can be adjusted to perform static compression of the midfoot, adjusting the external fixation to allow for partial weightbearing.

When using internal fixation, the external fixation is first removed. Under fluoroscopic guidance, minimally invasive arthrodesis is performed and then guidewires for large-diameter cannulated screws are inserted retrograde and percutaneously through the plantar skin into the metatarsal head by dorsiflexing the metatarsophalangeal joint. The medial column screw is advanced into the talus and the lateral column screw is directed into the calcaneus. The authors prefer using three large-diameter cannulated (7.0 or 8.0 mm) intramedullary screws inserted through the metatarsals. Predrilling or reaming is performed prior to screw insertion. Typically a first, second, and fourth metatarsal screw are placed. The medial and lateral column screws are partially threaded to allow for compression of the arthrodesis site and the centrally placed screw (second metatarsal) is fully threaded and is used for stabilization. These screws span the entire length of the metatarsals into the calcaneus and talus, respectively. The minimally invasive incisions are then closed, and a well-padded splint is applied. Before hospital discharge, the authors remove the patient's operative splint and apply a short leg cast. A non-weight-bearing short leg cast is maintained for 2–3 months, and then gradual progression to weightbearing in a cam boot is achieved. The entire treatment is completed in 4–5 months. The advantages of using external fixation combined with intramedullary fixation include obtaining an anatomic realignment of the foot, using a minimally invasive fixation technique, obtaining formal multiple joint fusions, adjacent joint fixation beyond the level of Charcot collapse, providing rigid interosseous fixation, preservation of foot length, and combining it with external fixation when necessary [19].

Alternatively, the external fixation can be used alone to obtain an arthrodesis of the midfoot. In this approach, medial and/or lateral incisions are still utilized to prepare the joints for a formal fusion. After skin closure, the external fixation is adjusted, adding a U-foot ring, for compression of the formal fusion via the bent wire technique. In addition, an external fixation walking ring is placed to allow for partial weightbearing with an assistive device (crutches/walker). (Figs. 13.1 and 13.2).

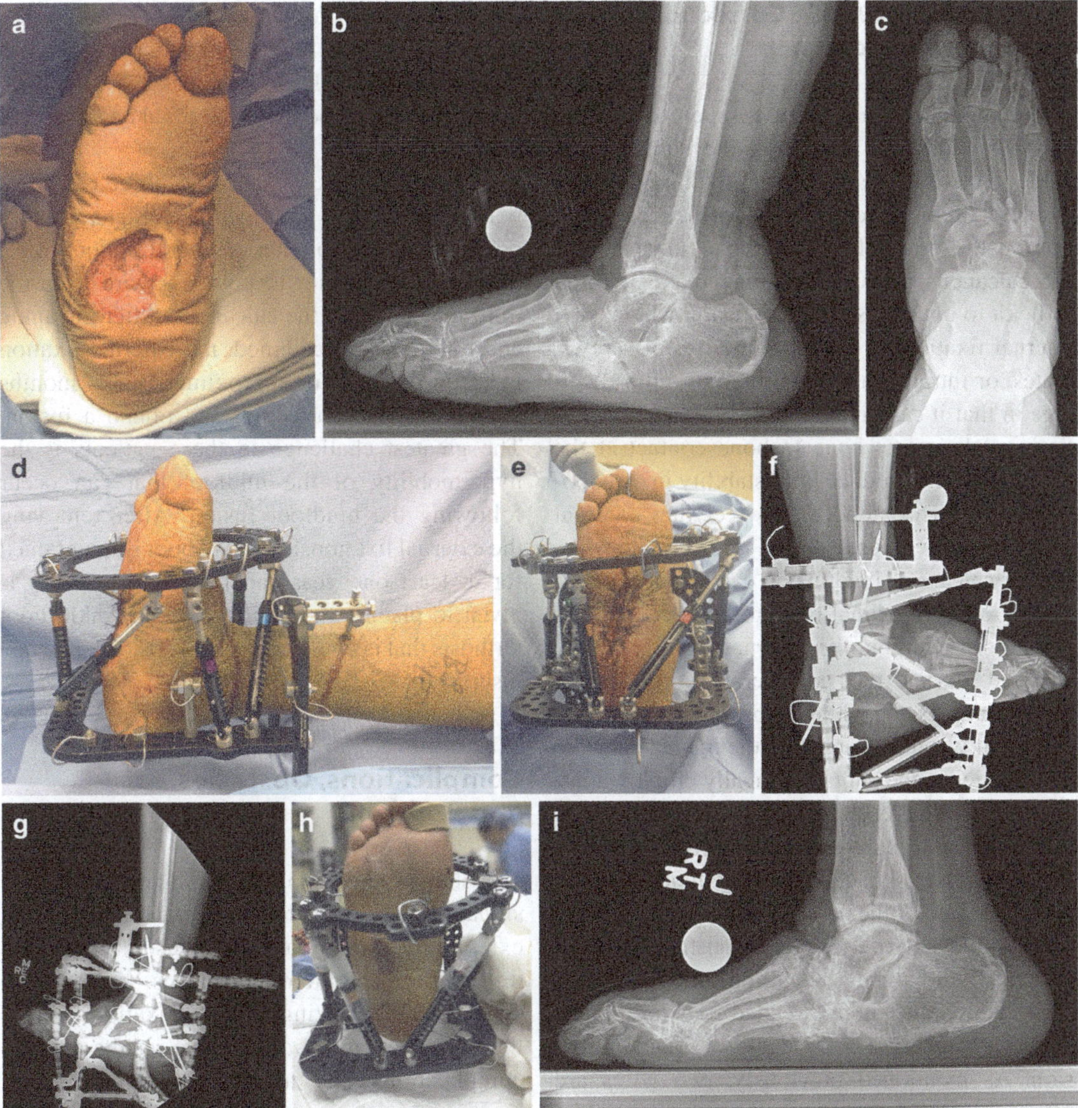

Fig. 13.2 (**a**) A patient who presented with a midfoot Charcot neuroarthropathy deformity (Eichenholtz stage II, unstable) along with a large plantar central ulceration. (**b**) Lateral weightbearing radiograph demonstrating midfoot collapse and equinus. (**c**) Anteroposterior weightbearing radiograph demonstrating a midtarsal Charcot deformity with superimposition of the tarsal bones and a varus deformity, indicating shortening of the foot. (**d**) Immediate postoperative lateral clinical picture shows application of Taylor Spatial Frame (6×6 butt) for gradual distraction of the midfoot Charcot dislocation. There were no open interventions other than an Achilles tendon lengthening. (**e**) Clinical image after acute excision of the plantar ulceration and closure were performed. (**f**) Immediate postoperative lateral radiograph shows application of Taylor Spatial Frame (Butt frame) for gradual distraction of the midfoot Charcot dislocation. Note that after the Achilles tendon lengthening an extra-articular temporary large diameter pin is traversing the calcaneus and tibia posterior and crosses the ankle and subtalar joints. (**g**) Postoperative lateral view after 2 weeks of gradual distraction of the midfoot with Taylor Spatial Frame. Note the realignment of the forefoot in relation to the hindfoot. A second minimally invasive joint fusion surgery was performed to achieve arthrodesis using external fixation compression. The compression frame was maintained for 2.5 months and the external fixation was then converted to a weightbearing frame with attachment of the walking ring. (**h**) A clinical image of the plantar surface of the foot at the time of external fixation removal, of note the plantar ulceration has completely healed. (**i**) The final 1 year postoperative lateral view weightbearing radiograph shows a stable midfoot fusion and a plantigrade foot

Acute Hindfoot/Ankle Correction with External Fixation

The authors feel that when a severe deformity and bone loss are present in the subtalar and ankle joints, the use of external fixation can be a viable fixation modality. The presence of the arthropathy often affects the bone substance of the calcaneus or talus and may make it more difficult to obtain a successful fusion when using internal fixation. In addition, the use of screws, plates, or intramedullary nailing has a disadvantage in that it can create more soft tissue dissection, result in less bone to bone contact at the fusion site, and produce limit stability in osteoporotic bone. The authors also feel that external fixation with compression of the tibiotalocalcaneal or calcaneal tibial fusion can provide stability and allow maximal bone to bone contact for healing. In addition, the external fixation can be adjusted during the postoperative course for added compression while the patient is allowed to be partial weightbearing. For the management of these patients, the authors typically employ a lateral transverse incision, at the level of the dorsal calcaneus, as seen on a lateral fluoroscopy image, to allow ease of skin closure that will occur due to the shortening of the osseous segments.

A stable external fixation construct is constructed. A tibial ring block and foot ring block are mounted and three threaded rods are placed between the ring blocks to allow for compression. As mentioned previously, two wires are placed in each bone segment (talus and calcaneus) and inserted with as much obliquity as possible. When performing a tibiotalarcalcaneal fusion, the subtalar joint is compressed first. To do this, the authors first apply the tibia fixation block, then apply to foot ring to the calcaneus with the two aforementioned tensioned calcaneal wires. Two talar wires are then inserted and, when attaching them to the foot ring, are arched down (insert them into a hole one closer to the foot ring than would be typical). By arching the talar wires down to the foot ring (tensioning the talar wires in such a way that forces the wire to straighten), this will compress the subtalar joint as the two calcaneal wires are already affixed to the foot ring. After subtalar compression has been achieved, the foot block is then compressed proximal against the tibial block by shortening the threaded rods between the tibial and foot ring fixation blocks.

For a tibial calcaneal fusion, three calcaneal wires are placed, the medial to lateral wire, posterior-medial to anterior-lateral oblique wire, and an axial anterior to posterior wire from the third metatarsal to the calcaneus. After the ankle and hindfoot are realigned, the external fixation is left in position for approximately 3–4 months to maintain the correction and obtain a fusion. The greatest challenge in these patients is the hypermobility of the midfoot that can occur following the hindfoot fusion. After removing the external fixation, a CROW boot is maintained for at least one year and then consideration is given to placing the patient into an Ankle Foot Orthosis that is combined with a custom shoe and insert (Fig. 13.3).

Complications, Obstacles, and Problems

The authors have published a standardized classification of difficulties that can arise during external fixation treatment. This classification differentiates problems, obstacles, and complications when utilizing external fixation [14] on the premise that not all adverse results are true complications that affect the final outcome. Furthermore, the authors feel that the problems and obstacles that arise may simply be hurdles to complete a successful treatment.

Adverse results can occur intraoperatively, perioperatively, or postoperatively. We have classified adverse results (undesirable outcomes) that occurred during treatment into problems, obstacles, and complications. Adverse results that can occur during surgical management include fixation failure, nonunion, vascular insult, pin site infections (superficial or deep), swelling, and delayed bone or soft tissue healing.

Problems are defined as anticipated adverse results that arise from the treatment but resolve without surgical intervention by the end of treatment.

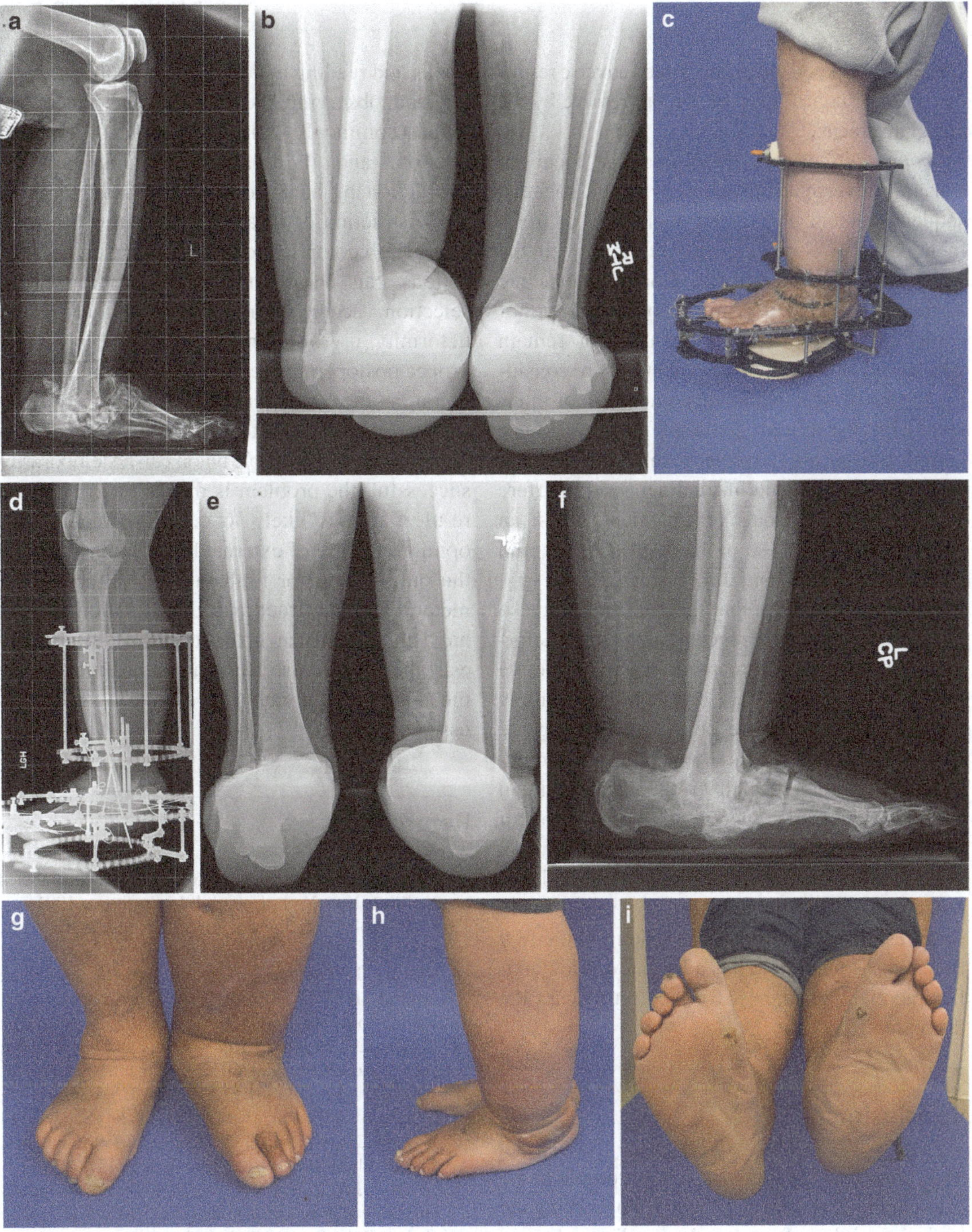

Fig. 13.3 (**a**) The lateral weightbearing radiograph demonstrating an unstable peritalar Charcot deformity. (**b**) A Saltzman weightbearing radiograph shows a varus and medial displaced left hindfoot. Note the enlarged soft tissue envelope of the left ankle and leg as compared to the right. (**c**) Postoperative lateral weightbearing clinical image shows a reinforced tibial and foot block with a static external fixator. Note the transverse lateral ankle incision, which provided for an ease of arthrodesis and closure. (**d**) Postoperative lateral weightbearing radiograph shows stable tibial and foot block external fixator for calcaneal tibial fusion. (**e**) The Saltzman weightbearing axial radiograph now shows a vertical and centralized hindfoot beneath the tibia. (**f**) A 3-year postoperative weightbearing lateral view radiograph shows consolidation of the calcaneal tibial fusion with a plantigrade foot. (**g**) A clinical anterior weightbearing view at 3 years postoperatively demonstrating good alignment. (**h**) A clinical weightbearing lateral view photo 3 years postoperatively. Note the well-healed lateral incision. (**i**) A clinical plantar view photo 3 years postoperatively demonstrating no plantar ulceration

Obstacles are described as anticipated adverse results that require surgical intervention but resolve by the end of treatment.

Complications are identified as local or systemic adverse results whereby their associated sequelae remain unresolved at the end of treatment. Not all complications interfere with the original goals of treatment. Complications are further subdivided into minor or major. Minor complications are adverse results that remain unresolved at the end of treatment but are considered to be of little significance and do not interfere with the initial goals of surgery. Major complications are adverse results that remain unresolved by the end of treatment and interfere with the original goals of treatment. Thus, an understanding of these problems, obstacles, and complications is essential for success.

One other problem that the authors have also observed is the reoccurrence of an equinus deformity that can occur months after reconstructive surgery. To address this problem in a timely manner, we routinely recommend checking the patient to make sure that no equinus has reoccurred. The authors feel that if there is no residual equinus component, there is less likelihood of collapse that can result in ulceration in the future. In the authors experience even if midfoot collapse reoccurs (due to broken hardware, partial/incomplete fusion, pseudoarthrosis), as long as the foot functions as a unit and has adequate ankle dorsiflexion, then the chances for recurrent ulceration decrease.

Conclusion

The Charcot foot and ankle are complex and challenging deformities to treat. By observing the basic principles of use, understanding when to utilize external fixation, learning how to construct a stable frame, and where to apply the external fixation is paramount to obtaining a good outcome. External fixation for treatment of Charcot arthropathy is not recommended for the inexperienced surgeon. To obtain adequate knowledge for use with this device may require going to courses, lectures, seminars, obtaining books and reading materials on this subject, visiting and observing these approaches at centers which commonly employ the use of external fixation, and if possible obtaining personal instruction by an experienced Ilizarov surgeon. Reconstruction of Charcot deformities has relatively high complication rates; however, complications can be minimized by proper patient selection, accurate preoperative evaluation of deformity, use of sound surgical principles, and proper postoperative care. Obtaining an osseous union is the standout factor for describing a successful surgical outcome. Although a pseudoarthrodesis or semi-stable union can be temporarily successful, the problem is that in the long run a re-ulceration is likely to occur. In the authors opinion, the use of external fixation may provide the only option for limb salvage. Although the method of reconstruction and the fixation utilized has a great influence on the success of the arthrodesis, the authors also feel that the health status of the host will ultimately determine a successful osseous union.

References

1. Frykberg RG, editor. The high risk foot in diabetes mellitus. New York: Churchill Livingstone; 1991.
2. Eichenholtz SN. Charcot joints. Springfield, IL: C. C. Thomas; 1966.
3. Shibata T, Tada K, Hashizume C. The results of arthrodesis of the ankle for leprotic neuroarthropathy. J Bone Joint Surg. 1990;72A:749–56.
4. Rogers LC, Frykberg RG, Armstrong DG, Boulton AJ, Edmonds M, Van GH, Hartemann A, Game F, Jeffcoate W, Jirkovska A, Jude E, Morbach S, Morrison WB, Pinzur M, Pitocco D, Sanders L, Wukich DK, Uccioli L. The Charcot foot in diabetes. J Am Podiatr Med Assoc. 2011;101(5):437–46.
5. Brodsky JW, Rouse AM. Exostectomy for symptomatic bony prominences in diabetic Charcot feet. Clin Orthop Relat Res. 1993;296:21–6.
6. Schon LC, Weinfeld SB, Horton GA, Resch S. Radiographic and clinical classification of acquired midtarsus deformities. Foot Ankle Int. 1998;19: 394–404.
7. Sanders LJ. The Charcot foot: historical perspective 1827–2003. Diabetes Metab Res Rev. 2004;20(Suppl): S4–8.
8. Pinzur M. The role of ring external fixation in Charcot foot arthropathy. Foot Ankle Clin N Am. 2006;11(4): 837–47.

9. Paley D. Principles of deformity correction. Revth ed. Berlin: Springer; 2005.

10. Lamm BM, Paley D. Charcot neuroarthropathy of the foot and ankle. In: Rozbruch SR, Ilizarov S, editors. Limb lengthening and reconstructive surgery. New York: Informa Healthcare; 2007. p. 221–31.

11. Jolly GP, Zgonis T, Polyzois V. External fixation in management of Charcot neuropathy. Clin Pediatr Med Surg. 2003;20:741–56.

12. Cooper PS. Application of external fixators for management of Charcot deformities of the foot and ankle. Foot Ankle Clin N Am. 2002;7:207–54.

13. Lamm BM, Paley D, Herzenberg JE. Gastrocnemius Soleus recession: a simpler, more limited approach. J Am Podiatr Med Assoc. 2005;95(1): 18–25.

14. Paley D. Problems, obstacles, and complications of limb lengthening by the Ilizarov technique. Clin Orthop Relat Res. 1990;250:81–104.

15. Wang JC, Le AW, Tsukuda RK. A new technique for Charcot's foot reconstruction. J Am Podiatr Med Assoc. 2002;92:429–36.

16. Bevilacqua NJ, Stapleton JJ. Advanced foot and ankle fixation techniques in patients with diabetes. Clin Podiatr Med Surg. 2011;28(4):661–71.

17. Sammarco VJ. Superconstructs in the treatment of Charcot foot deformity: plantar plating, locked plating, and axial screw fixation. Foot Ankle Clin N Am. 2009;14(3):393–407.

18. Crim BE, Lowery NJ, Wukich DK. Internal fixation techniques for midfoot Charcot neuroarthropathy in patients with diabetes. Clin Podiatr Med Surg. 2011;28(4):673–85.

19. Lamm BM, David Gottlieb H, Paley D. A two-stage percutaneous approach to Charcot diabetic foot reconstruction. J Foot Ankle Surg. 2010;49(6):517–22.

20. Lamm BM, Siddiqui NA, Nair AK, LaPorta G. Intramedullary foot fixation for midfoot Charcot neuroarthropathy. J Foot Ankle Surg. 2012;51:531–6.

Appendix

Table 1 Table discussing physical, laboratory, and radiologic studies used to differentiate patients presenting with Charcot arthropathy from those presenting with an infection

	Charcot	Infected Charcot
Physical findings		
Skin	Edema, erythema, warm	Edema, erythema, warm
Leg elevation	Resolves edema/erythema	Edema/erythema persist
Ulcer	Non-draining	Draining, extends to bone
Temperature	Afebrile	Febrile
Discomfort	Painless	Painful
Lab findings		
Glucose	No change	Out of control
WBC[a]	Normal	Elevated
CRP[b]	Normal	Elevated
X-ray exam	Fracture/dislocation, periosteal reaction	Same, *Air Present*
99m-TC bone scan[c]	Positive	Positive
Indium-111 bone scan	Negative (usually)	Positive
MRI scan[d]	Soft tissue and bony edema, joint destruction	Fluid Collections; Air

[a]White blood cells
[b]C-reactive protein
[c]Technetium-99m
[d]Magnetic resonance imaging

© Springer International Publishing Switzerland 2016
D. Herscovici, Jr. (ed.), *The Surgical Management of the Diabetic Foot and Ankle*,
DOI 10.1007/978-3-319-27623-6

Table 2 Wagner system for grading diabetic ulcers

Dysvascular foot breakdown - Natural history

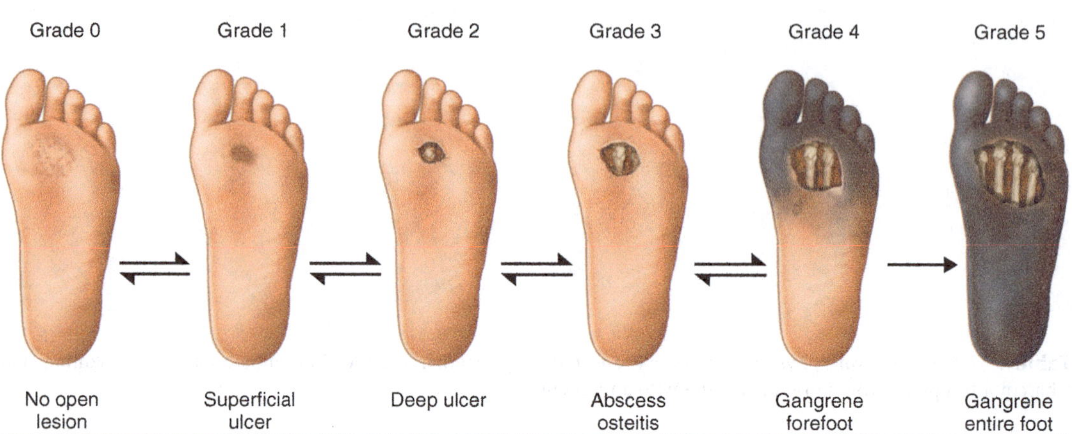

Glossary

Adaptive Immune System Immune system that responds into action against pathogens that are able to evade or overcome the Innate Immune System.

Allele One of a number of alternative forms of the same gene or genetic locus.

Alpha Stage Indicating mild to moderate deformities in patients with Charcot arthropathy of the midfoot and based on the classification by Schon et al.

Anatomic Classification System Describes the location of a disease about an anatomic location in the foot or ankle.

Ankle Brachial Index (ABI) A ratio of the measured systolic pressure at the ankle (dorsalis pedis or posterior tibial) over the measured systolic brachial (arm) blood pressure.

Ankle Foot Orthosis (AFO) A custom-fabricated or commercially available, well-padded ankle-foot appliance that extends from the toes up to the proximal tibia, which helps to support and limit ankle, subtalar and midtarsal joint movement.

Ankylosis Immobility and consolidation of a joint due to disease, injury, or a surgical procedure. Seen in Eichenholtz stage III, of a Charcot joint, and demonstrated radiographically with bony union of bones and joints due to a proliferation of bone cells.

Angiopathy Indicating a disease of the blood vessels.

Antigen A substance that is capable of inducing the formation of antibodies and reacting in some detectable manner when these antibodies are produced.

Apoptosis A normal, genetically regulated process leading to the death of cells and triggered by the presence or absence of certain stimuli, such as DNA damage.

Apropulsive Gait Opposite of propulsive (or toe-lift) phase. Indicates that the foot cannot be propelled off of the toes, when transitioning from stance to toe-lift, due to the absence of one or more anatomic structures.

Astragalectomy A complete excision of the talus.

Atherogenesis Conducive to or causing the formation of a thickened, mass of yellowish material, containing cholesterol, lipoid material, and lipophages (plaque), that is deposited within the degenerative arterial walls of the tunica intima and media.

Arthrodesis Also known as artificial ankylosis, it is surgical fixation between two or more bones designed to accomplish a fusion of the joint surfaces by promoting the proliferation of bone cells.

Autonomic Dysfunction Neuropathy due to sympathetic denervation resulting in a loss of vasomotor control, producing anhidrosis (lack of sweating), an increase in blood flow, and the loss of normal skin temperature regulation in the lower extremities, resulting in hyperemia with elevated skin temperatures and stiff, dry, scaly skin that cracks easily.

Axial Fixation Involves the placement of intraosseous screws through the metatarsal shafts, in which the screws act as load sharing devices similar to steel rebar in concrete, which span the

© Springer International Publishing Switzerland 2016

D. Herscovici, Jr. (ed.), *The Surgical Management of the Diabetic Foot and Ankle*,

DOI 10.1007/978-3-319-27623-6

area of deformity fixing the proximal and distal fusion segments.

Bayonet Apposition Arthropathy which causes breakdown of the midfoot leading to a lateral radiographic appearance in which the dorsally displaced forefoot sits on the top of the hindfoot (e.g., as seen with a bayonet attached to a rifle).

Beta Stage Indicating a severe deformity in patients with Charcot arthropathy of the midfoot and based on the classification by Schon et al.

Calcaneus Gait Gait pattern in which the major weight-bearing area is the heel, often seen with an inability of the Achilles to provide push-off (heel lift) after the stance phase.

Cantilever (bending load) A loading situation in which one end of a long structure has support or rigid fixation (side a) while the other free end (side b) is loaded (e.g., a diving board).

Charcot Arthropathy (disease) A painless disintegration of the joints often seen in diabetic patients presenting with prolonged neuropathy.

Charcot Restraint Orthotic Walker (CROW) A custom, bivalved, total contact AFO with full foot enclosure, a rocker bottom sole modification, and a custom orthosis that is made from a casted model of the patient's foot and ankle.

Chopart Amputation A disarticulation of the foot, through the talonavicular and calcaneocuboid joints, leaving only the talus and calcaneus.

Claudication A complex of symptoms consisting of no pain or discomfort when the limb is at rest, initiation of pain and weakness when activity begins, which intensifies as the activity increases, and which disappears after a period of rest. Often seen in occlusive arterial diseases of the limb.

Coagulopathy Any disorder that affects the ability of blood to coagulate (i.e., clot)

Coalescence Used to describe stage II of Eichenholtz's classification and refers to a radiographic appearance demonstrating sclerosis and absorption of fine debris, with a fusion of most of the large fragments.

Cytokines Molecules of protein that help regulate the body's immune response to infections and trauma. Some promote the healing of wounds and some increase inflammation (proinflammatory cytokines) causing diseases to progress.

Dysvascular Indicating an abnormally poor or insufficient circulation, often of an extremity.

Eichenholtz Classification The only pure temporal classification system used to describe the different stages of Charcot's disease.

Epigenetic Development of an organism, from an undifferentiated cell, into the successive formation and development of organs and parts that do not preexist in the fertilized egg.

Equinus Also known as talipes equinus, it describes a deformity in which the foot is plantar flexed, causing the person to walk on their toes without touching the heel to the ground.

Exostosis(es) Benign bony growth(s) projecting outward from the surface of the bone.

Foot Block Also know as a "bumper," is used to describe two completed rings that are placed around the foot during the use of small wire fixation.

Fragmentation A division of bone into small pieces; frequently used to describe stage I of Eichenholtz's classification and refers to a radiographic appearance of bony destruction seen with multiple pieces of bone and cartilage leading to joint subluxations or dislocations.

Gangrene Tissue necrosis, which can be considerable in size and is often followed by infection and putrefaction, usually associated with a loss of the vascular supply.

Glycation The result of typically covalent bonding of a protein or a lipid molecule with a sugar molecule, without the controlling action of an enzyme (e.g., glycated hemoglobin is also know as hemoglobin A1c).

Haplotype A combination of alleles or to a set of single nucleotide polymorphisms found on the same chromosome.

Hyalinization Refers to the transformation or tissue degeneration of a substance into a glasslike (hyaline) or transparent state.

Hyperemia An excess of blood or engorgement of the extremity, due to an increase in peripheral blood flow, producing elevated skin temperatures and changes in skin color.

Immunocompetence The ability or capacity to develop an immune response following an antigenic challenge.

In-Depth Shoe Also known as an extra-depth shoe, it is an oxford-type or athletic shoe with an additional 1/4- to 1/2-in. of depth throughout the shoe to allow extra volume for the inserts or orthoses, as well as to accommodate for any deformity associated with a diabetic foot.

Indurated Indicating that some soft tissue has hardened or has been rendered hard.

Innate Immune System A collection of cells and proteins which are always present and ready to mobilize and fight microbes at the site of an infection.

Leukocytosis A transient increase in the number of leukocytes (white blood cells) in the blood, may be due to a number of causes, e.g., infection, inflammation, and fever.

Ligamentotaxis Technique used to describe the concept of restoring length to a comminuted fracture by applying distraction through the capsuloligamentous structures that are connected to fracture fragments, using either internal or external fixation.

Ligand An organic molecule that donates the necessary electrons needed to form coordinated covalent bonds with metallic ions (e.g., oxygen bound to the iron atom of hemoglobin).

Lipophage A cell that ingests or absorbs fat.

Lisfranc (Tarsometatarsal) Amputation Disarticulation of the foot at the tarsometatarsal joints.

Matrixectomy A partial or complete resection of the nail and nail bed (matrix) that is performed using a carbon dioxide laser, phenol and alcohol or sodium hydroxide, usually after failure of conservative care for chronically infected or deformed toenails.

Meary's Angle Also known as the Meary-Tomeno axis, it is identified on a lateral radiograph of the foot by drawing a line parallel to the midshaft axis of the first metatarsal that bisects a parallel line drawn along the axis of the talar neck and body.

Mercaptan(s) Any compound(s) containing a sulfur hydrogen radical group bound to carbon.

Neuropeptides A class of compounds which yield two or more amino acids on hydrolysis; forms the constituent part of proteins of the nerves.

Nitrosylation Any chemical reaction that incorporates a nitric oxide (NO) moiety into another (usually organic) molecule.

Orthosis(es) A removable insole which provides pressure relief and shock absorption. May be pre-made or custom-made (made from a cast model of the foot) which are commonly prescribed for patients with diabetes.

Osteomyelitis An inflammation and infection of the bone frequently caused by a pyogenic (pus producing) organism.

Osteoprotegerin Also known as osteoclastogenesis inhibitory factor (OCIF), it is a glycoprotein and a member of the tumor necrosis factor receptor superfamily that regulates bone resorption by reducing the production of osteoclasts, inhibiting the differentiation of osteoclasts precursors, and regulates the resorption of osteoclasts *in vivo* and *in vitro*.

Paracrine Factors Proteins that are synthesized by one cell and are secreted into the immediate extracellular environment that diffuse over small distances to induce changes in neighboring cells.

Pedorthist An individual who is trained in foot anatomy and the construction of shoes and foot orthotic devices, who fits and dispenses footwear according physicians' prescription.

Peptides Biologically occurring molecule consisting of two or more short chains of amino acid monomers linked by peptide (amide) bonds that are formed then the carboxyl group of one amino acid reacts with the amino acid of another.

Phenotype The entire physical, biochemical, and physiologic makeup of an individual as determined both genetically and environmentally.

Pillar One of several lines of a weight-bearing force identified by Harris and Brandt and described as either a posterior (calcaneus), central (talus), or an anterior (navicular) pillar.

Polymorphism The occurrence together, in the same population, of two or more genetically determined phenotypes in such proportions that the rarest of them cannot be maintained merely by recurrent mutation.

Prothrombotic Describing any agent or condition that leads to or has a predisposition for thrombosis.

Pseudoarthrosis Type of nonunion in which the fracture site results in the formation of a false joint where a fibrocartilagenous cavity is lined with synovium producing synovial fluid.

Putrefaction Enzymatic decomposition of tissues producing foul-smelling compounds such as hydrogen sulfide, ammonia, and mercaptans.

Ring Fixation Block Used to describe circular ring fixation; after small fixation wires and/or half-pins have been inserted into bone and attached to a ring fixator, the wires, pins, and ring will act as one unit (block).

Rocker Bottom Foot A deformity of the foot, due to collapse and reversal of the longitudinal arch, which gives the foot the appearance of the curved strut as seen on the bottom of a rocking chair.

Reconstruction or Reconstitution Used to describe stage III of Eichenholtz's classification and refers to a radiographic appearance demonstrating less sclerosis, a rounding of major fragments and an attempt at reformation of joint architecture.

Scintigraphy A radiologic modality that detects the distribution in the body of a radioactive agent, most often technetium-99m or indium-111, after it is injected into the vascular system. Often used in the evaluation of patients suspected of having a bony infection.

Sclerosis (Bony) Also known as eburnation and indicates the conversion of bony fragments into a denser, ivory-like mass. When it occurs at the joint, eburnation describes the loss of articular (hyaline) cartilage resulting in exposure of the subchondral bone.

Semmes-Weinstein Monofilaments Also known as an esthesiometer, these are nylon monofilaments precisely calibrated and of equal lengths (38 mm) used to measure the lower thresholds of touch and pain. The force needed to cause the monofilament to "buckle" determines the tactile reading.

Silversköld Test Physical maneuver used to differentiate gastrocnemius from gastrosoleal equinus. With knee extended, the foot is supinated and unable to be dorsiflexed (gastrocnemius equinus) and with the knee flexed to ninety degrees, there is 10° or less of dorsiflexion of the foot (gastrosoleal equinus).

Superconstruct Term used to describe fixation techniques that have been developed to increase the stability of the repair for Charcot arthropathy, which reduces the risk of fixation failure.

Syme Amputation Described in 1843 by James Syme, it is an ankle disarticulation with preservation of the heel flap to permit weight-bearing on the end of the stump.

Synovia Also known as synovial fluid, it is a transparent alkaline viscid fluid, resembling the white of an egg, that is secreted by the synovial membrane and is contained in joint cavities, bursae, and tendon sheaths.

Temporal Classification (Staging) System Used to describe the stage of disease and varied characteristics of the disease over time as explained in the Eichenholtz classification system.

Toe Pressure(s) An objective vascular test used to evaluate for peripheral arterial disease (PAD), it obtains the systolic pressures of the greater and lesser toes.

Trophic Pertaining to late changes such as shiny or cool, pale skin, nail changes, contractures, osteoporosis, and muscle atrophy.

Upregulation An increase in the number of receptors on the surface of target cells, making the cells more sensitive to a hormone or another agent.

Wagner-Meggitt A five-point grading scale that was developed to describe and classify diabetic foot ulcers and infections.

Wedge Resection A bi-planar, plantar-based, closing medial wedge resection of bone performed at the apex of the deformity, often in patients presenting with Charcot arthropathy of the midfoot, which is used to correct a rigid rocker bottom deformity.

Index

© Springer International Publishing Switzerland 2016

D. Herscovici, Jr. (ed.), *The Surgical Management of the Diabetic Foot and Ankle*,
DOI 10.1007/978-3-319-27623-6

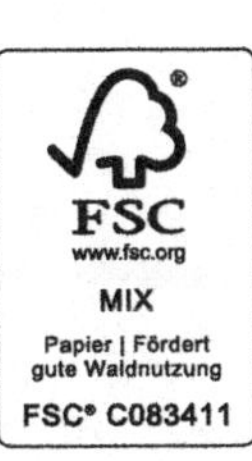